AF583826

Keto

THE ULTIMATE COLLECTION

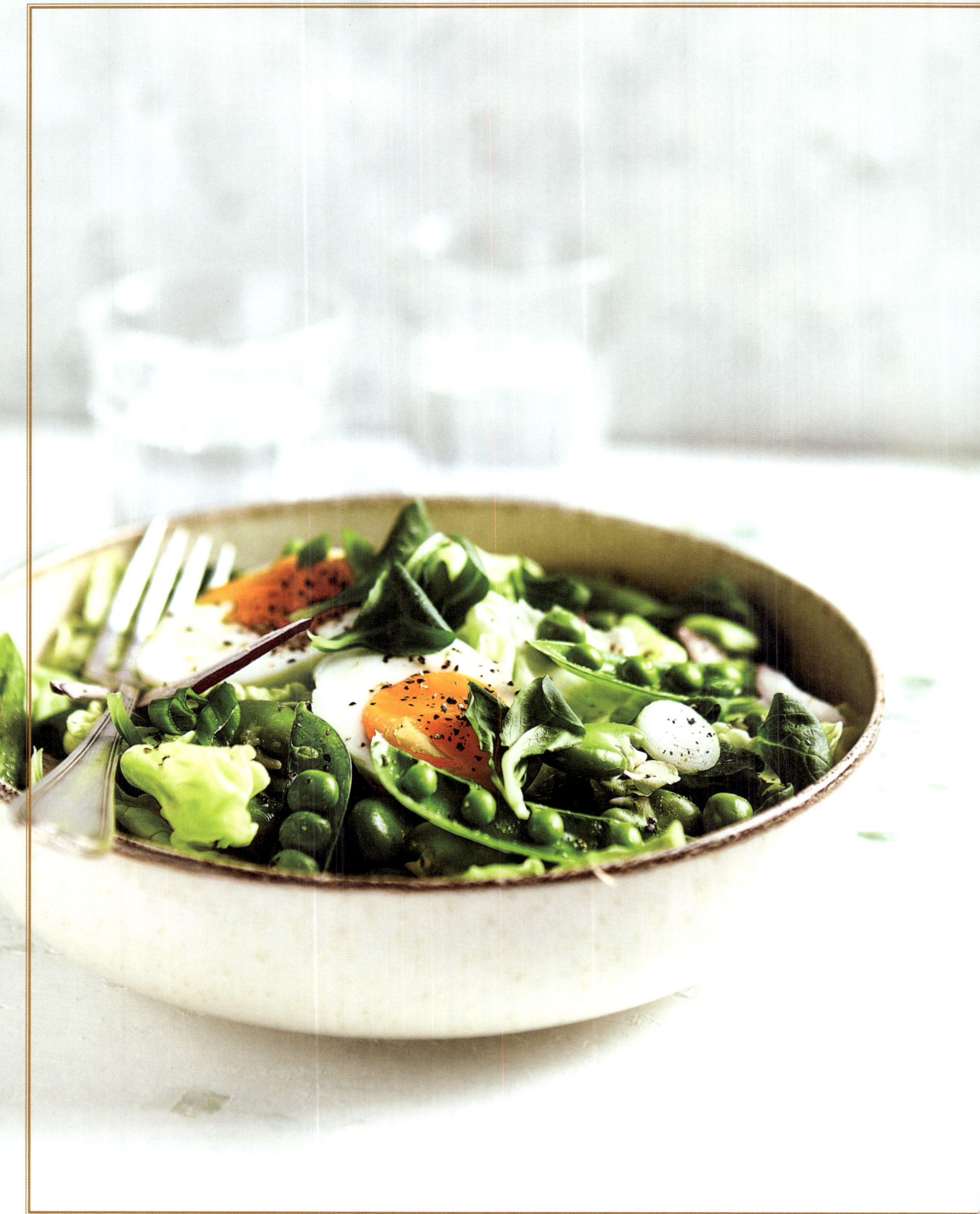

Keto

THE ULTIMATE COLLECTION

The absolute best recipes, so you can get the most out of your meals.

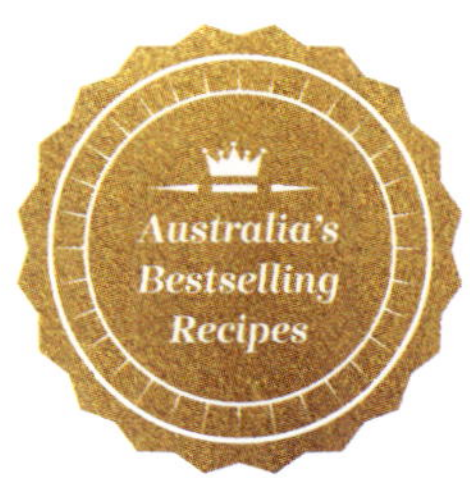

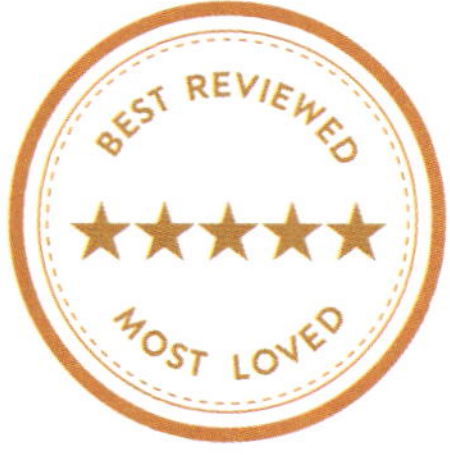

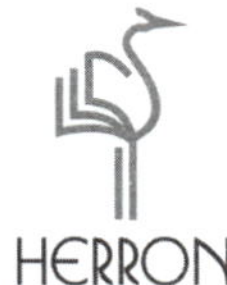

Contents

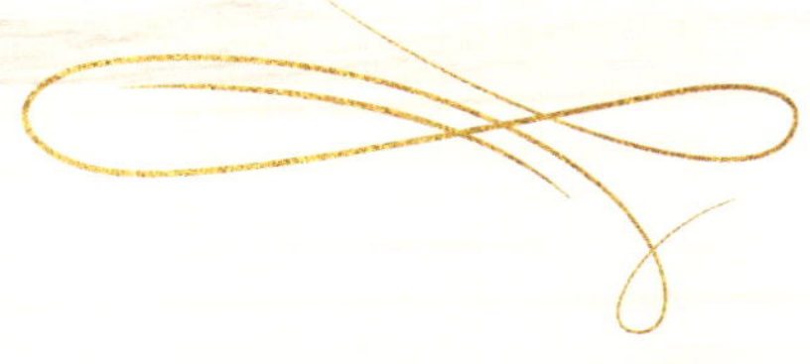

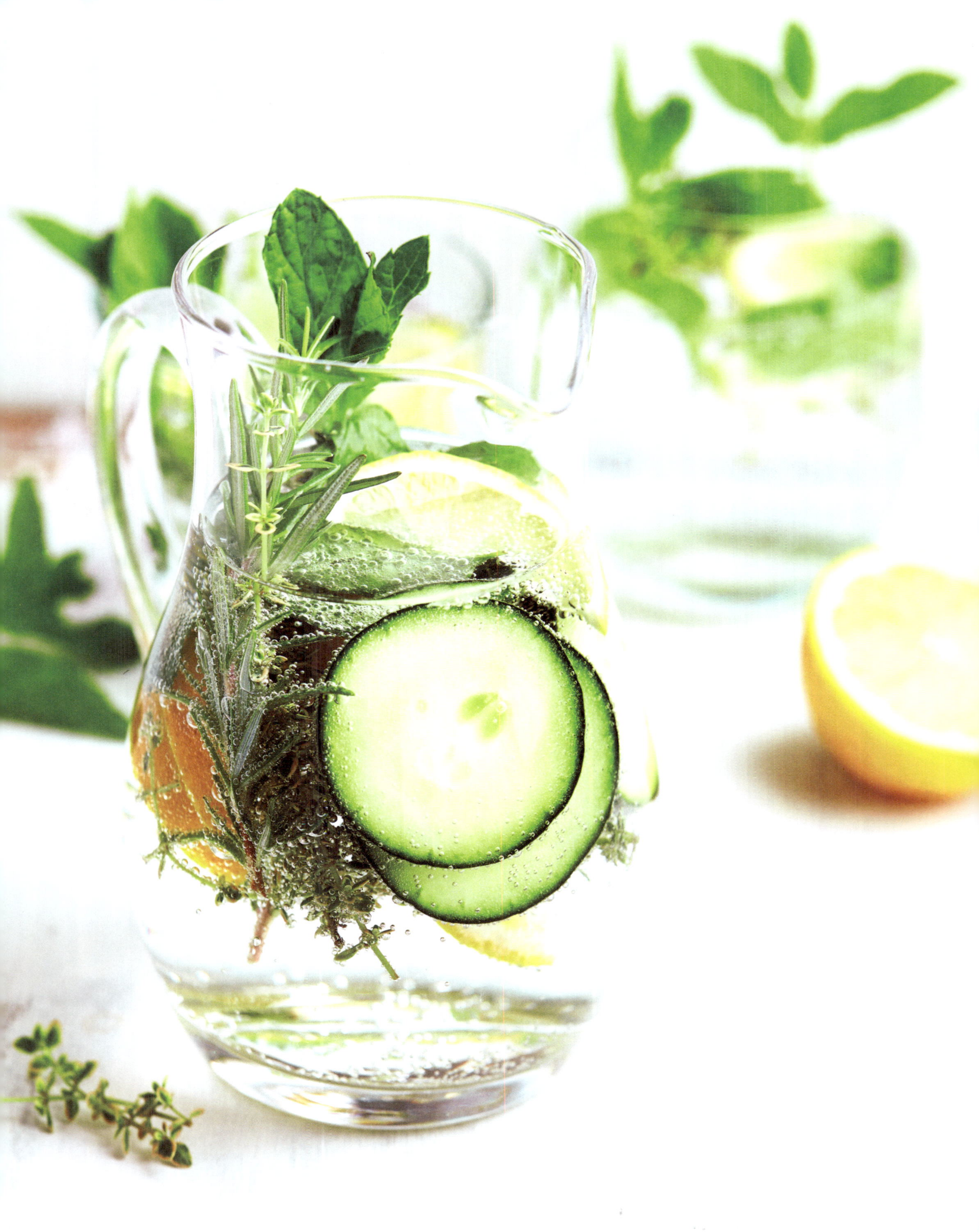

Welcome to the Ultimate Collection of Keto Recipes.

The recipes in this book are the best of the best. They have been handpicked from a selection of Australia's bestselling keto cookbooks, so that you have the most useful, versatile and successful collection of recipes in one place. Packed full of inspiration, ideas and practical tips, they will set you on track to eating keto-style with ease.

Although there are restrictions, eating a keto-inspired diet doesn't have to be hard. The recipes in this book present low-carb, high-fat options that anyone can use. They avoid the keto no-no ingredients and focus on the yes-yes instead.

Understanding the principles of keto and setting them at the heart of meal planning is the focus of this book. A good rule of thumb is that keto eating will consist of about 75% fat, 20% protein and only 5% carbohydrates, which is less than 50g of carbs per day. Strict keto diets focus on net carbs, which is the number of grams of total carbs in a portion of food minus the fibre. Mathematics aside, what this tells you is that it's a balancing act – plenty of good fat, a decent amount of protein and a little bit of carb – that's the golden line you want to try to tread in order to feel the benefits of the keto diet.

The goal of keto is to edge the body away from using glucose (from carbs) as an energy source towards using stored fat instead. This is thought to have many health benefits such as increased mental clarity, weight loss, greater energy and even reduced risk of certain diseases.

In this book you'll find recipes that will help you shift the balance away from carbs, with clever and tasty substitutes for pasta (zoodles!), rice (cauliflower) and bread (make your own – it's easy, or use veggies instead), so you don't need to miss out on your favourite classic dishes like bolognaise, lasagne or pizza. You'll also discover here an easy keto-friendly salad, soup, stew, roast, barbecue or baked dish to suit every mood. And there are even recipes for cakes, brownies and bliss balls that you can eat guilt-free.

Although the recipes in this book are organised around standard daily meal times, you can eat whatever you want whenever you want! 'Intuitive eating' is all about tuning into your body to identify what your body is telling you that it needs. So listen to your body, learn a few new culinary tricks from the recipes in this book, and feel the benefits of your keto-inspired diet.

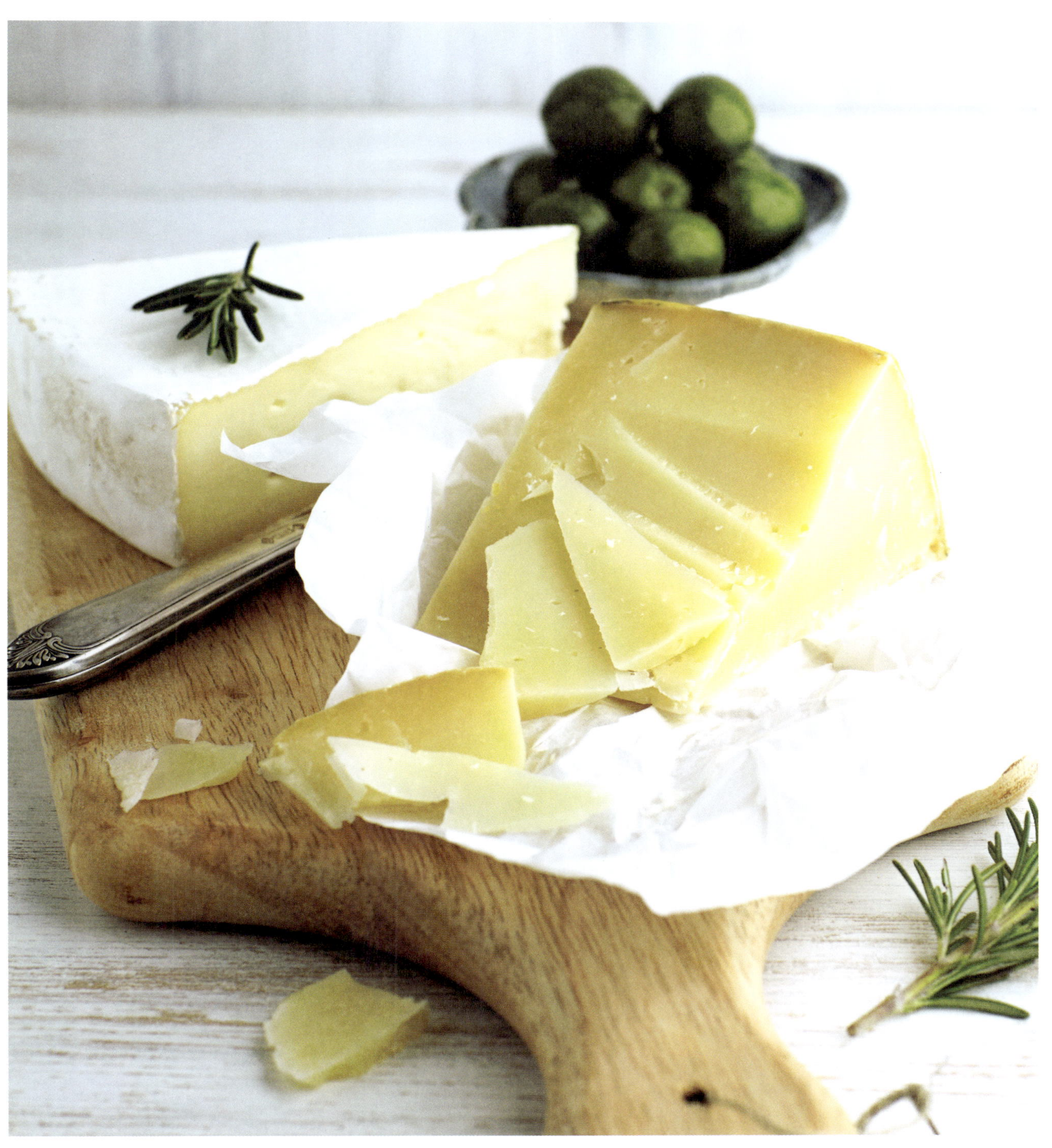

Keto Principles.

WHAT IS KETO?

In the keto diet you 'eat fat to burn fat'. The goal is to get the body to make a shift from using the glucose (sugar) that comes from carbohydrates for energy to using stored fat. This only happens when the body reaches a metabolic state known as ketosis. Getting to this state is different for everybody – because we all have different bodies.

Keto diets feature a low-carb, moderate-protein and high-fat dietary intake. The amount you need to eat of each of these groups depends on your 'macros'. Macros (short for macronutrients) refers to the balance of carbohydrates, protein and fat that your body needs to enter the state of ketosis. The easiest way to understand the ratio you need is to hop online and search for a keto calculator. You'll punch in some basics such as your height, weight, activity level and body-fat percentage, and be given a personalised ratio of daily carbs, protein and fats to aim for. You can then track your consumption by analysing the values of the foods you consume.

When cutting carbs from your diet it is important to focus on net carbs, which is the number of grams of total carbohydrates in a portion of food minus the grams of fibre. Fibre is deducated because the body does not absorb it well. Unlike other carbs, it doesn't get transformed into glucose, or influence blood sugar in the same way. (It's still important to get enough fibre, however, so don't neglect your greens, nuts and seeds.)

KETO AND THIS BOOK

The recipes in this book feature low-carb, high-fat options that anyone can use. If are tracking your macros carefully, it would be helpful to create meal plans using these and other recipes so that you can monitor your daily intake. You'll find plenty of tools online to help support you in this too.

Of course, you don't have to keep track. For many people it's enough to know that keto diets contain healthy foods and following the basic principles may bring benefits. If that's you, then follow the recipes in this book and enjoy.

PLEASE NOTE: ***the keto diet is not without its critics, who point to possible negative side effects associated with entering ketosis. If this is your goal, as with any extreme diet, it is best to do it under medical supervision.***

FOODS ARE NOT KETO, YOU ARE

Remember that particular foods aren't 'keto' or 'not keto', because ketosis is the state triggered by the absence of carbs. If a food fits within your personal macros limit then it's fine to enjoy.

PORTION SIZE MATTERS

Portion size matters more than ever on a keto diet. You can eat generous amounts of low-carb foods, but if you'd like to have some fruit, for example, then it is important to keep the amount you eat within your daily limit.

ALL VEGETABLES ARE NOT CREATED EQUAL

Vegetables have quite different carb contents so research the detail if you are counting carefully. A good rule of thumb is that 'above ground' veggies are okay, but 'below ground' vegetables should be consumed in moderation or not at all. Dark and leafy green veggies are best of all. Onions are high in carbs but generally only used in small amounts. You can cut up and freeze onion in small portions to use in recipes that need it. A whole onion is not often required. If it is, choose a small onion.

LEGUMES

Legumes are a healthy source of fibre and even protein – which makes them popular on a vegetarian diet – but they are high in carbs. Some have a higher ratio of protein to carb than others, so do your research. A good rule of thumb is to go by size: the smaller the bean, the higher the ratio. Lentils, for example, have more protein than chickpeas.

SOY SAUCE

Soy sauce can be used in a keto diet, but many followers of the diet prefer to substitute with the widely available wheat-free version, tamari, which we have used in the recipes in this book, or coconut aminos, which is gluten-free and low in salt by comparison. You can freely substitute soy sauce, tamari or coconut aminos as you prefer.

CHECK THE LABELS

Pre-made dressings, sauces, nut butters and spreads often contain added sugar. You can also use food labels to calculate the net carb allocation per serving size.

NUT BUTTERS

Nut butters are awesome keto fat bombs and it's easy to make your own. If you buy them pre-made check the label for added sugar.

KETO BAKING POWDER

Regular baking powder contains cornflour which is not ideal on a keto diet. It's easy to make your own using a combination of bicarbonate of soda and cream of tartar in a ratio of 1:2 (ie 1 tablespoon of bicarbonate of soda and 2 tablespoons of cream of tartar). It doesn't keep well so make it when you need it, and use whenever regular baking powder is called for.

BUTTER AND GHEE

On the keto diet, butter is good but ghee is better. The reason for this is that it contains a slightly higher percentage of short- and medium-chain fats. These are more easily digestible and therefore more accessible as an energy source, all aiding the body's journey to ketosis. For the uninitiated ghee might sound a bit strange, but it tastes even more buttery than butter itself making it a really flavoursome option. It also has high smoke point, so it's ideal for cooking with at high temperatures. Depending on your preference, ghee can be used in place of butter and vice versa in the recipes in this book.

SUGAR AND SWEETENERS

The goal is to avoid any form of crystal or liquid sugar – white sugar, coconut sugar, honey and maple syrup included – while on the keto diet and longer term to reduce your desire for sweet foods. You'll still need to find ways to flavour certain meals, however, and that's where sweeteners come in. In this book, we have generally used stevia because it's a keto-friendly choice that's widely available. It's very sweet and only a little is required, so it can't be like-for-like switched with sugar. Be aware that brands vary, meaning the stevia-to-sugar ratio can also vary. This information is usually available on the packaging. Use the quantities in the recipes as a guide and cross check with the stevia that you purchase. Sugar alcohols erythritol and xylitol are user-friendly because they are granulated, taste like sugar and can be used in similar measurements. They are okay keto choices, and more closely mimic sugar so they are preferred in some desserts and baked goods, but require extra effort to source. Some people have adverse reactions to these sweeteners, too. The best idea is to source the different options and experiment.

GLUTEN AND THE KETO DIET

The keto diet doesn't allow bread, grains or grain-based products, which means that it is largely gluten-free, and all the recipes in this book are gluten-free with the usual caveat that gluten can pop up in the strangest of places. So if you are following a strict gluten-free diet be sure to check the ingredients label on any pre-packaged sauces or marinades. If you are a coeliac, follow your usual dietary precautions.

LOW-CARB FOOD CHOICES

A fundamental part of the keto diet is choosing to eat low-carb foods. Generally, this means avoiding processed foods, most fruit and grains and eating more veggies and protein. For most of us there will probably be some disappointments (what, no fruit, popcorn, beer?) and surprises (beetroot, peas and pumpkin may need to be eaten in moderation or not at all depending on your macros) to get used to. The next page provides a simple guide to foods that you should consider avoiding and foods to embrace on the keto diet. If you are not sure, do your own research and make sure you eat to suit your personal goals. There is no one-size-fits-all in keto.

Red Flag Foods

PROCESSED & 'LOW-FAT' FOODS
Low-fat cheese and dairy, low-fat ice cream and diet soft drink.

BEER, SUGARY MIXED DRINKS AND JUICES

PRE-MADE DRESSINGS & SAUCES
Such as barbecue sauce, salad dressings and dipping sauces. Check the labels for added sugar.

STARCHY VEGETABLES
Potatoes (even sweet potatoes), squash, pumpkin and corn.

BEETROOT
(But feel free to eat the leaves!)

MOST FRUIT
Especially bananas, grapes, red apples, watermelon, mango, peaches, oranges and plums. Dried fruit.

VEGETABLE OILS & MARGARINE
Including canola and soybean oils.

CASHEW NUTS

LEGUMES
Including beans, chickpeas and peas.

GRAINS & GRAIN PRODUCTS
Including bread, tortillas, rice (white, brown, wild), pasta and oats and most breakfast cereals. Wheat flour, cornflour, baking powder.

SUGARS
Such as maple syrup, agave syrup and coconut sugar.

POPCORN

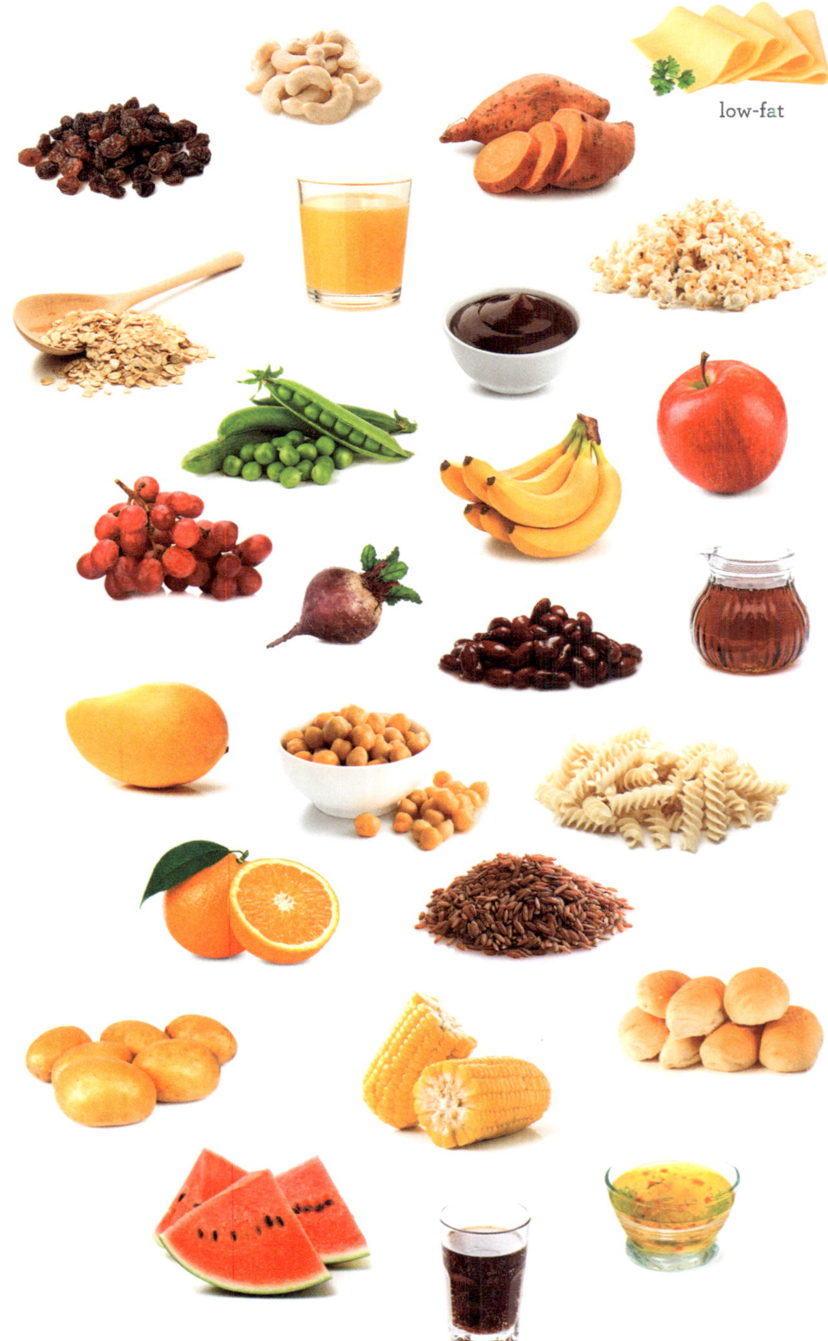

Bottom line: restrict your consumption of processed foods, grains, unhealthy fats & fruits.

Green Light Foods

MEAT AND POULTRY

Beef, chicken, turkey and pork (if budget allows buy organic, pasture-raised options).

FISH AND SHELLFISH

Fatty fish like salmon, sardines, mackerel and herring. Oysters, prawns and scallops.

EGGS

(If budget allows, buy organic, omega-3-enriched eggs.)

FULL-FAT DAIRY

Yoghurt (check it's sugar-free), butter, ghee, heavy cream and sour cream.

CHEESE

Brie and camembert, ricotta, cream cheese, Cheddar and goat's cheese.

OILS

Coconut, avocado, olive oil.

AVOCADOS

BERRIES

Blueberries, raspberries, blackberries.

NUTS AND NUT BUTTERS

Macadamia nuts, almonds, pecans, pistachios. Almond butter, peanut butter.

SEEDS

Pumpkin seeds, sunflower seeds, chia seeds.

VEGETABLES

Mushrooms, cauliflower, capsicums, tomatoes. Use fresh or frozen.

GREENS

Zucchini, Brussels sprouts, broccoli, kale, spinach, pak choy, bok choy, asparagus, celery.

CONDIMENTS

Sea salt, pepper, salsa, herbs, garlic, vinegars, mustard, olives and spices.

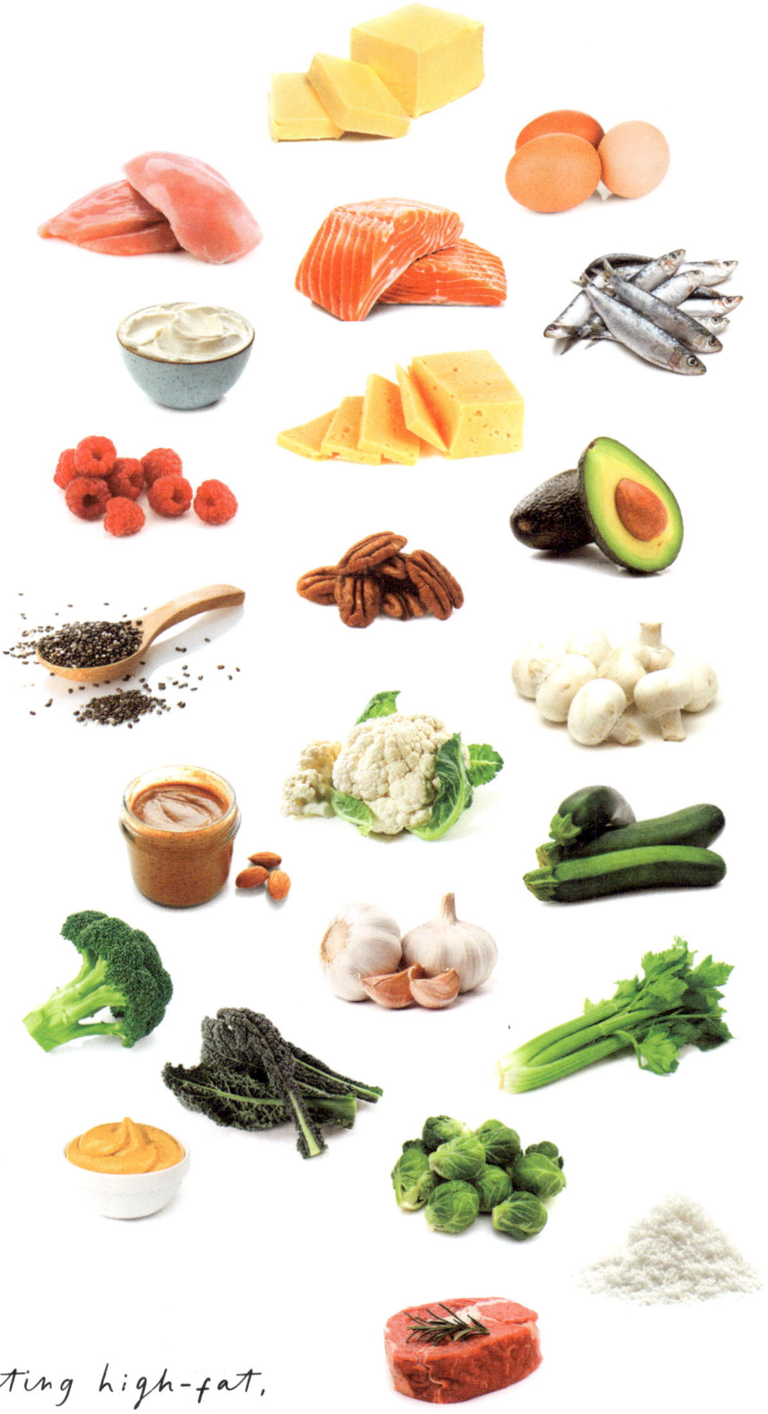

Bottom line: focus on eating high-fat, low-carb foods including meat, fish, dairy, eggs & vegetables.

Chapter One

Mornings

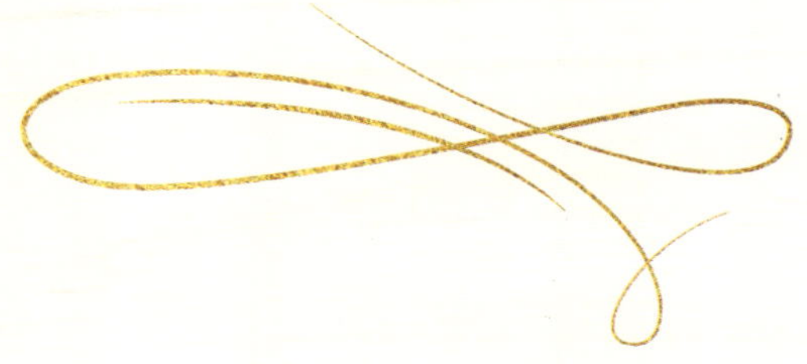

SALMON & SPINACH EGG MUFFINS

10 large eggs
½ tsp lemon zest
1 tbsp lemon juice
1 tbsp finely chopped fresh dill
Salt and pepper to taste
1 cup (40g) packed spinach, chopped
125g smoked salmon, cut into 12 even pieces

Preheat the oven to 180°C. Grease a 12-hole muffin tin.

In a medium jug, whisk together eggs, lemon zest, lemon juice and dill. Season with salt and pepper.

Distribute the spinach evenly between the prepared muffin cups. Add a piece of salmon to each cup, then pour in the egg mixture until each cup is about halfway full.

Bake for 18-22 minutes or until the eggs are set. Remove from the oven and cool slightly before serving.

Season once more with pepper, then serve.

BREAKFAST BOWL

2 cups (60g) tightly packed mixed salad leaves
200g smoked salmon
1 small avocado
4 eggs
White vinegar
1 radish, thinly sliced
1 tbsp black sesame seeds
1 tbsp white sesame seeds
2 lemon wedges

Split the salad leaves between two serving bowls.

Place half the smoked salmon on top in each bowl.

Slice the avocado and place half in each bowl.

To poach the eggs, add a small dash of vinegar to a pan of steadily simmering water – about 5cm deep.

Crack each egg gently into a small shallow dish and use this to slide them into the water one at a time.

Cook for 2½-3 minutes for a runny yolk. Cook for 3½-4 minutes for a set yolk.

Gently lift the eggs out with a slotted spoon and drain on a paper towel.

Place two eggs in each bowl to the side of the avocado. Place the sliced radish on top. Garnish with the sesame seeds and lemon wedges.

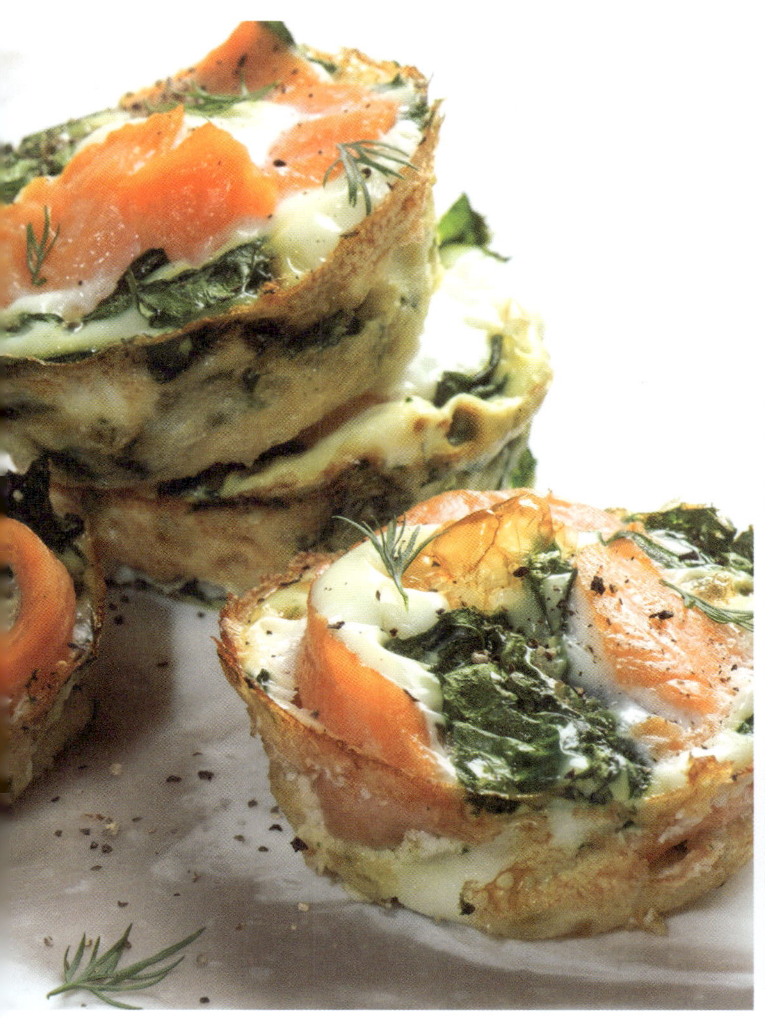

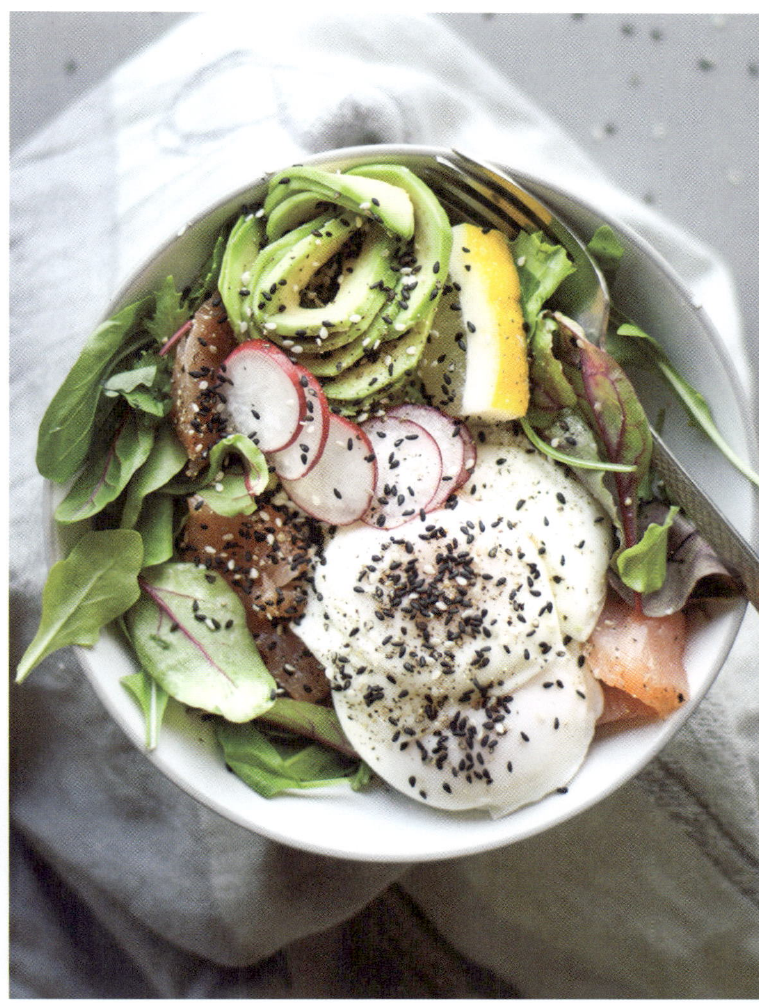

Salmon & Spinach Egg Muffins

MAKES 12

PREP + COOK TIME: 30 MINS

GLUTEN FREE

Breakfast Bowl

SERVES 2

PREP + COOK TIME: 20 MINS

GLUTEN FREE • DAIRY FREE

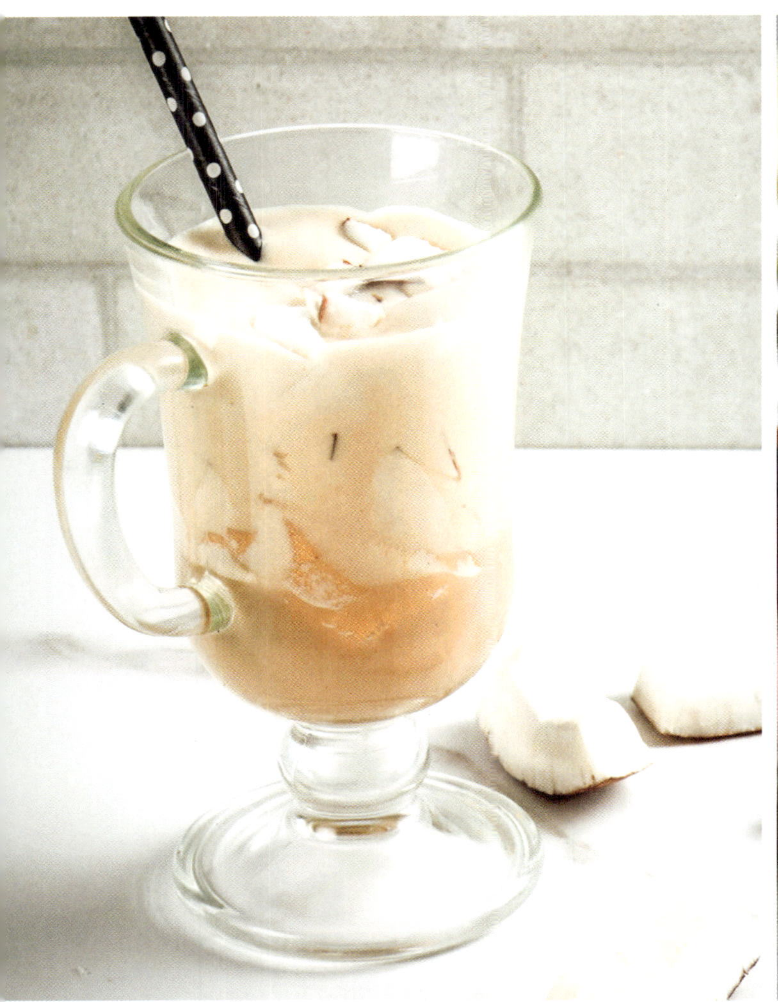

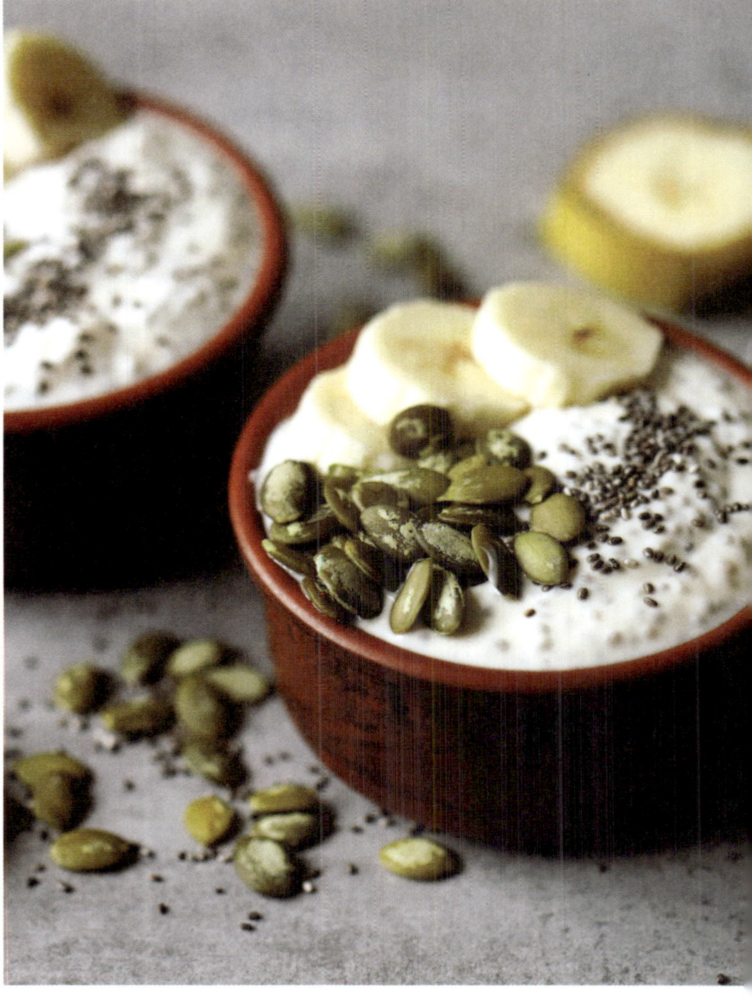

Coconut Latte Smoothie

SERVES 2

PREP TIME: 10 MINS

VEG • GLUTEN FREE • DAIRY FREE

Vanilla Cream Chia Pots

SERVES 2

PREP + COOK TIME: 5 MINS + CHILLING

VEG • GLUTEN FREE • DAIRY FREE

COCONUT LATTE SMOOTHIE

¼ tsp ground cinnamon
2½ tsps raw cacao powder
1 cup (250ml) coffee, frozen into ice cubes
1 tbsp almond butter
Pinch of stevia powder, to taste
1 tbsp coconut oil
1¼ cups (300ml) coconut milk
Shaved coconut pieces, to garnish

Place everything except the shaved coconut in a blender and puree until smooth and creamy.

Serve garnished with shaved coconut.

VANILLA CREAM CHIA POTS

4 tbsps chia seeds + ½ tsp to serve
1 tbsp monkfruit sweetener
1 tsp vanilla extract
¾ cup (185ml) full-fat coconut milk (from a can)
¼ cup (60ml) water
2 tbsps pumpkin seeds
½ small banana, sliced (optional)

Add 4 tablespoons chia seeds, sweetener, vanilla extract, coconut milk and water to a bowl and whisk to combine.

Cover the bowl and place in the fridge for at least 1 hour, or overnight.

Remove from the fridge and spoon into bowls. Top with pumpkin seeds, additional chia seeds and sliced banana if desired.

Serve immediately.

Tip:

Bananas are a high-carb food with 23g of carbs on average per banana. They are not recommended on a keto diet; however, three slices of banana on a pudding will not kick you out of ketosis. You can always choose to omit the banana on this pudding if you prefer though.

Green Salad & Mayo

SERVES 4

PREP + COOK TIME: 15 MINS

VEG • GLUTEN FREE

MAYONNAISE

2 large egg yolks, room temperature

¼ tsp salt + more to taste

1 tbsp Dijon mustard

1 cup (250ml) avocado oil

1 tbsp red or white wine vinegar

1 tsp lemon juice

SALAD

4 bunches asparagus, trimmed

1 cup (115g) sugar snap peas

⅔ cup (150g) crumbled feta cheese

Handful of fresh mint leaves

Handful of fresh basil leaves

POACHED EGGS

4 eggs

Salt and pepper to taste

To make the mayonnaise, whisk together the egg yolks, salt and mustard in medium bowl. Gradually add oil, in a thin, steady stream, whisking constantly until the mixture thickens. Stir vinegar and lemon juice into the mixture.

Blanch the asparagus in a pan of simmering water for 2 minutes, then remove with a slotted spoon and set aside.

Swirl the water in the pan with a wooden spoon to create a whirlpool then crack the eggs into the whirlpool and simmer gently for 3 minutes until the whites are cooked and the yolks are still runny. Remove with a slotted spoon and drain on paper towels.

Divide the asparagus between four plates. Scatter with sugar snap peas and crumbled feta. Sprinkle with mint and basil leaves, then top each plate with a poached egg.

Season with salt and pepper and serve with mayonnaise.

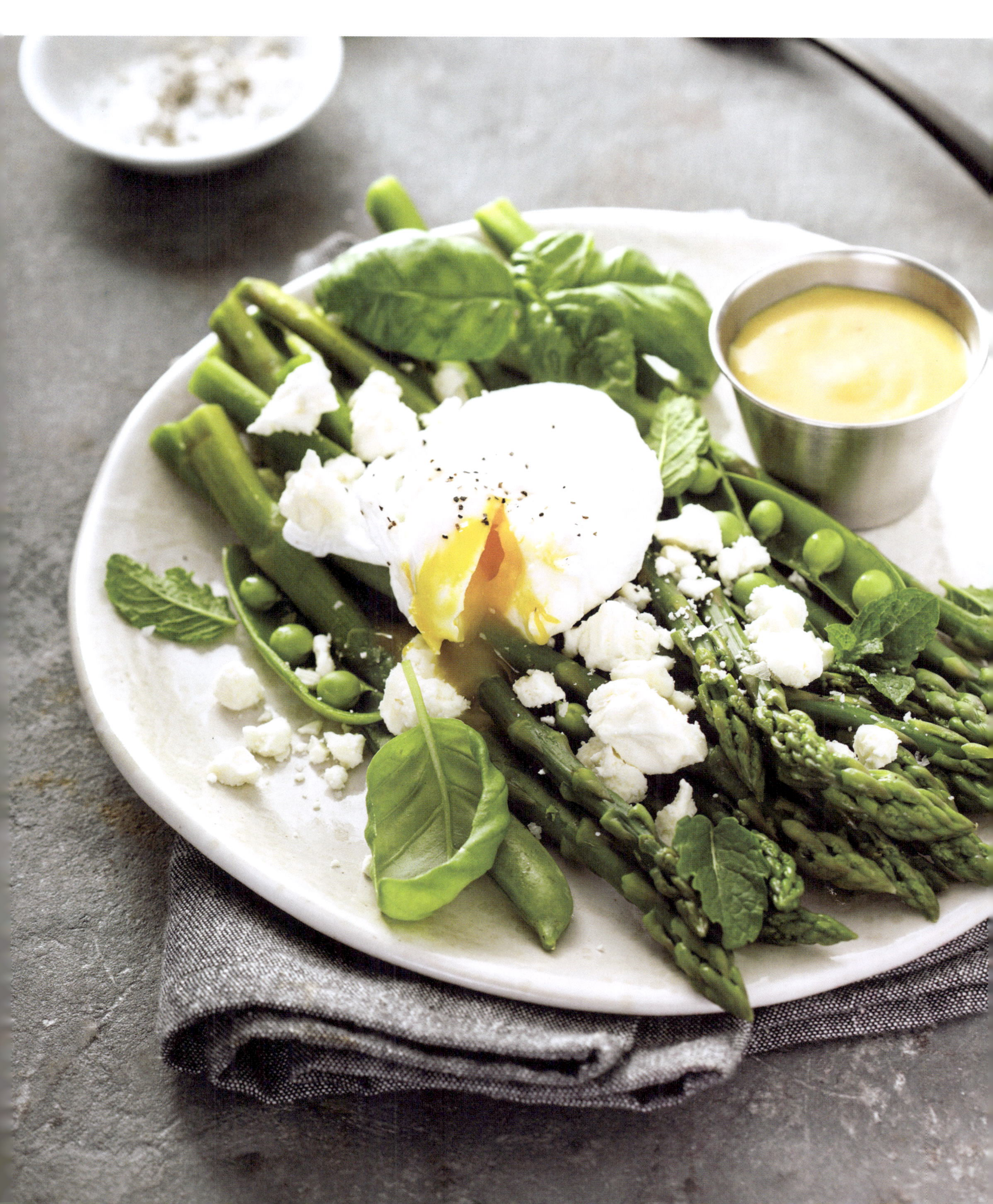

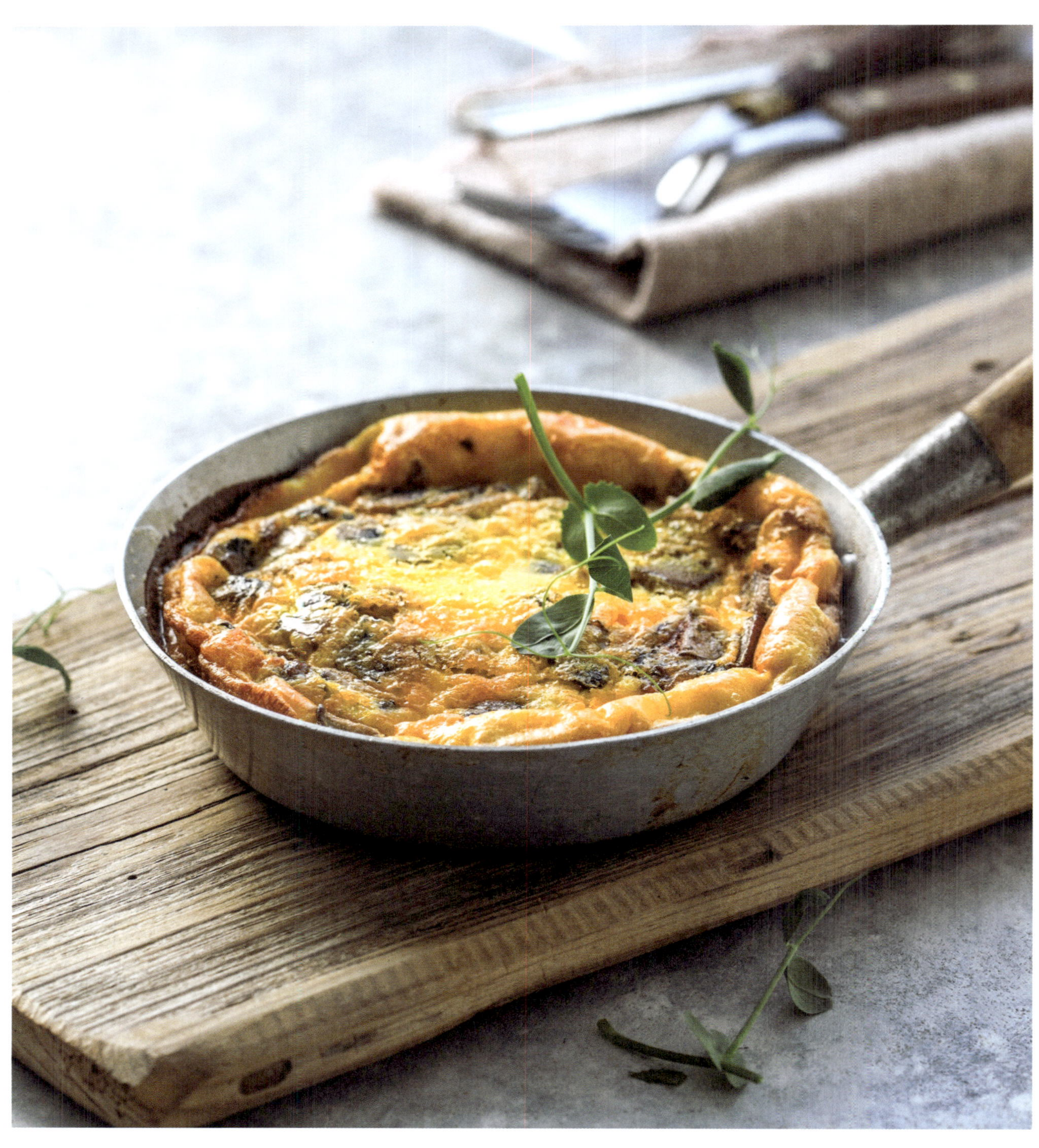

Mushroom Frittata

SERVES 4

PREP + COOK TIME: 45 MINS

GLUTEN FREE • DAIRY FREE

MUSHROOM FRITTATA

1 tbsp olive oil
450g button mushrooms, sliced
8 large eggs
¼ cup (60ml) sour cream
¼ tsp salt
¼ tsp pepper
¼ tsp dried thyme
½ cup (50g) chopped spring onions, green parts only
½ cup (50g) grated Parmesan cheese

Preheat oven to 200°C.

Heat the olive oil in a large ovenproof frying pan over medium heat. Add the mushrooms and cook for 8-10 minutes until tender and all liquids have evaporated.

In a medium bowl beat the eggs with the sour cream, salt, pepper and thyme. Add the spring onions and cheese and stir to combine.

Pour the egg mixture into the frying pan, then transfer to the oven.

Bake for 30 minutes until the edges are brown, the frittata is golden brown and puffy, and a knife inserted in centre comes out clean.

Tip:

Try adding sliced zucchini or other low-carb veg for a variation to the mushroom frittata.

ULTIMATE GREEN SMOOTHIE

2 tbsps chia seeds
½ small Lebanese cucumber, roughly chopped
1¼ cups (35g) spinach leaves, roughly chopped
1 medium avocado, diced
1 cup (250ml) coconut water
1 cup (250ml) water

Place the half the chia seeds,a all the cucumber, spinach, avocado, coconut water and water in a blender and process until smooth. Let sit for 5 minutes to thicken.

Divide the smoothie between serving glasses and serve garnished with remaining chia seeds.

BROCCOLI CHEESE

500g broccoli, cut into florets
250g cream cheese
¼ cup (60g) mayonnaise
1 cup (125g) grated Cheddar cheese
Salt and pepper to taste
¼ cup (25g) Parmesan, grated

Preheat oven to 180°C.

Steam the broccoli over a pan of boiling water for 4-5 minutes until tender. Add the cream cheese, mayonnaise, and Cheddar to a small bowl. Season with salt and pepper and mix well to combine.

Stir the cream cheese mixture into the steamed broccoli. Transfer broccoli to one large or four individual baking dishes and sprinkle over the Parmesan. Transfer to the oven and bake for 10 minutes until golden brown.

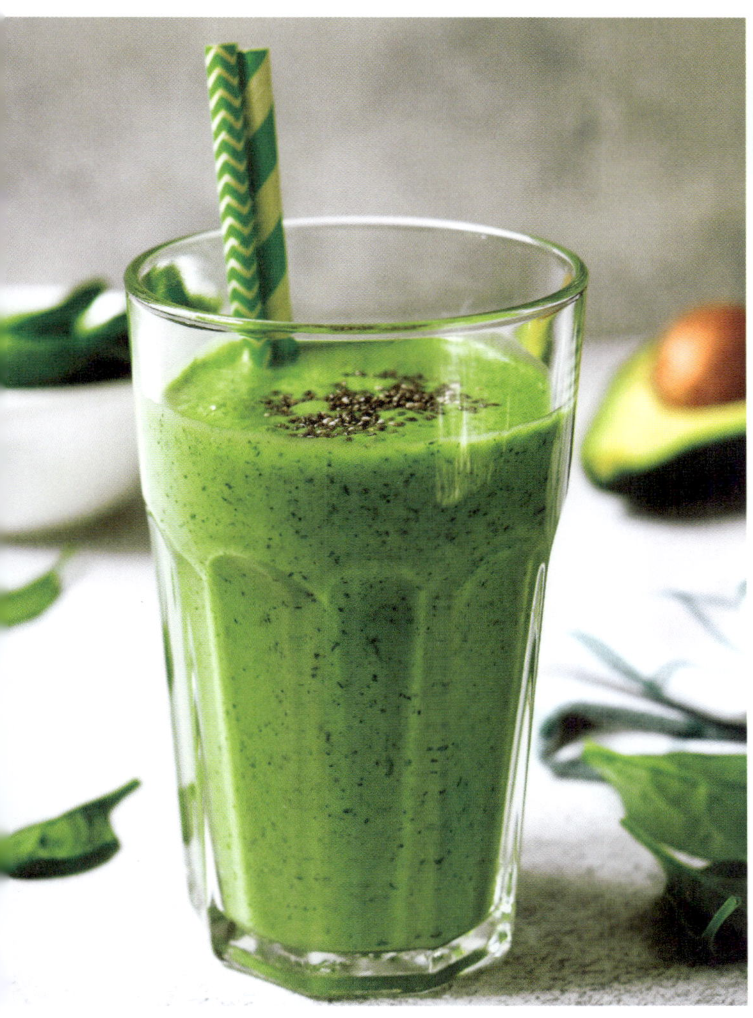

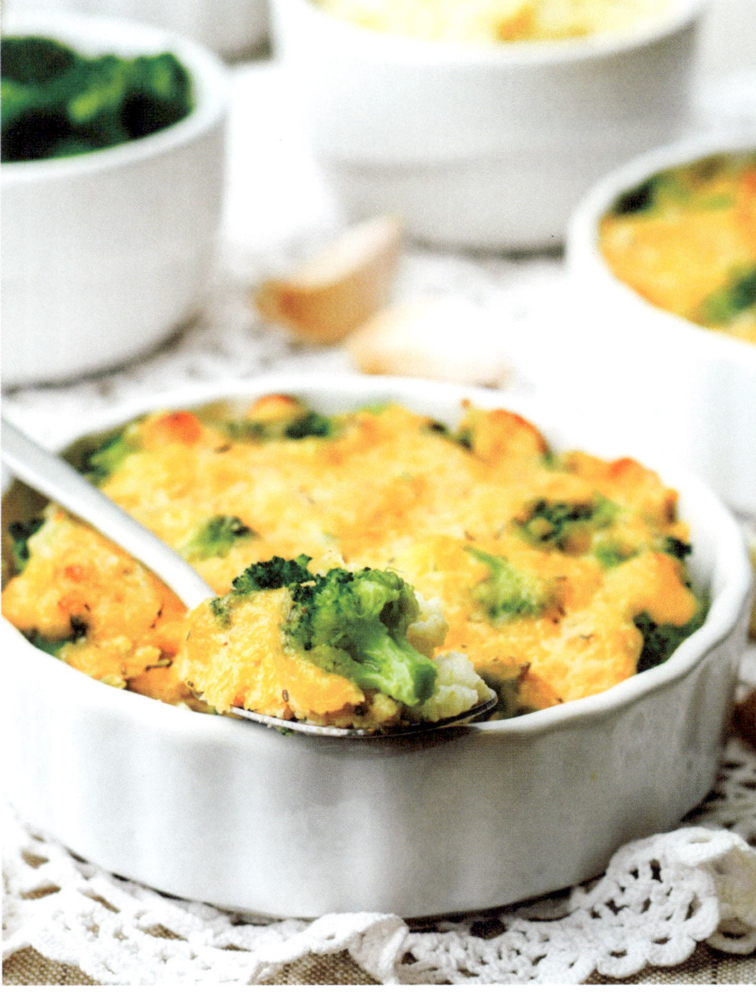

Ultimate Green Smoothie

SERVES 2

PREP: 15 MINS

VEG • GLUTEN FREE • DAIRY FREE

Broccoli Cheese

SERVES 4

PREP + COOK TIME: 20 MINS

VEG • GLUTEN FREE

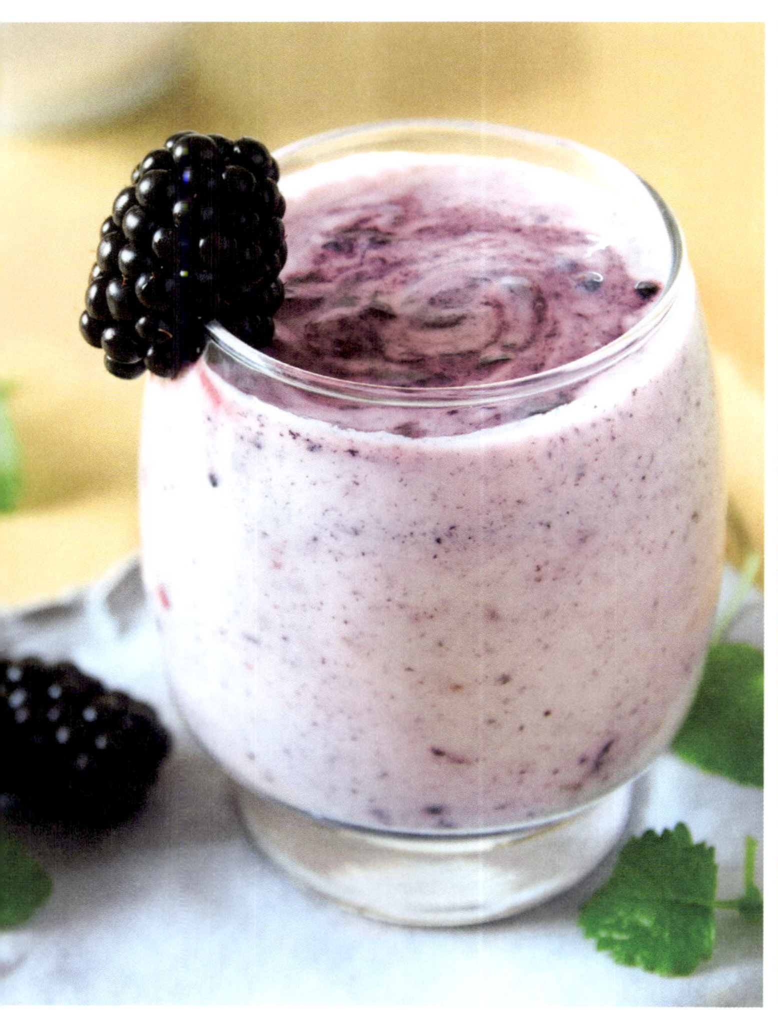

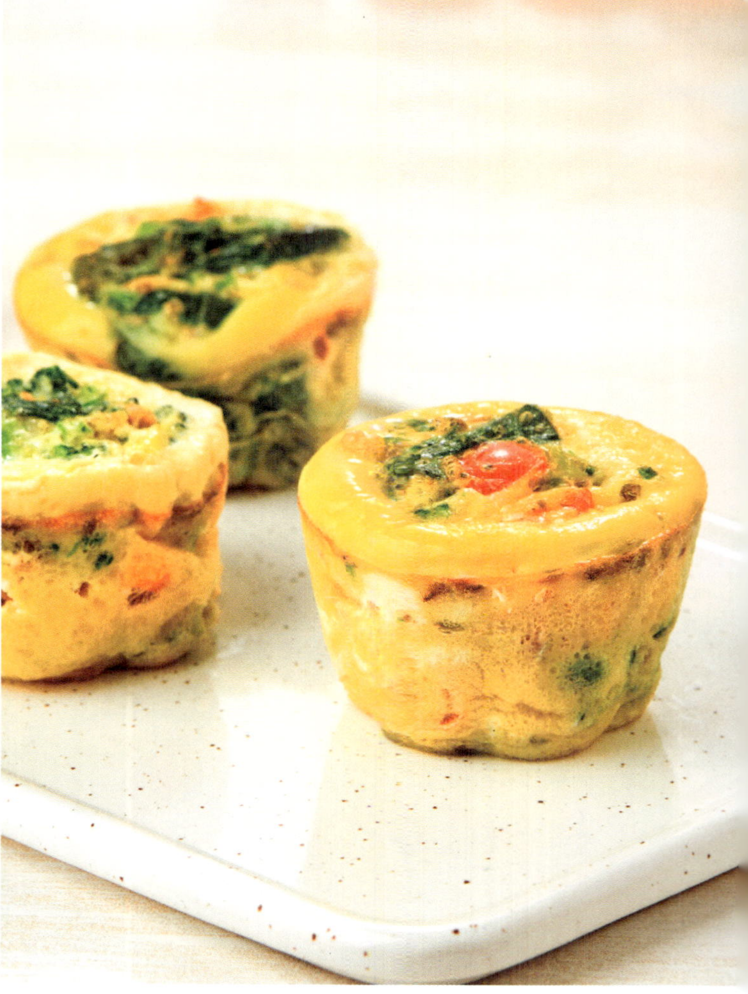

Blackberry Smoothie

SERVES 2

PREP + COOK TIME: 5 MINS

VEG • GLUTEN FREE • DAIRY FREE

Spinach Egg Cups

MAKES 8

PREP + COOK TIME: 20 MINS

VEG • GLUTEN FREE

BLACKBERRY SMOOTHIE

½ cup (60g) frozen blackberries

2 cups (500ml) coconut milk

½ cup (125ml) coconut cream (or double cream if dairy is ok)

½ tsps cinnamon

Place all ingredients into a high-speed blender. Blend on high for 30 seconds until well combined.

Pour into bottles or glasses to serve.

SPINACH EGG CUPS

3 tbsps olive oil

1 cup (30g) spinach leaves, chopped

8 eggs

1 cup (125g) grated Cheddar cheese

⅓ cup (75g) cherry tomatoes, chopped

Preheat oven to 200°C. Grease eight cups of a muffin tin with the oil. Place chopped spinach leaves in the bottom of each muffin cup.

In small bowl, whisk together the eggs and cheese. Add the tomatoes and gently mix through.

Pour egg mixture into each muffin cup, filling about two-thirds full.

Bake in oven for 10-12 minutes, until egg has set and the tops are golden. Serve warm or cold.

Asparagus in Bacon

SERVES 4

PREP + COOK TIME: 40 MINS

GLUTEN FREE

500g asparagus spears, trimmed

1 tbsp olive oil

Salt and pepper to taste

8 rashers thick-cut bacon

1 tsp dried mixed herbs (optional)

⅛ tsp dried chilli flakes (optional)

1 tbsp fresh parsley, chopped, to serve

YOGHURT AND DILL DRESSING

½ cup (125ml) Greek yoghurt

4 tbsps mayonnaise

1 tsp fresh dill, finely chopped

1 tsp lemon juice

Salt and pepper to taste

Preheat the oven to 200°C. Line a baking tray with greaseproof paper.

Place asparagus on baking tray. Drizzle with olive oil and sprinkle with salt and pepper. Toss to coat.

Divide asparagus into 8 bundles and wrap each bundle with a piece of bacon. Place seam side down on the baking tray. Sprinkle with the herbs and chilli flakes, if using.

Transfer to the oven. Bake for 20-25 minutes until bacon is cooked and asparagus is tender.

Mix together the dressing ingredients in a small bowl until well combined.

Sprinkle asparagus with parsley and serve warm with the dressing.

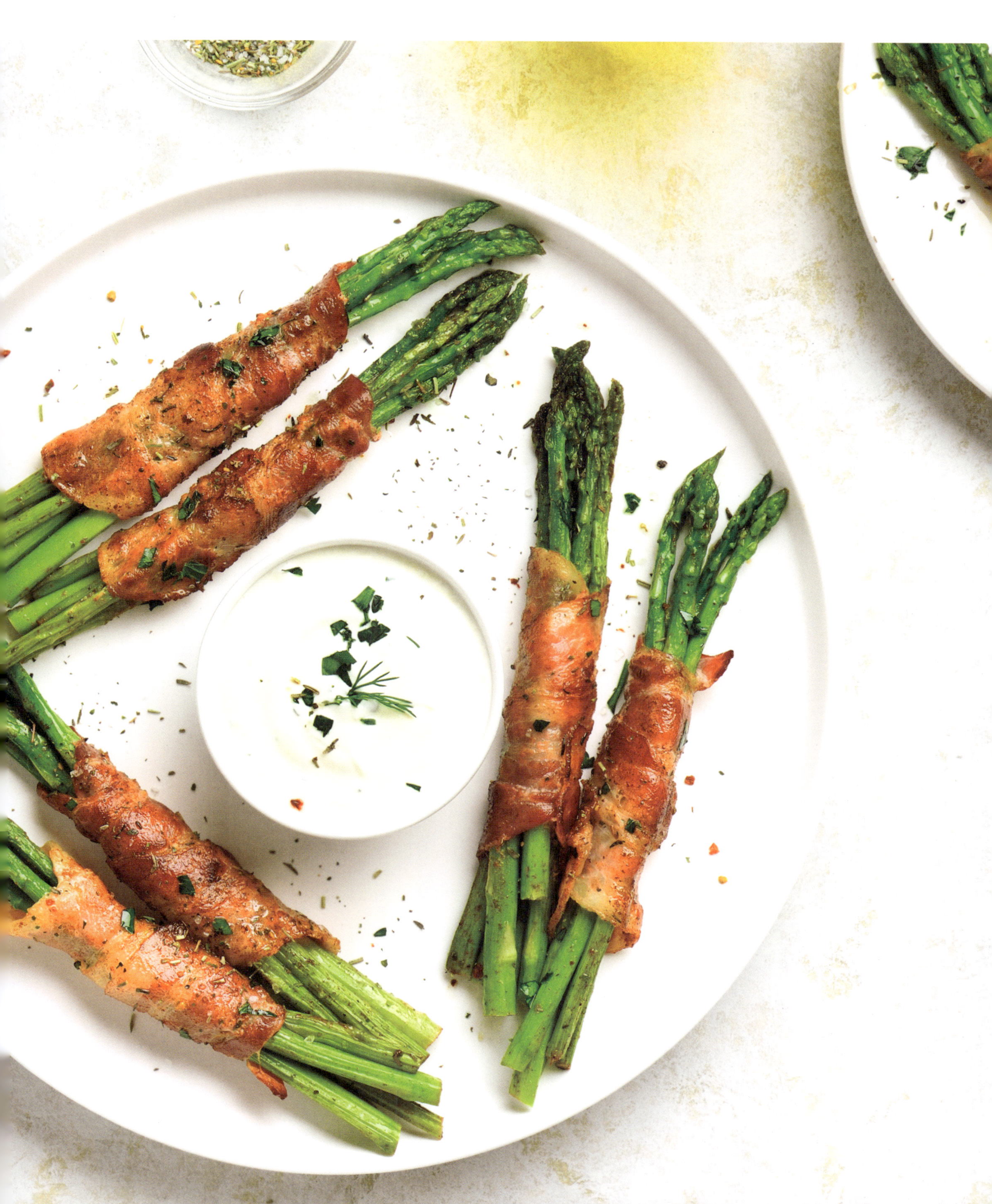

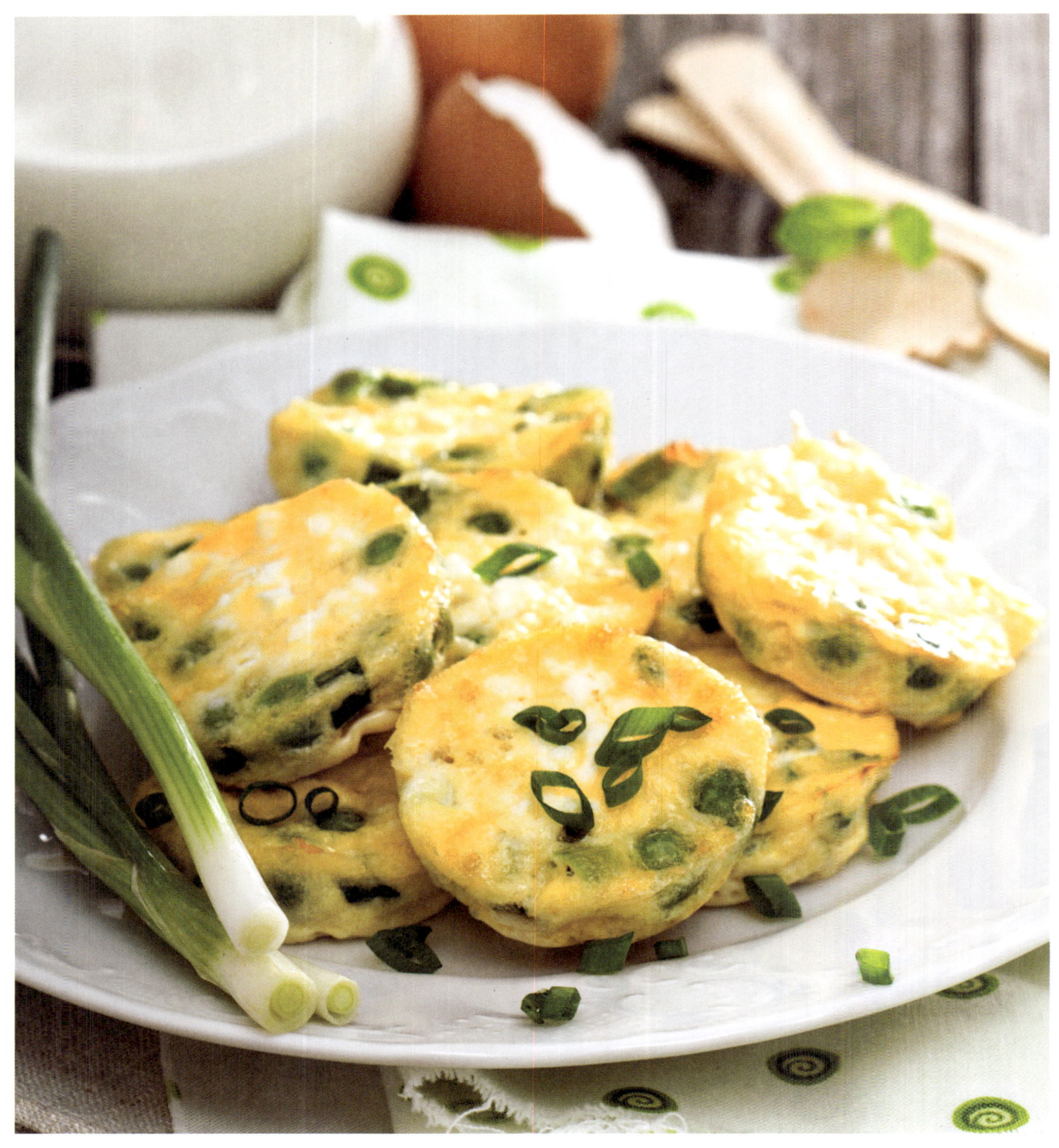

Egg & Feta Muffins

MAKES 12

PREP + COOK TIME: 30 MINS

VEG • GLUTEN FREE

EGG & FETA MUFFINS

18 eggs
¼ cup (60ml) cream
⅓ cup (80g) crumbled feta cheese
⅛ tsp garlic powder
⅛ tsp onion powder
3 spring onions, chopped
Salt and pepper to taste

Preheat the oven to 180°C. Grease a 12-hole muffin tin.

In a large bowl beat the eggs with the cream until frothy.

Place the feta, garlic powder, onion powder, spring onions, salt and pepper to the bowl with the beaten eggs. Fold until all the ingredients are well incorporated.

Pour the mixture halfway up into each well of the prepared muffin tin.

Bake for 20 minutes or until eggs are fully set.

Serve immediately or store in the fridge for up to 5 days.

Note:

If you have a 6-hole muffin tin this can be used in place of the 12-hole tin to yield 6 muffins. Simply halve the quantities in this recipe and follow the method in the same way.

Yoghurt Parfait with Nutty Granola

SERVES 2

PREP + COOK TIME: 45 MINS

VEG • GLUTEN FREE

GRANOLA

½ cup (60g) pecans
½ cup (60g) walnuts
2 tsps coconut oil, melted
2 tsps xylitol
1 tsp cinnamon
½ tsp vanilla extract

PARFAIT

½ cup (125ml) full-fat Greek yoghurt
¼ cup (60ml) double cream
1 tsp vanilla extract

Preheat oven to 140°C. Line a baking tray with greaseproof paper.

Finely chop the nuts leaving a few pieces still chunky.

Add the chopped nuts to a mixing bowl along with the melted coconut oil, xylitol, cinnamon and vanilla. Stir well to combine.

Arrange the nuts in an even layer across the lined baking tray and transfer to the oven to bake for 30-35 minutes until fragrant and golden brown. Allow to cool completely.

In a mixing bowl, add the yoghurt, cream and vanilla. Whisk together until thick and creamy.

Divide the yoghurt between two glasses. Top with the nutty granola and serve.

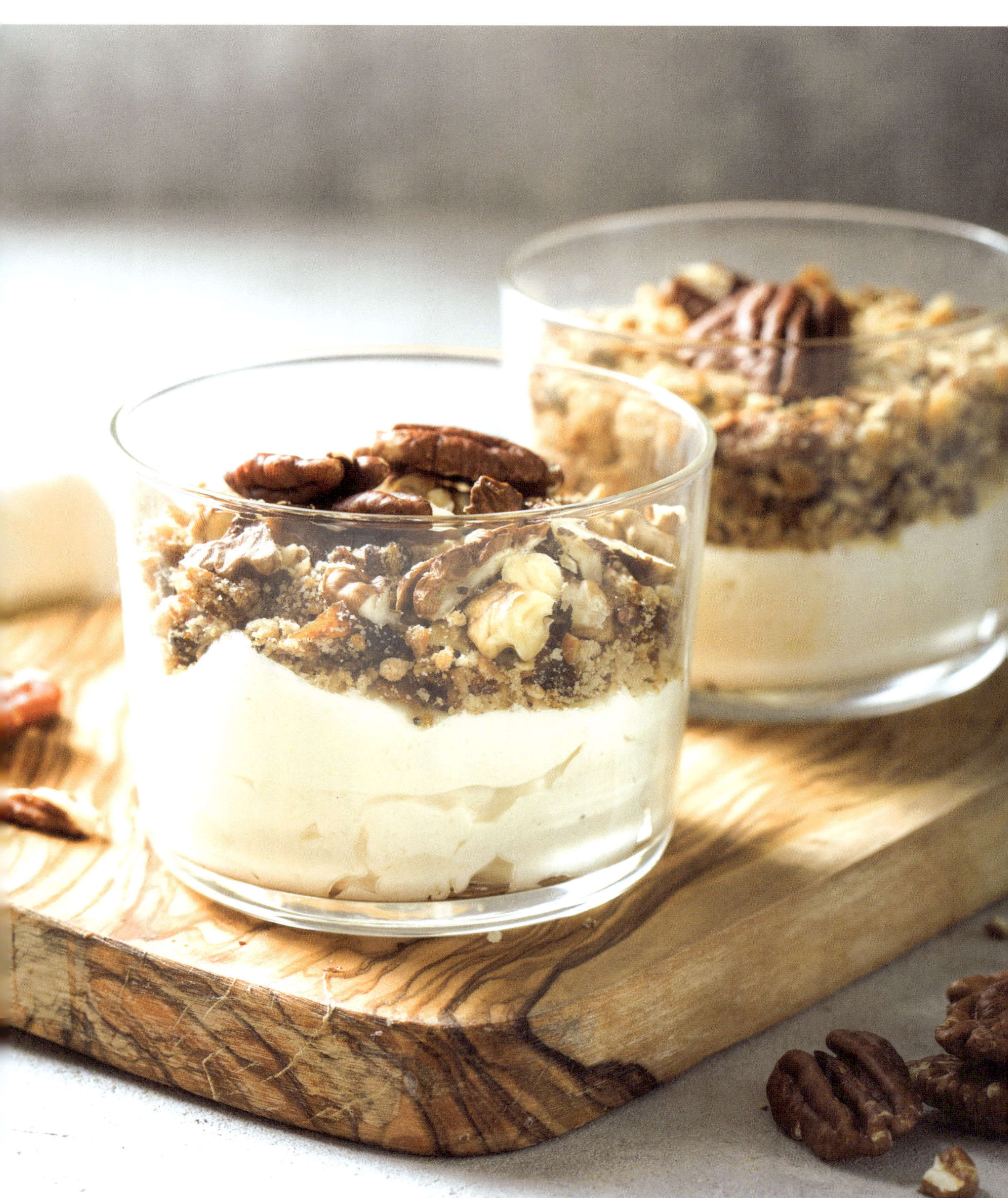

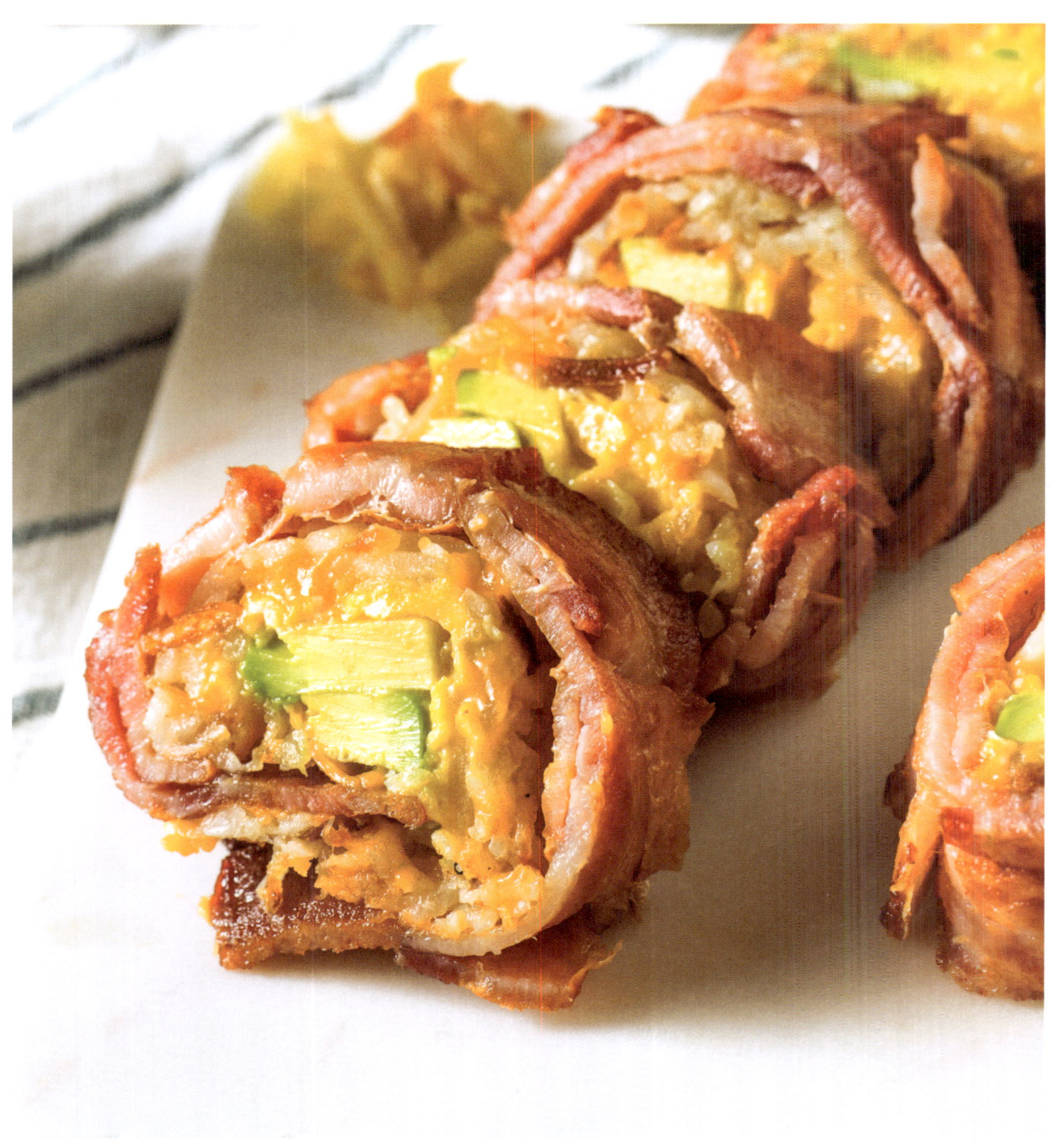

Breakfast Sushi

SERVES 4

PREP + COOK TIME: 20 MINS

GLUTEN FREE

BREAKFAST SUSHI

1 tbsp butter
½ onion, chopped
7 large eggs, room temperature
1 cup (125g) grated tasty cheese
2 large avocados, sliced and chopped
18 rashers middle bacon
Salt and pepper to taste

Heat the butter in a large nonstick frying pan over medium heat and fry the onion for 4 minutes until softened. Whisk the eggs together and add to the pan. Scramble for 3 minutes, then remove to a large mixing bowl. Wipe down the pan for reuse.

Mix the cheese and avocado gently into the eggs and season lightly.

On a flat workspace, lay out three strips of bacon, slightly overlapping. Spread out one-sixth of the egg mixture along one side of the strips. Roll them up and place seam-side down in the pan over medium-high heat. Repeat with the remaining strips of bacon and egg. Fry each roll until crispy all over.

Cut into bite-size sushi-style rolls and serve hot.

Stuffed Buckwheat Pancakes

SERVES 4

PREP + COOK TIME: 20 MINS + RESTING

GLUTEN FREE

PANCAKES

100g unsalted butter

¾ cup (90g) buckwheat flour

¼ cup (30g) coconut flour

3 eggs

½ tsp salt

1⅓ cups (400ml) soy or almond milk

FILLING

½ cup (60g) Parmesan, grated

2 cups (500g) cherry tomatoes, halved

400g prosciutto

2 cups (60g) loosely packed baby spinach

2 cups (60g) loosely packed rocket

¼ cup (10g) parsley, roughly chopped

Preheat the oven to 60°C for keeping the cooked pancakes warm.

Melt half the butter and combine in a medium bowl with the flours, eggs, salt and half the milk. Whisk together and add the rest of the milk a small amount at a time until the mixture is smooth.

Let mixture sit for at least 30 minutes.

Melt 1 tablespoon of the remaining butter in a large nonstick frying pan and pour a quarter of the mixture into the pan.

Cook the pancake on one side for 2 minutes or until the edges start to brown and come away from the pan.

Carefully flip over and sprinkle a quarter of the Parmesan over the pancake. Cook for another 30 seconds then carefully transfer to a serving plate. Place one quarter of the remaining filling ingredients over one half of the pancake, then fold the other half of the pancake over the filling.

Place in the oven to warm while you repeat the steps with the remaining batter and ingredients.

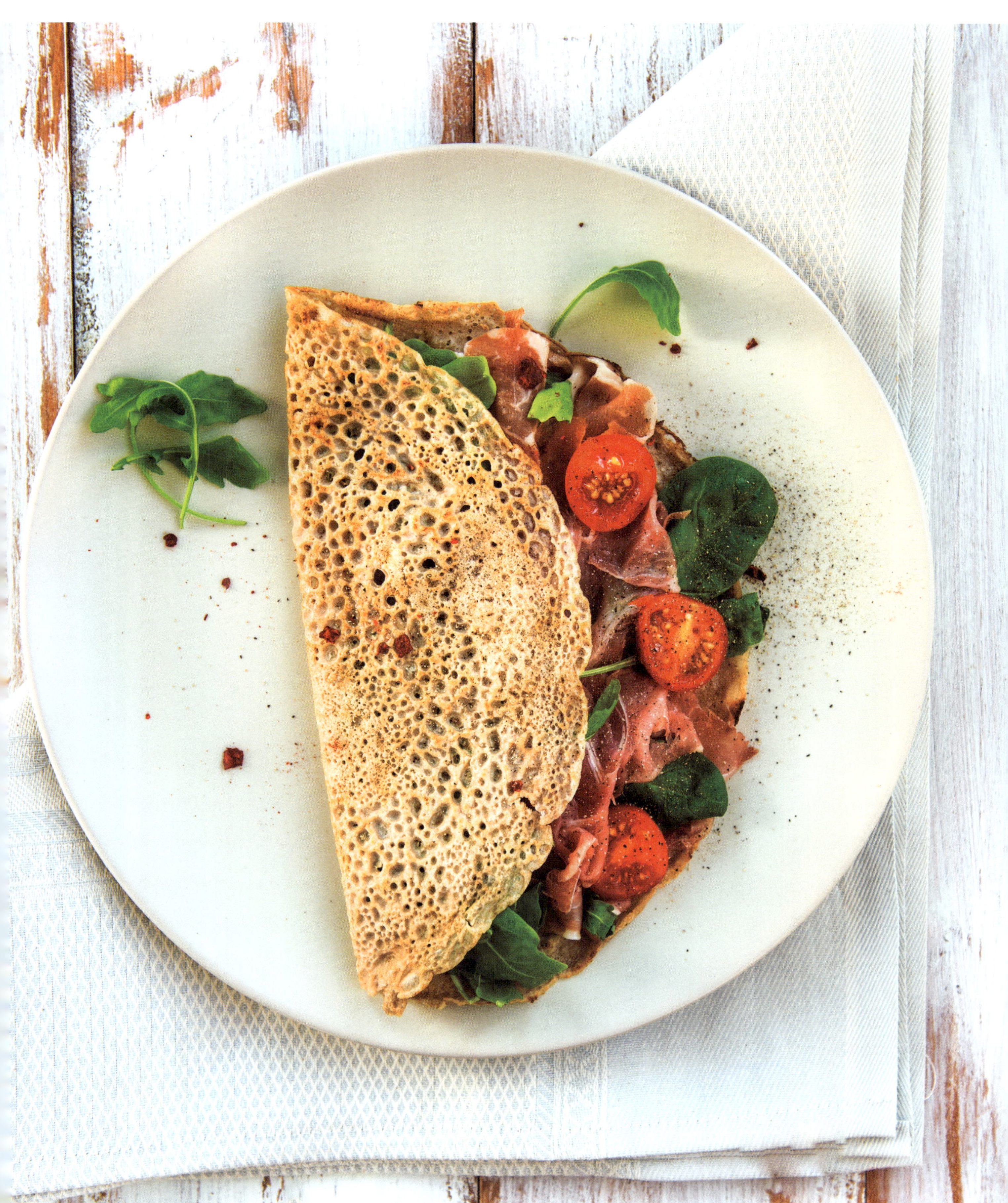

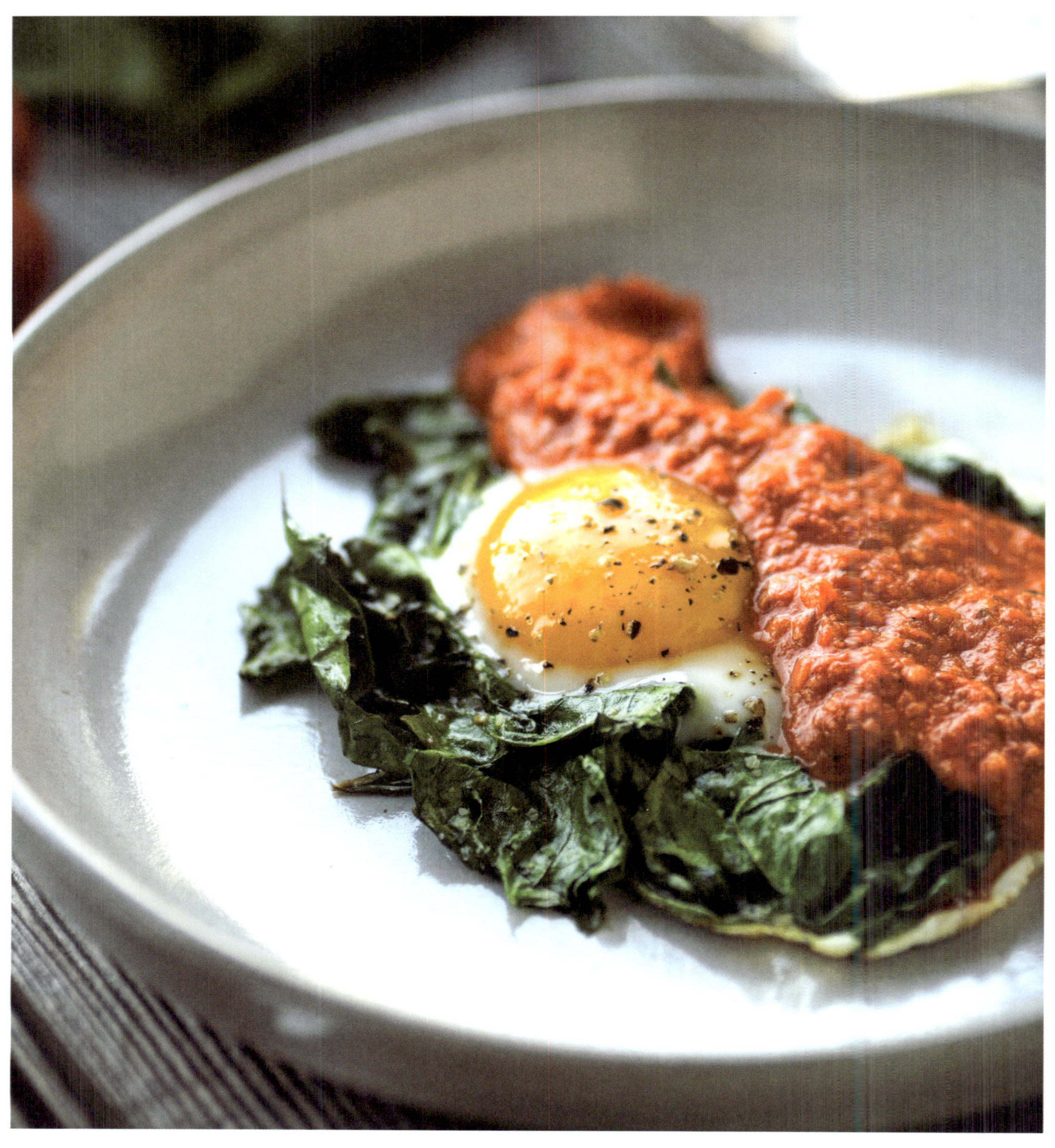

Fried Egg & Spinach with Romesco Sauce

SERVES 4

PREP + COOK TIME: 15 MINS

VEG • GLUTEN FREE • DAIRY FREE

FRIED EGG & SPINACH WITH ROMESCO SAUCE

- 3 tbsps olive oil
- 1 onion, finely diced
- 500g baby spinach
- Salt and pepper to taste
- 4 eggs

ROMESCO SAUCE

- ¾ cup (100g) blanched almonds
- 200g roasted capsicum from a jar, drained
- 1 clove garlic
- 1 tbsp sherry vinegar
- 1 tsp smoked paprika
- ¼ cup (50ml) olive oil

To make the romesco sauce, toast the almonds in a dry frying pan over medium-low heat, shaking often, for 3-4 minutes until fragrant and starting to turn golden. Remove from the pan and leave to cool.

Drain the capsicums and add to a food processor with the almonds, garlic, vinegar and smoked paprika, then blitz to a chunky paste.

With the motor still on, slowly drizzle in the olive oil and keep blending until combined. Set aside until ready to serve.

Heat olive oil in a large frying pan, over medium heat. Add onion and cook, stirring regularly, for 5-7 minutes until soft and translucent.

Add the spinach and season with salt and pepper. Cook, stirring gently, until the spinach leaves wilt and the liquid evaporates.

Make four wells in the spinach mixture and crack an egg into each well. Cook for 3-4 minutes until the egg whites are set.

Sprinkle salt and pepper on each egg.

Serve immediately with romesco sauce.

Tip:

Save leftover romesco sauce to serve with fish or chicken.

BLUEBERRY SMOOTHIE BOWL

½ cup (50g) frozen chopped cauliflower

½ cup (50g) frozen blueberries, plus a few extra to garnish

⅓ cup (80ml) almond milk

2 tbsps chopped walnuts, to garnish

2 tbsps flaked almonds, to garnish

Place the cauliflower, blueberries and milk into a high-speed blender and process until smooth, scraping down the sides as needed.

Spoon into a bowl. To serve, garnish with extra berries, walnuts and flaked almonds, if desired.

KETO BREAD

3 large eggs, separated

⅛ tsp cream of tartar

90g mascarpone or cream cheese (softened)

⅛ tsp salt

Preheat the oven to 150°C. Line a baking tray with greaseproof paper.

In a large bowl, use an electric mixer to beat the egg whites and cream of tartar until stiff peaks form.

In a second large bowl, use the mixer to beat the mascarpone, egg yolks and salt until smooth.

Carefully fold a third of the egg whites into the mascarpone mixture with a spatula. Then fold in the remaining egg white mixture. Scoop the mixture into six discs onto the prepared baking tray.

Bake for 25-35 minutes, until golden.

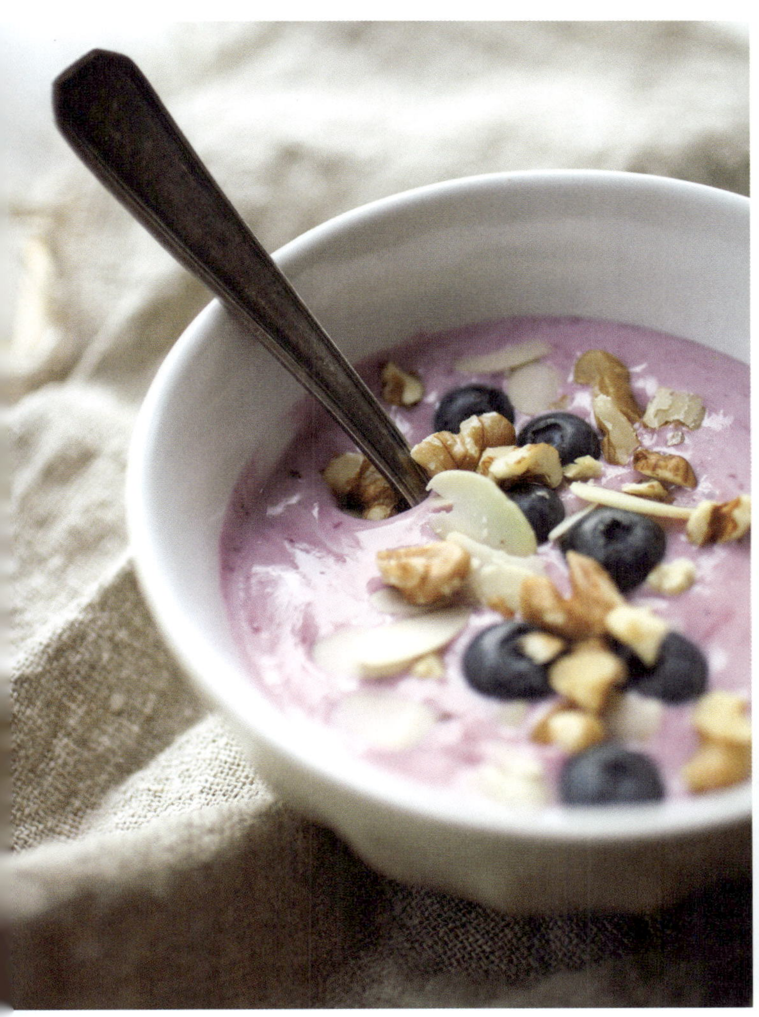

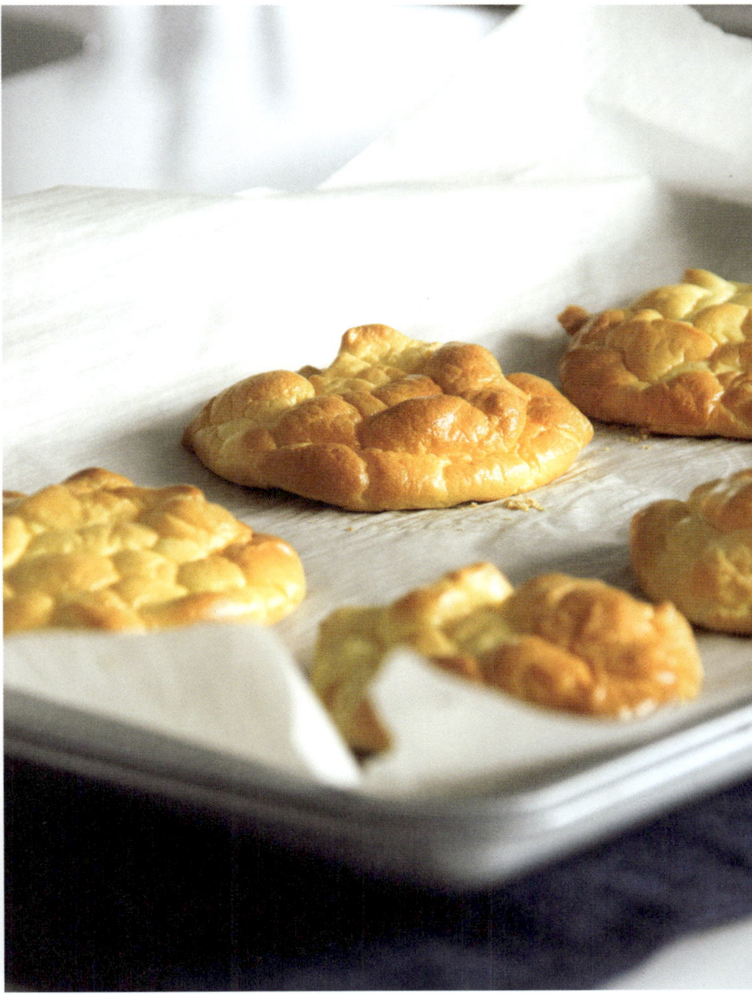

Blueberry Smoothie Bowl

SERVES 1

PREP + COOK TIME: 10 MINS

VEG • GLUTEN FREE • DAIRY FREE

Keto Bread

SERVES 6

PREP + COOK TIME: 35 MINS

VEG • GLUTEN FREE

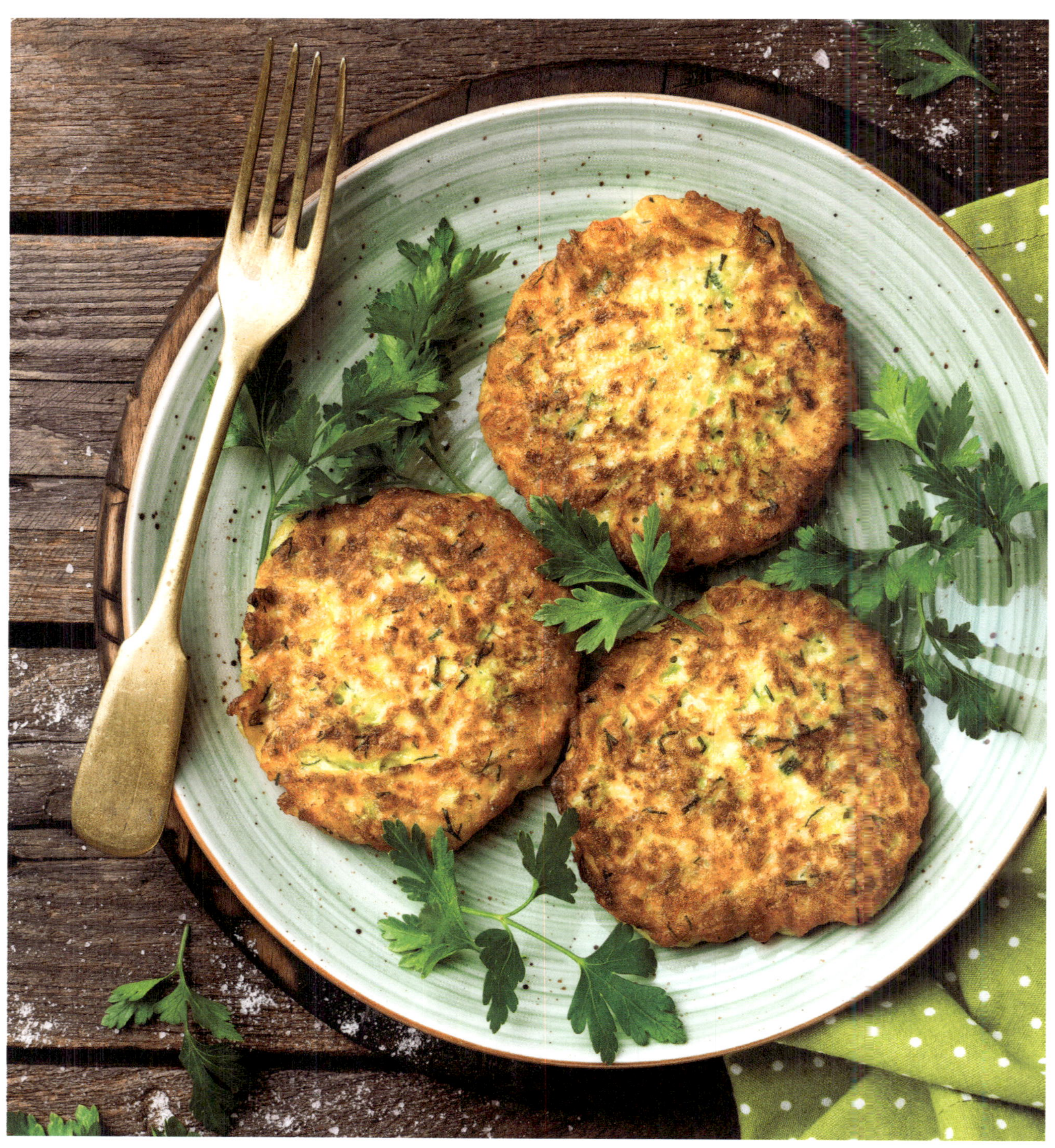

Zucchini Pancakes

SERVES 4

PREP + COOK TIME: 30 MINS

VEG • GLUTEN FREE • DAIRY FREE

ZUCCHINI PANCAKES

75g cream cheese
3 large eggs, room temperature, lightly whisked
4 medium zucchinis, grated, squeezed to remove excess liquid
¼ cup (10g) fresh parsley, finely chopped
¼ cup (25g) grated Parmesan
½ tsp onion powder
1 tsp baking powder
⅓ cup (30g) coconut flour
Salt and pepper to taste
3 tbsps butter

Whisk together the cream cheese and eggs in a large bowl. Add the zucchini, parsley, Parmesan, onion powder, baking powder and coconut flour as well as a couple of grinds of salt and pepper.

Heat half the butter in a large non-stick frying pan over medium heat.

Drop ⅓ cup portions of the zucchini mix into the pan and fry for 4 minutes. Carefully flip over and fry for another 3 minutes. Repeat with the rest of the batter and add more butter as needed.

Drain on paper towels and serve warm.

Buckwheat Bake with Spinach & Egg

SERVE 2

PREP + COOK TIME: 30 MINS

VEG • GLUTEN FREE

2 cups (500ml) water

Salt and pepper to taste

½ cup (85g) buckwheat groats

2 tbsps butter

1 onion, chopped

1 cup (30g) spinach

150g feta cheese

1 cup (125g) grated Cheddar cheese

¼ cup (30g) walnuts, chopped and toasted

2 eggs

Preheat oven to 180°C.

Pour water into a small pan with a pinch of salt. Bring to a boil and add the buckwheat groats. Cover and reduce heat to low. Cook for about 15 minutes, until water is absorbed and the groats are creamy.

Meanwhile heat butter in a frying pan over medium heat. Cook onion, stirring regularly, for 3-5 minutes until soft and translucent. Add spinach, season with salt and pepper and cook for 2-3 minutes until wilted. Remove from heat.

In a large bowl combine the buckwheat, spinach and onion mixture, the feta, Cheddar and walnuts. Mix to combine, and divide between two ovenproof dishes.

With a spoon, make a well in the centre of each portion. Crack an egg into each well.

Transfer to the oven and bake for 15 minutes until the cheese is melted and the egg is cooked.

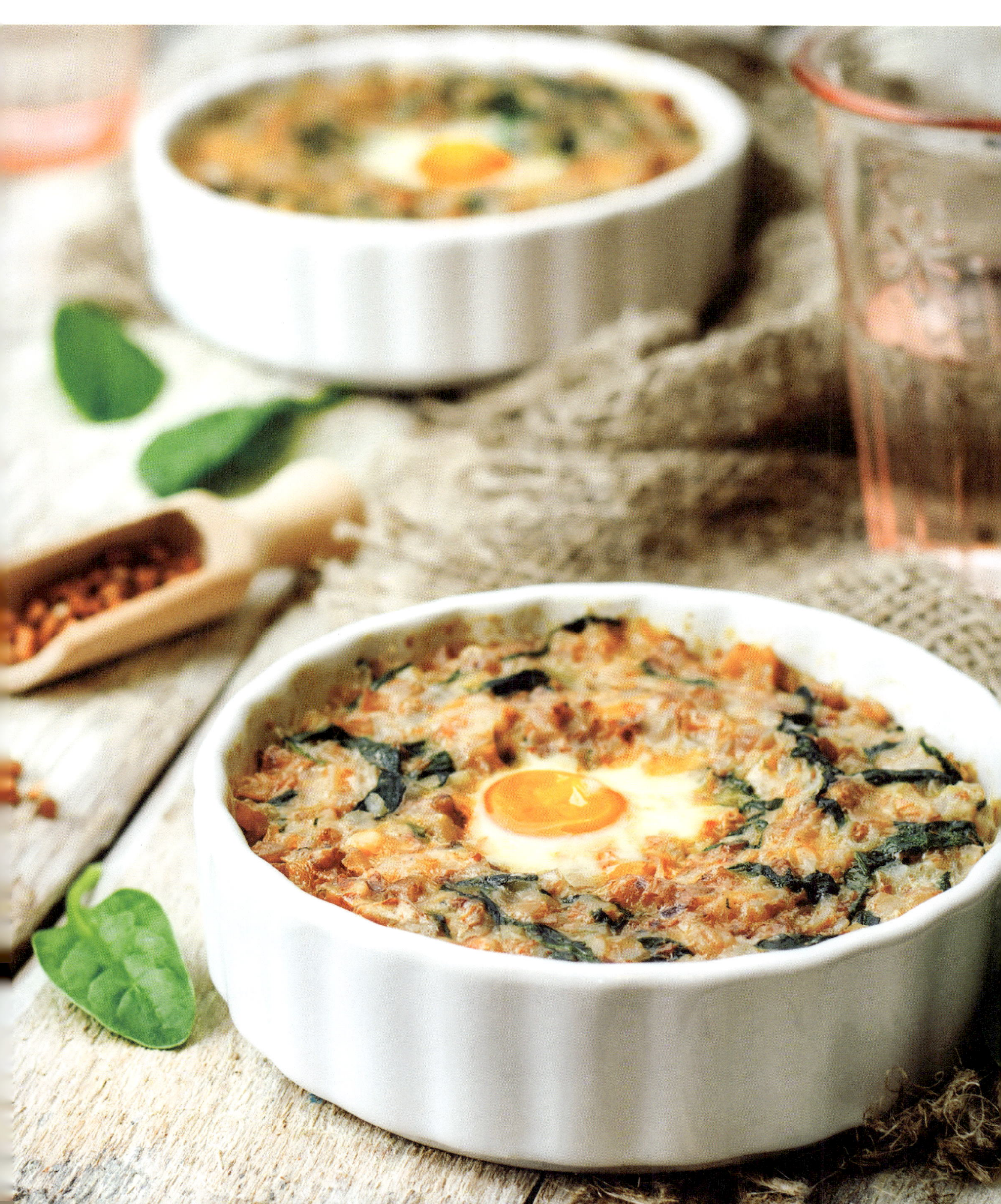

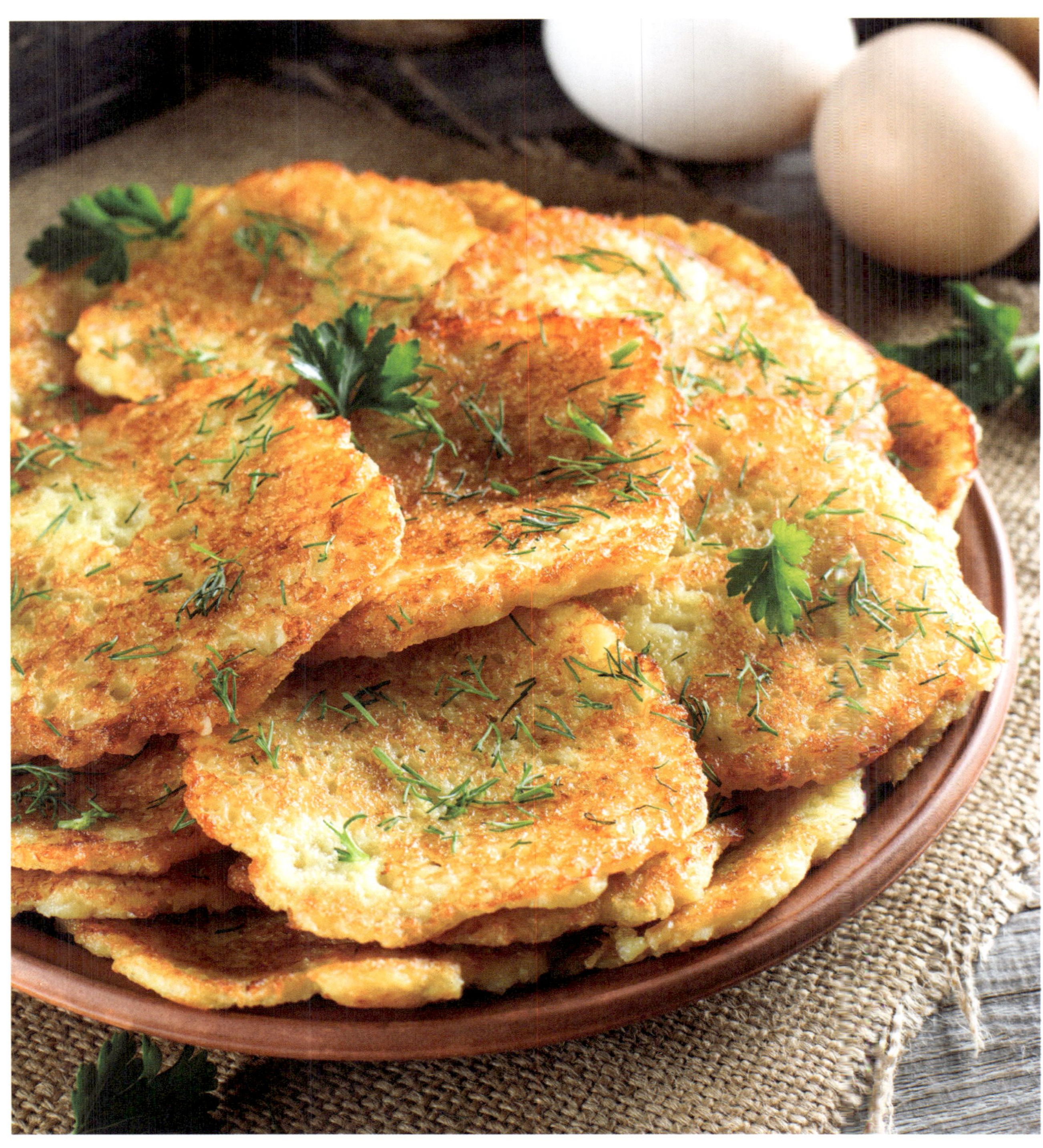

Cauliflower Fritters

SERVES 4

PREP + COOK TIME: 30 MINS

VEG • GLUTEN FREE

CAULIFLOWER FRITTERS

500g cauliflower
1 cup (125g) grated Cheddar cheese
2 large eggs
2 tbsps coconut flour
Salt and pepper to taste
Olive oil for frying
2 tbsps chopped dill to serve
Parsley leaves to serve

Shred the cauliflower with a food processor or large cheese grater. Steam cauliflower for 3-4 minutes until just tender.

Drain to remove any excess liquid.

Transfer cauliflower to a large bowl and stir in the cheese until it melts.

Add eggs and coconut flour. Season with salt and pepper and mix to combine.

Heat 2 tablespoons of olive oil in a large, nonstick frying pan over medium heat. Use a ¼ cup to scoop cauliflower batter. Drop the cauliflower batter into the pan and press down slightly with a spatula to form a disc. Cook for 2-3 minutes on each side until crispy. Make sure the bottom side is completely browned and cooked before attempting to flip the fritters.

Repeat with remaining batter. Add more oil to the pan if needed.

Scatter with fresh dill and parsley to serve.

Avocado Burger

SERVES 4
PREP + COOK TIME: 20 MINS
GLUTEN FREE • DAIRY FREE

AVOCADO BURGER

4 large avocados
1 tsp + 2 tbsps olive oil
8 rashers shortcut bacon
4 eggs
¼ cup (60g) mayonnaise
4 frisee lettuce leaves
1 large beef tomato, sliced
½ red onion, sliced
2 tbsps black sesame seeds

Cut the avocados in half then use a large soup spoon to carefully scoop out each half from the skin in one piece. Set the avocado halves aside.

Heat 1 teaspoon oil in a large frying pan over medium-high heat. Cook bacon for 3-4 minutes each side or until cooked to your liking. Transfer to a plate. Keep warm.

Heat 1 tablespoon oil in a large frying pan over medium heat. Crack two eggs into the pan. Let the eggs cook, gently tilting the pan occasionally to redistribute the oil, until the edges are crisp and golden and the yolk is cooked to your liking, about 2 minutes for runny yolks or 3 minutes for medium yolks. Use a spatula to transfer to a plate.

Repeat with the remaining two eggs.

Take four avocado halves. Spread each one with mayonnaise, then top with lettuce leaves, tomato, red onion and bacon. Gently lay the fried eggs on top and finish with the remaining avocado halves.

Sprinkle with black sesame seeds to serve.

Tip:

To make your own mayo see the recipe on page 22. If using a store-bought mayo, check the label carefully and avoid 'light' versions which often contain less fat and more sugar.

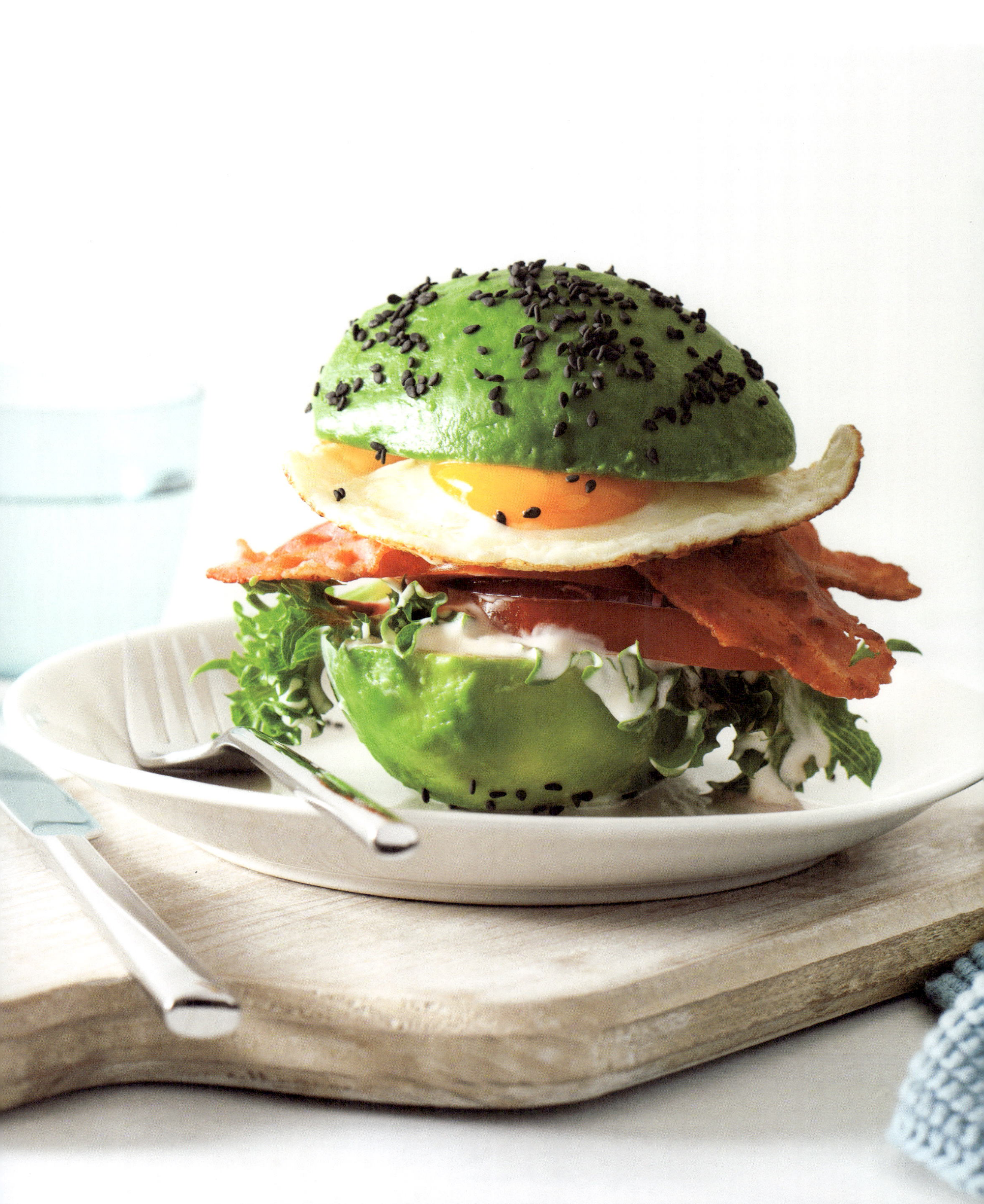

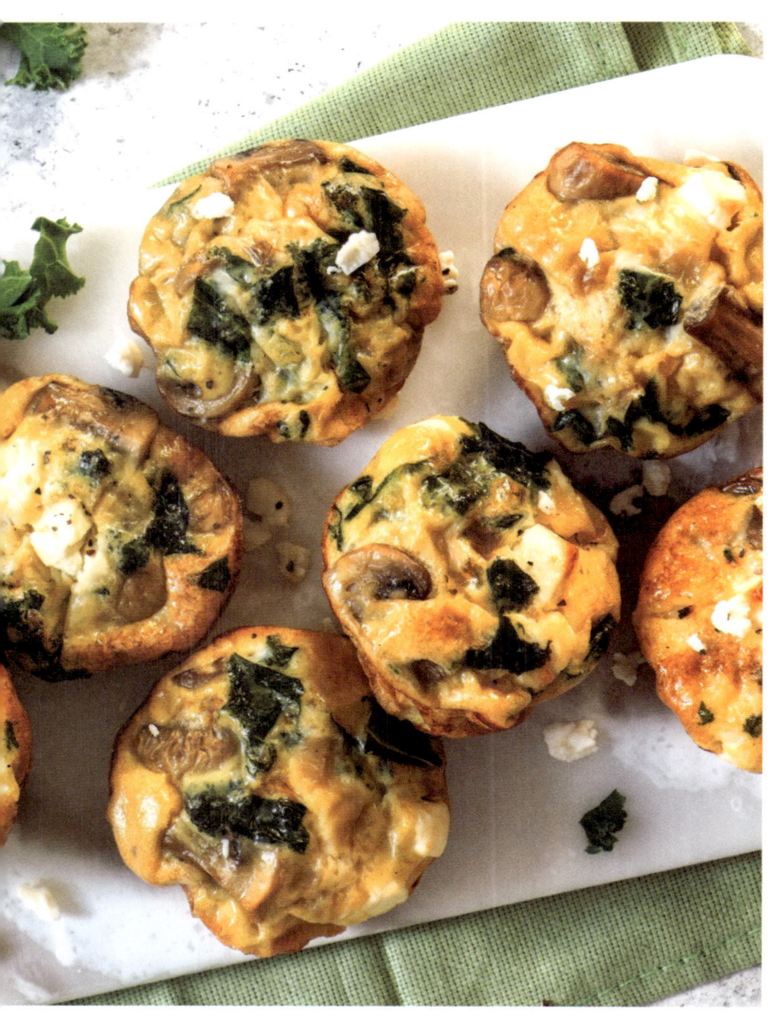

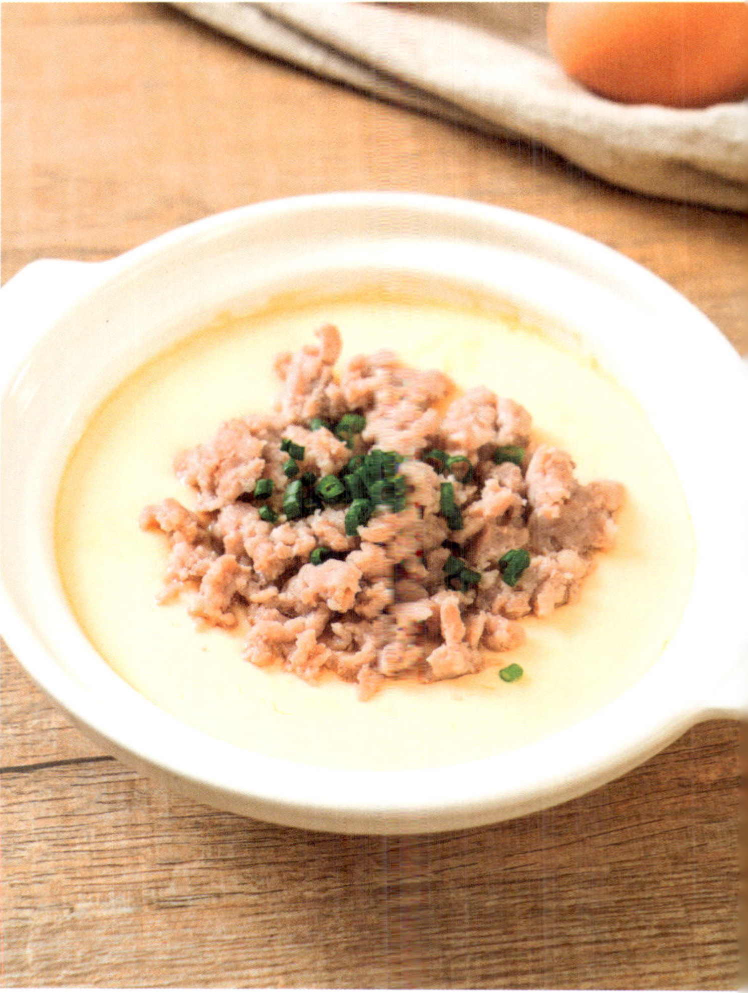

Egg Muffins with Mushrooms, Kale & Feta

MAKES 12

PREP + COOK TIME: 50 MINS

VEG • GLUTEN FREE

Chinese-Style Egg Custard with Minced Pork

SERVES 4

PREP + COOK TIME: 30 MINS

GLUTEN FREE • DAIRY FREE

EGG MUFFINS WITH MUSHROOMS, KALE & FETA

1 tbsp olive oil

1 medium onion, finely chopped

3 cloves garlic, minced

350g mushrooms, sliced

2 cups (140g) chopped kale

250g feta cheese, crumbled

6 eggs

Preheat oven to 180°C. Grease a 12-hole muffin pan.

Heat olive oil in a large frying pan over medium-high heat. Add onion and cook, stirring regularly, for 3-5 minutes until soft and translucent. Add garlic and cook for 1 minute until fragrant. Add mushrooms and cook for 5 minutes until tender. Add kale and cook for about 2 minutes, stirring, until it wilts slightly. Remove from the heat then stir in feta. Divide the mixture evenly between the muffin cups.

Whisk the eggs in a small jug, then pour equal amounts of egg into each cup, filling to just below the rim.

Bake for 25-30 minutes until the eggs are set.

Serve immediately or store in an airtight container in the fridge for up to 4 days.

CHINESE-STYLE EGG CUSTARD WITH MINCED PORK

3 large eggs, whisked, room temperature

2 tbsps sesame oil

Salt and pepper to taste

1 tbsp fresh ginger, finely grated

2 small spring onions, green and white parts finely sliced and separated

700g pork mince

3 cups (800ml) bone broth

½ tbsp fish sauce

Heat 1 tablespoon of the sesame oil in a wok over medium-high heat. Add half the ginger, the white part of the chopped spring onion and the pork. Stir-fry for 8 minutes until the pork is cooked through. Season to taste and set aside.

Bring the broth and the rest of the ginger to a simmer. Stir in the remaining sesame oil, fish sauce and salt as needed.

Pour ¼ cup of the broth into the eggs and whisk through. Then pour the egg mixture into the broth in a thin stream, stirring the broth the whole time. Cook for a further 1 minute but do not let it boil.

Serve immediately with a portion of the pork on top, garnished with the green spring onion.

SPICY FRITTERS

1 small head cauliflower, cut into florets
2 eggs
¾ cup (90g) almond meal
2 tbsps fresh coriander, chopped
¼ tsp garlic salt
1 tsp chilli flakes
½ cup (60g) mozzarella, grated
3 tbsps olive oil
Lime wedges to serve

Place the cauliflower into a food processor and pulse until finely chopped.

Measure 2½ cups of the cauliflower and place into a large mixing bowl.

Add eggs, almond meal, coriander, garlic salt, chilli flakes and grated cheese.

Mix until well combined.

Use your hands to shape small fritters.

Heat the oil in a large frying pan over medium heat.

When the oil is hot, cook the cauliflower fritters in batches. Cook for 3-5 minutes on each side or until golden brown. Transfer to a plate lined with paper towels.

Repeat until all the fritters are cooked.

Squeeze over lime wedges to serve.

SAUSAGE & TOMATOES

8 Italian sausages
2 tbsps olive oil
1 onion, thinly sliced
1 red capsicum, sliced
3 cloves garlic, chopped
2 tsps dried thyme
1 x 400g can chopped tomatoes
2 cups (500ml) chicken stock
Salt and pepper to taste

Heat a large frying pan over medium heat. Cook sausages for 8 minutes or until golden.

Remove from the pan and thickly slice, then set aside.

Heat olive oil in a large pan over medium heat. Add the onion and cook for 3-5 minutes, stirring occasionally, until soft and translucent.

Add the capsicum and cook, stirring occasionally, for a further 4-5 minutes until tender.

Add the garlic and thyme and cook for 1 minute more until fragrant.

Add the tomatoes and stock. Bring to the boil. Reduce heat to medium-low. Simmer for 20 minutes.

Add the sliced sausage. Cook for 10 minutes or until sausage is heated through. Season with salt and pepper and serve.

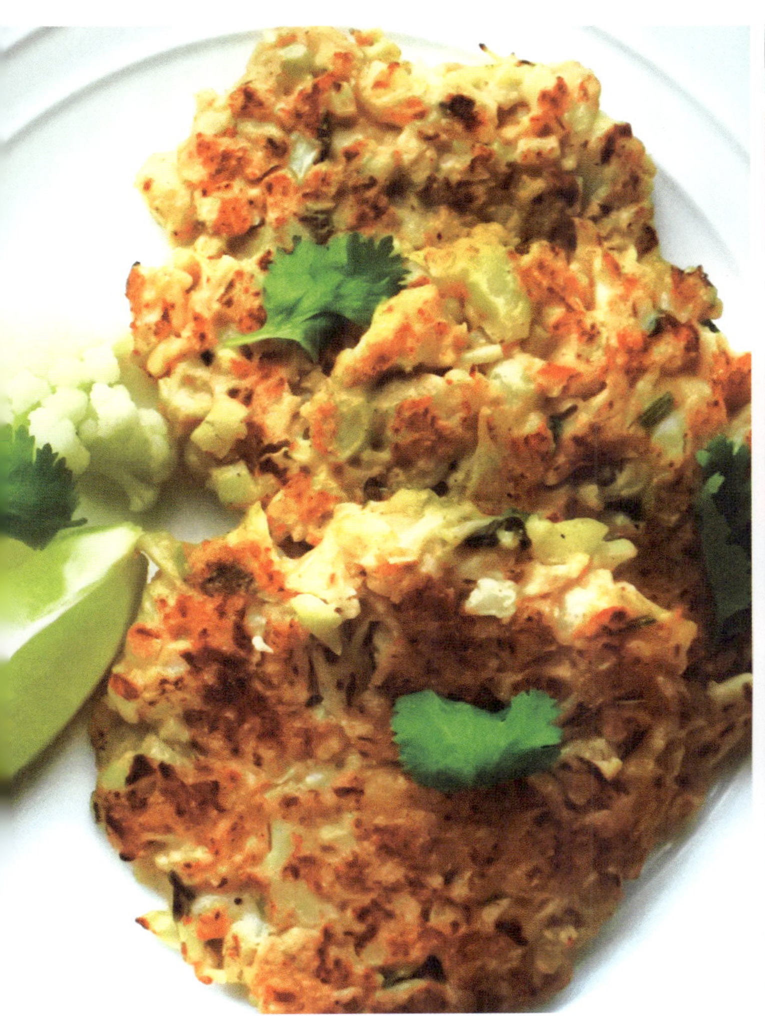

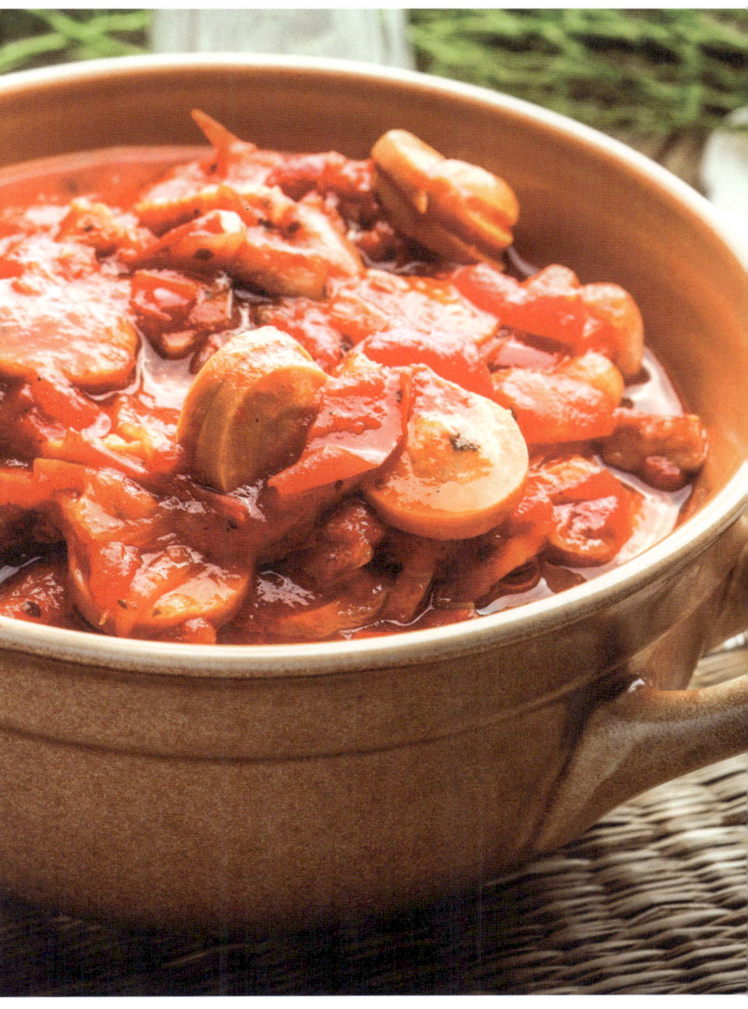

Spicy Fritters

SERVES 4

PREP + COOK TIME: 30 MINS

VEG • GLUTEN FREE

Sausage and Tomatoes

SERVES 4

PREP + COOK TIME: 55 MINS

GLUTEN FREE • DAIRY FREE

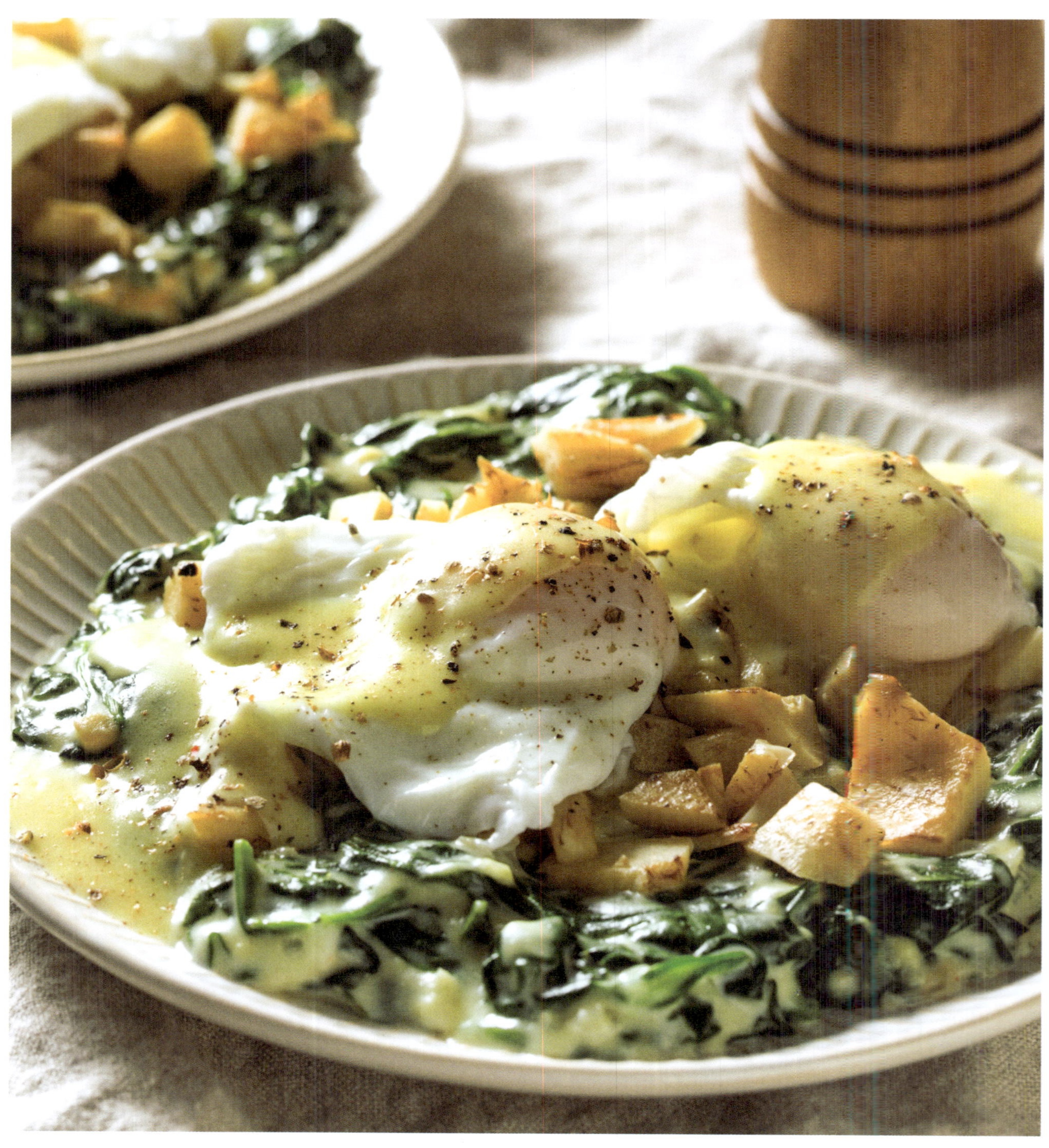

Eggs Sardou

SERVES 4

PREP + COOK TIME: 20 MINS + RESTING

VEG • GLUTEN FREE

EGGS SARDOU

4 tbsps butter

1 clove garlic, minced

1 small shallot, finely chopped

300g fresh spinach leaves, roughly chopped

Salt and pepper to taste

½ cup (125ml) cream

⅓ cup (30g) finely grated Parmesan cheese

8 canned or jarred artichoke hearts, roughly chopped

8 large eggs

Pinch of dried chilli flakes (optional)

HOLLANDAISE

2 egg yolks

1 tsp water

1 tsp lemon juice

Pinch of salt

8 tbsps butter

2 dashes Tabasco sauce

Prepare the hollandaise and add a dash of Tabasco.

Melt 2 tablespoons butter in a saucepan over medium heat. Add garlic and shallot and cook, stirring, for 3 minutes until soft and translucent. Add spinach and stir until wilted. Season with salt and pepper, then add another tablespoon of butter along with the cream. Heat for 2-3 minutes until the cream thickens, then add the Parmesan. Cook for another 2 minutes, stir in a dash of Tabasco and keep warm until ready to use.

Meanwhile melt the remaining butter in a small frying pan over medium heat. Add artichokes and cook, stirring, for about 5 minutes until heated through. Keep warm until ready to serve.

Bring a large pan of water to boil then reduce heat to low. Swirl the water to create a vortex, then break the eggs one at a time into the water. Poach eggs for 3 minutes each until whites are set but yolks are still runny. Remove with a slotted spoon.

Divide creamed spinach between four plates. Top with artichokes and two poached eggs per plate. Pour the hollandaise sauce over the eggs and season with pepper and dried chilli flakes, if desired.

Halloumi, Eggs & Avocado

SERVES 2
PREP + COOK TIME: 15 MINS
VEG • GLUTEN FREE

180g halloumi, sliced
1 tsp olive oil
1 egg
1 cup (75g) cos lettuce, roughly torn
1 avocado
1 tsp black and white sesame seeds

TAHINI DRESSING

2 tbsps tahini
⅓ cup (100ml) Greek yoghurt
Juice of ½ lemon
Salt, to taste

Brush the slices of halloumi with olive oil. Place in a frying pan over a medium heat and cook for 2-3 minutes each side until golden brown.

Meanwhile place the egg in a small pan of cold water.

Place the pan over a medium heat. Bring to a gentle simmer then cook for a further 4 minutes.

Drain, rinse under cold water then peel and remove shell.

Combine the dressing ingredients in a small bowl and mix well.

Arrange the lettuce in two serving bowls. Top with the fried halloumi and half an egg and half an avocado in each bowl.

Drizzle over the dressing and sprinkle over the sesame seeds.

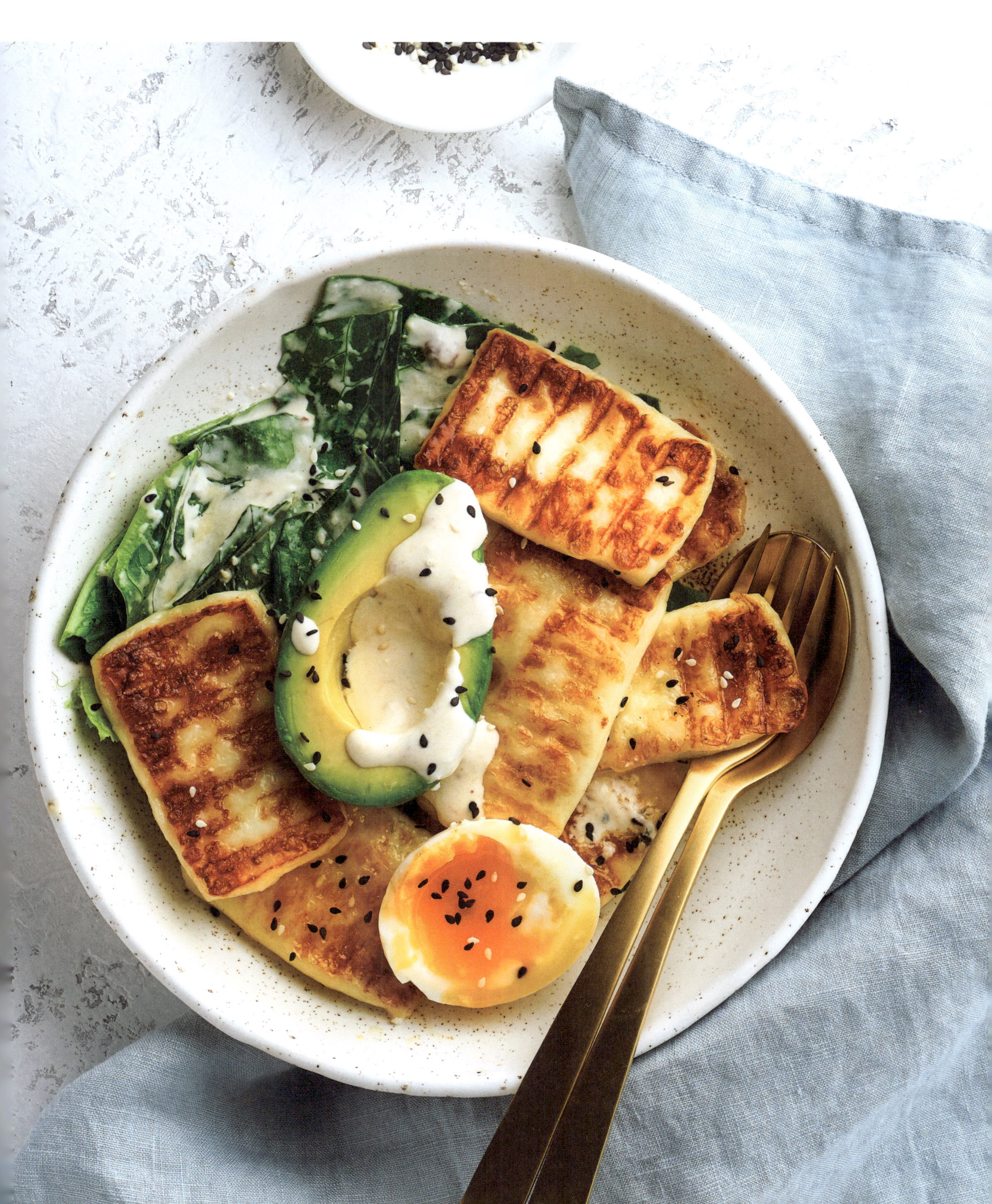

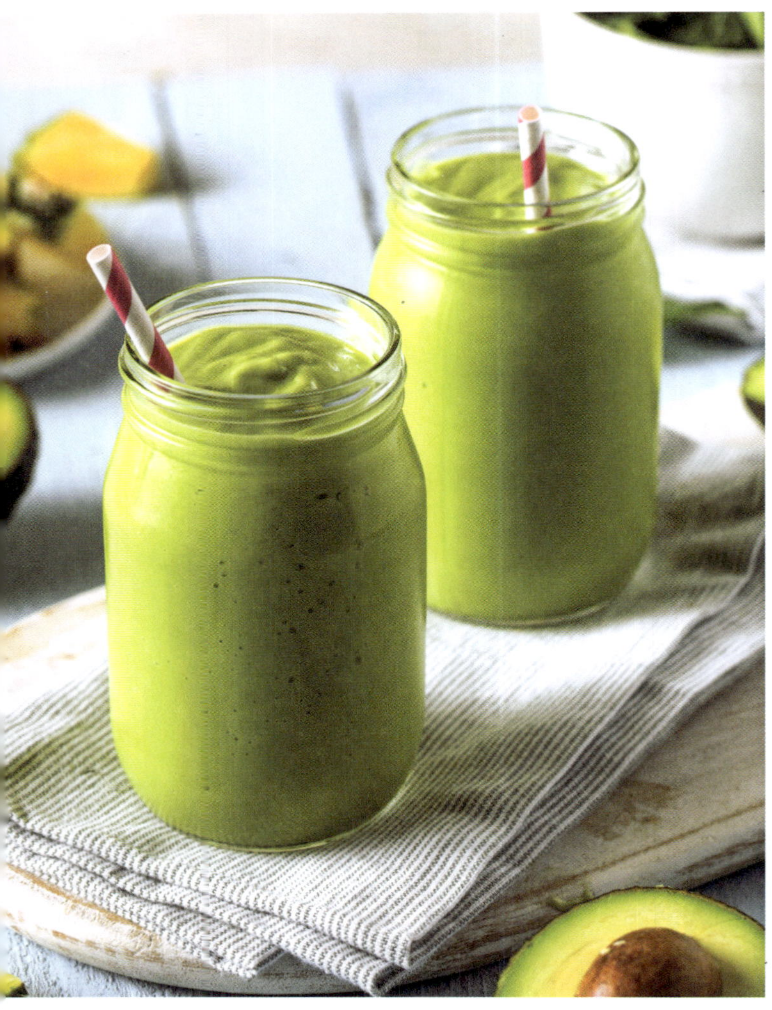

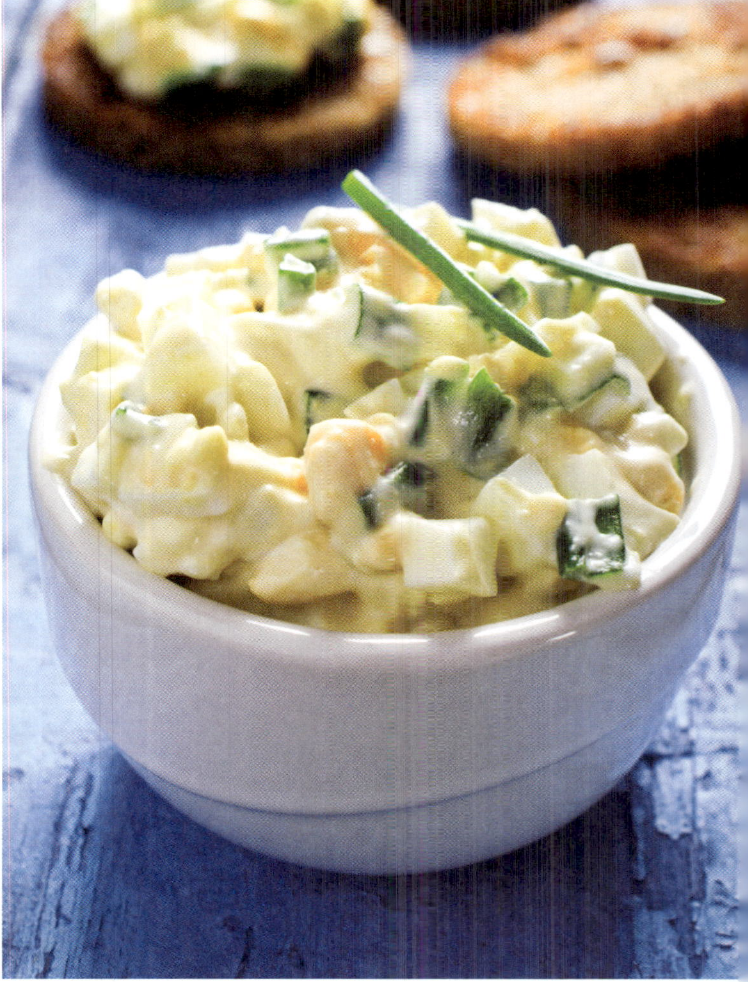

Avocado Smoothie with Spinach

SERVES 2

PREP + COOK TIME: 5 MINS

VEG • GLUTEN FREE • DAIRY FREE

Egg Salad

SERVES 4

PREP + COOK TIME: 20 MINS

GLUTEN FREE

AVOCADO SMOOTHIE WITH SPINACH

1 avocado

1 cup (30g) spinach

½ cup (75g) crushed ice

1 cup (250ml) coconut milk

1 tsp vanilla extract

2 tbsps MCT oil

4 tbsps granulated stevia

Scoop the avocado flesh into a blender along with all the remaining ingredients. Blend until completely smooth.

Serve immediately.

EGG SALAD

8 eggs

½ cup (120g) mayonnaise

1 tsp Dijon mustard

1-2 spring onions, chopped

Salt and pepper to taste

Place eggs in a saucepan and cover with cold water. Bring water to a boil and immediately remove from heat. Cover and let eggs stand in hot water for 10-12 minutes.

Remove eggs from hot water. Run under a cold tap, then peel and chop into 1cm dice.

Place the chopped eggs in a bowl and stir in the mayonnaise, mustard and spring onion. Season with salt and pepper and stir gently to combine.

Serve on its own or on keto bread or crackers.

Tip:

To make your own mayo see the recipe on page 22. If using a store-bought mayo, check the label carefully and avoid 'light' versions which often contain less fat and more sugar.

TURKISH EGGS WITH HALLOUMI

2 tbsps olive oil
Salt and pepper
2 large cloves garlic, crushed
2½ tsps smoked paprika
2 tsps ground cumin
2½ cups (550g) tinned diced tomatoes
6 large eggs, room temperature
200g halloumi, sliced

Heat the oil in a large, deep-sided frying pan over medium heat. Add the garlic and fry for 1 minute. Add the paprika, cumin and tomatoes and cook for a further 10 minutes, stirring frequently, until the tomato has softened.

Make six small wells in the tomato mix and gently break the eggs into the wells. Turn the heat down to low and scatter the halloumi over the top. Cover and cook for 10 minutes, until the eggs are cooked to your liking.

Season to taste and serve hot.

PUMPKIN MUFFINS

Avocado oil, for liners
4 large eggs
½ cup (110g) cooked and mashed pumpkin
4 tbsps melted butter
1 tsp stevia glycerite
2 tsps vanilla extract
2 tsps ground cinnamon
6 tbsps coconut flour
1 tsp baking powder

Preheat oven to 180°C. Line six muffin cups with foil or silicone liners and spray the liners with oil.

In a medium bowl, whisk together the eggs, pumpkin, melted butter, stevia, vanilla and cinnamon. Whisk in the coconut flour until very smooth. Finally, mix in the baking powder. Pour the batter into the prepared muffin cups.

Bake for 20 minutes until set and an inserted skewer comes out clean. Transfer the muffins to a cooling rack and allow to cool completely.

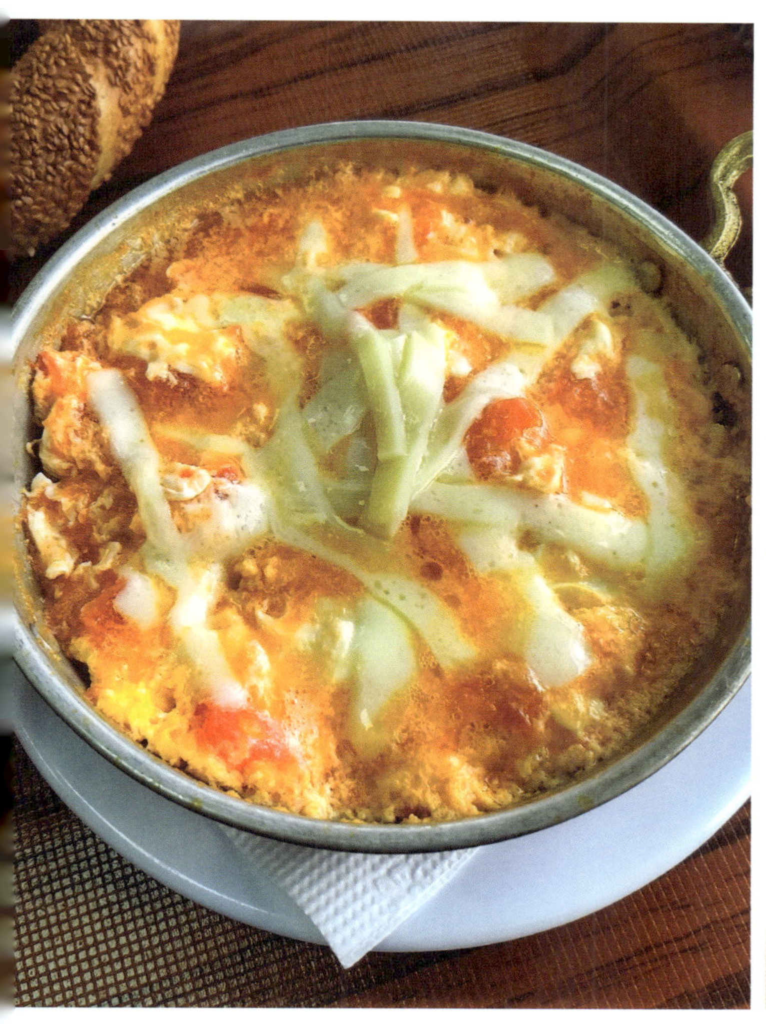

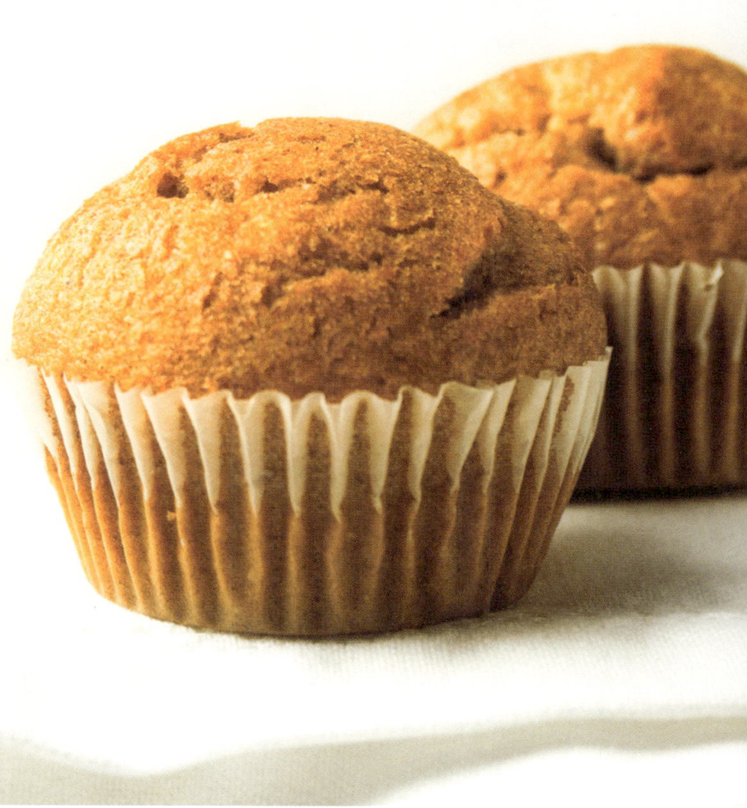

Turkish Eggs with Halloumi

SERVES 6

PREP + COOK TIME: 35 MINS

VEG • GLUTEN FREE

Pumpkin Muffins

MAKES 6

PREP + COOK TIME: 35 MINS

VEG • GLUTEN FREE

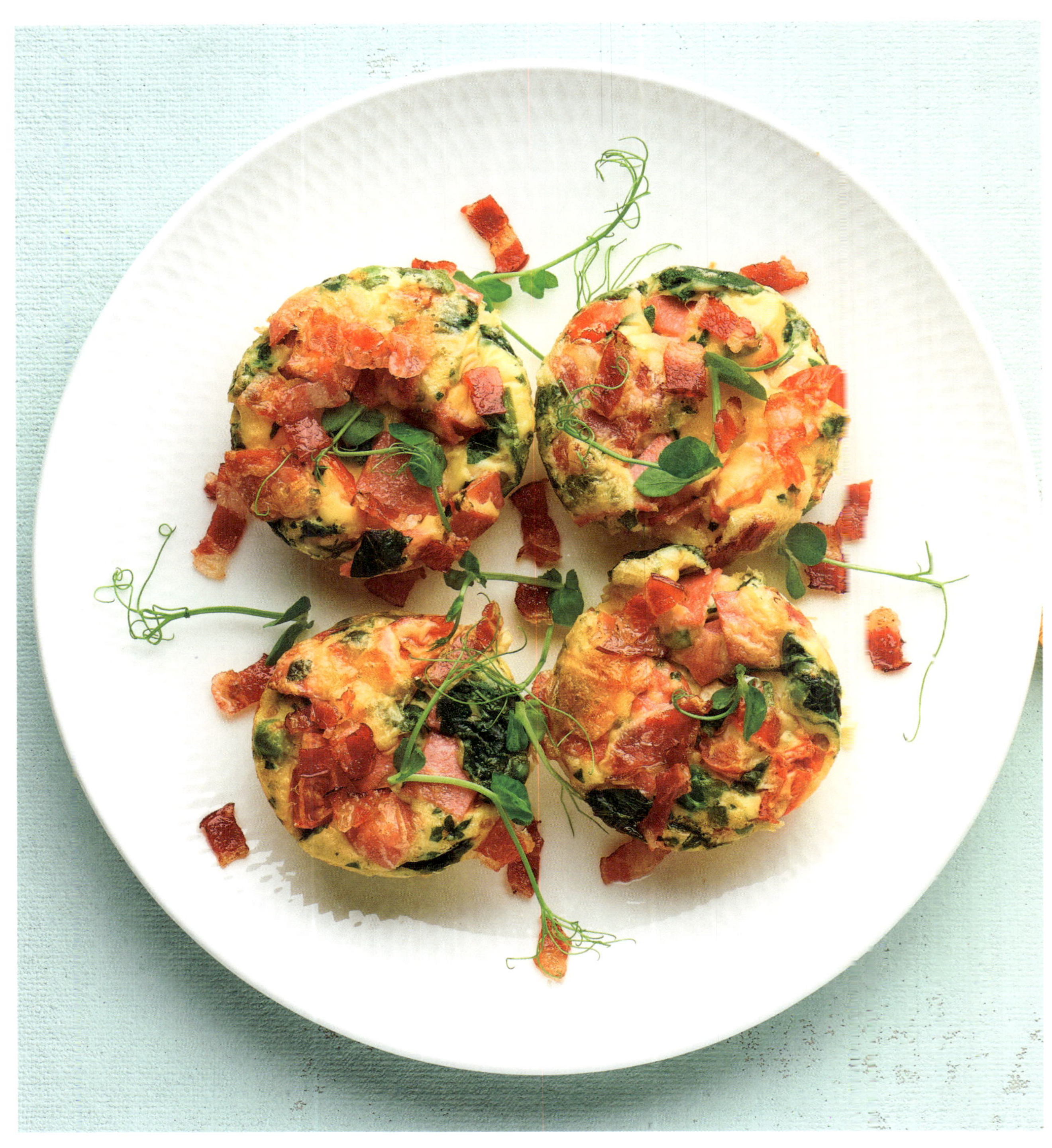

Spinach, Egg & Bacon Muffins

SERVES 12

PREP + COOK TIME: 30 MINS

GLUTEN FREE

SPINACH, EGG & BACON MUFFINS

6 bacon rashers

6 eggs

½ tsp salt

¼ cup (60ml) cream

2 cups (250g) grated tasty cheese

1 cup (250g) spinach, cooked, excess moisture squeezed out (frozen is fine)

10 cherry tomatoes, cut into quarters

Preheat oven to 180°C and lightly grease 12 muffin tin holes.

Cook the bacon in a frying pan over medium heat. Drain off excess fat and cut into pieces.

In a large mixing bowl, beat the eggs until smooth. Add the cream, salt, cheese and stir to combine, then add the spinach, tomato and cooked bacon and stir. Spoon the egg mixture into the prepared tin holes.

Place in the oven and bake for 20 minutes until cooked.

Remove from the oven, and allow the muffins to cool before removing them from the pan.

Keto Arepa Reina

SERVES 4

PREP + COOK TIME: 45 MINS

VEG • GLUTEN FREE

DOUGH

4 tbsps cream cheese

4 tbsps ground chia seeds

⅔ cup (75g) finely ground almond meal

4 tsps coconut oil + more for greasing

1 egg

½ tsp salt

FILLING

3 large ripe avocados

Juice of 1 lemon

4 tbsps mayonnaise

¼ cup (10g) chopped coriander

½ red onion, finely chopped

1 jalapeno, seeds removed and finely chopped

Salt and pepper to taste

Combine the cream cheese, ground chia seeds, almond meal, coconut oil, egg and salt in a large bowl. Mix well to combine then let stand, covered, for 5 minutes.

Lightly grease a large nonstick pan with a small amount of oil. Divide the dough into 4 small rounds. The dough will be quite moist and sticky. Place the dough rounds into the pan. Flatten the dough rounds until about 1½cm thickness. Place the pan over a very low heat. Cook, covered, for 7-9 minutes until the bottoms of the discs are golden brown. Flip the discs over and cook for about 7 minutes on the other side until both sides are golden brown. Remove the arepas from the pan and let them rest for a minute.

Meanwhile mash the avocado flesh with lemon juice and mayonnaise. Stir in the chopped coriander, red onion and jalapeno. Season with salt and pepper to taste.

Cut the discs in half and fill with the filling. Serve immediately.

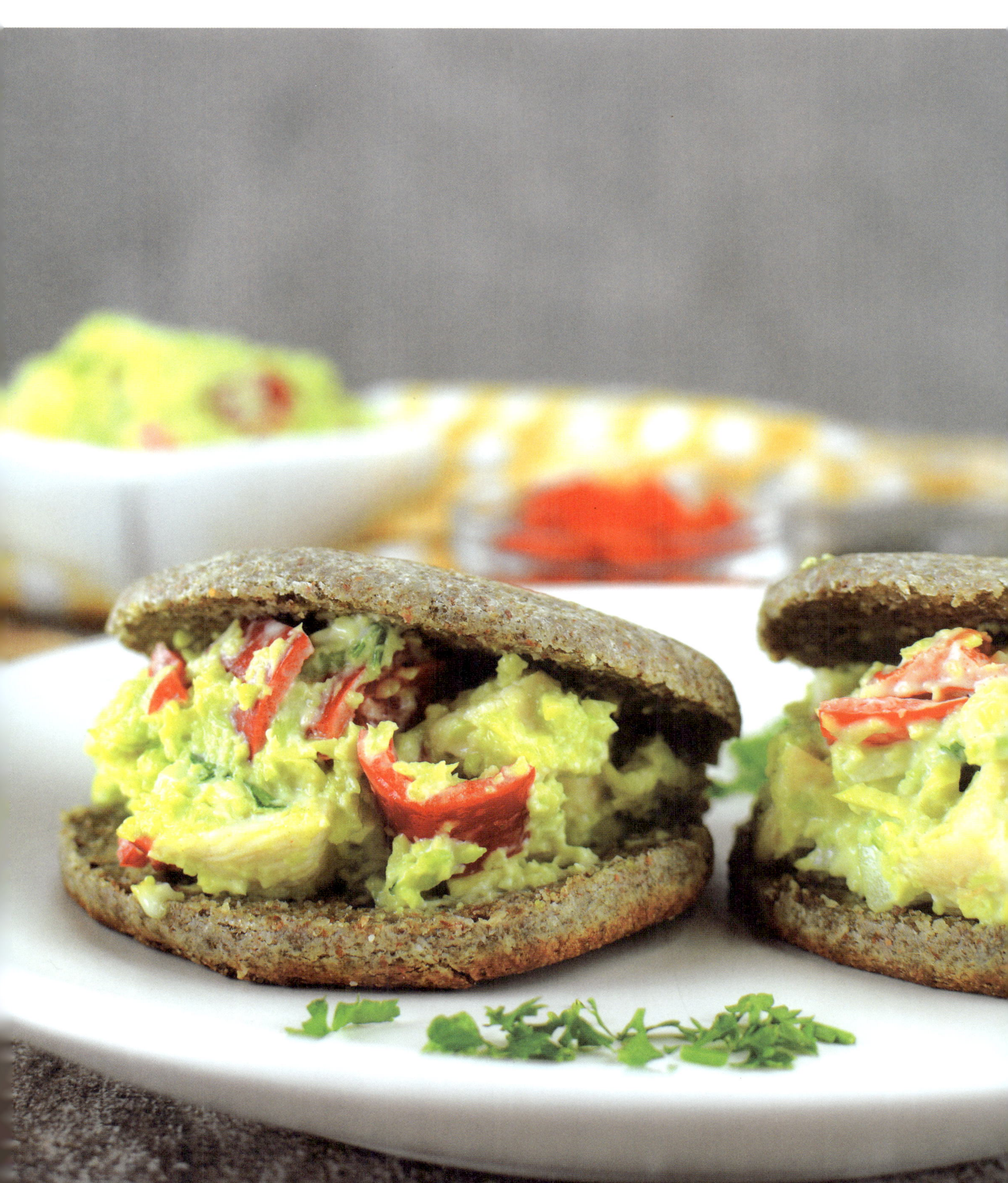

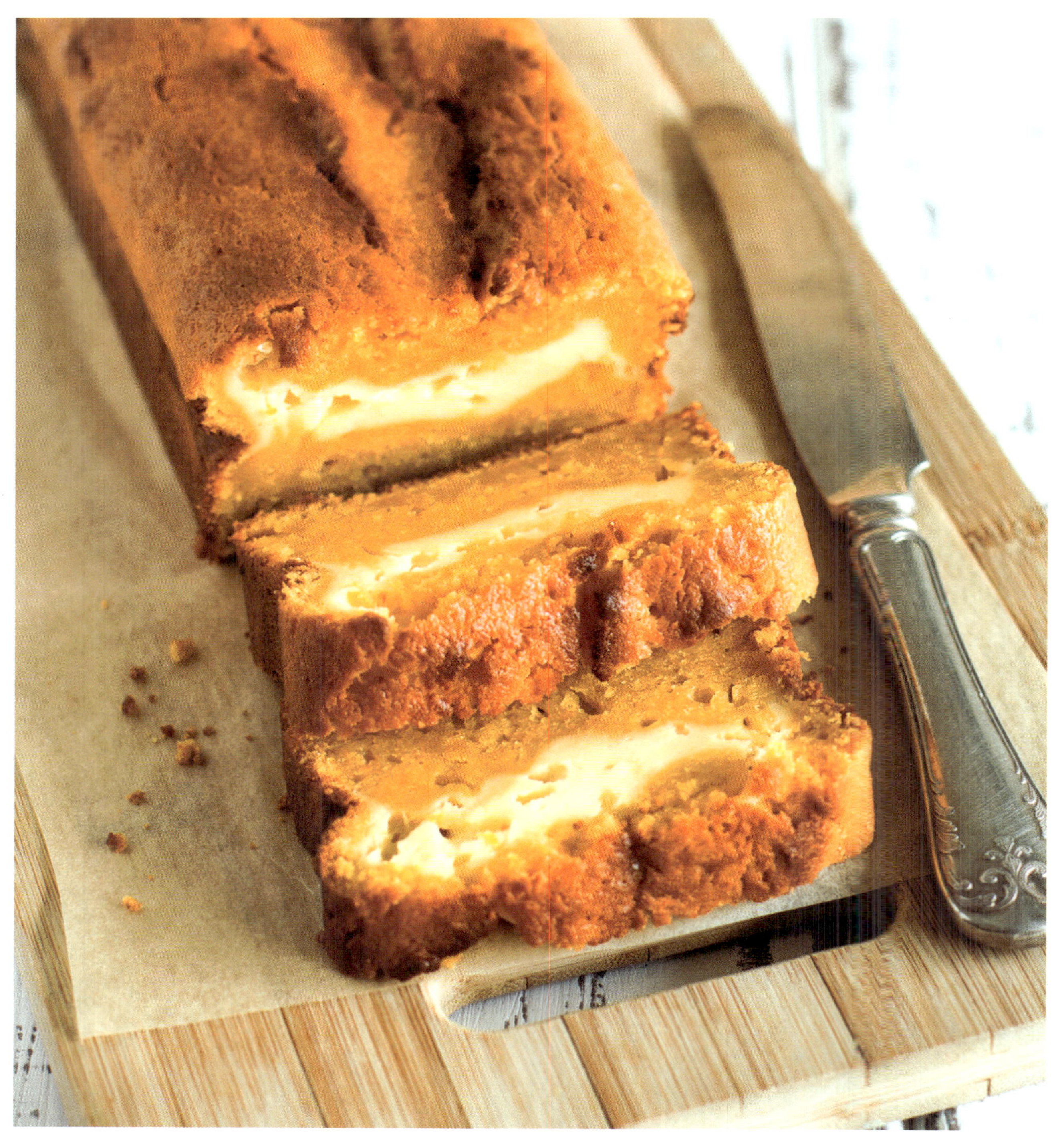

Pumpkin Loaf with Cream Cheese Filling

SERVES 10

PREP + COOK TIME: 1 HOUR 30 MINS

VEG • GLUTEN FREE

PUMPKIN LOAF WITH CREAM CHEESE FILLING

¼ cup (60ml) sour cream
250g cream cheese
⅓ cup (65g) + ¾ cup (150g) erythritol
5 large eggs, room temperature
1¼ cups (275g) pumpkin, cooked and mashed
½ tsp baking powder
85g butter
½ cup (50g) coconut flour
2½ cups (250g) almond flour
Pinch of salt
2½ tsps allspice

Preheat oven to 160°C and grease and line a 23 x 13cm loaf tin with baking paper.

Beat together the sour cream, cream cheese, ⅓ cup erythritol and 1 egg until combined then set aside.

Place the rest of the ingredients in a large mixing bowl and mix until combined.

Spread half the pumpkin mixture in the bottom of the loaf tin. Spoon the cream cheese filling over the top and smooth over.

Pour the rest of the pumpkin over the top.

Bake for 70 minutes or until a skewer inserted into the middle comes out clean.

Let cool for 10 minutes in the pan before removing to a wire rack to cool.

Tip:

Due to the pumpkin content, this recipe may not be suitable for those on a very low-carb diet.

SPINACH PANCAKES

4 eggs
30g frozen spinach, thawed and squeezed
½ cup (50g) coconut flour
1½ tbsps arrowroot flour
½ cup (125ml) almond milk
Pinch of salt
½ tsp olive oil
½ cup (125ml) low-sugar cranberry jam, to serve

Place the eggs, spinach, coconut flour, arrowroot, almond milk and salt into a blender and blend until smooth.

Heat a medium frying pan over a medium heat. Brush with olive oil.

Pour ¼ cup batter into the pan and swirl to distribute.

Cook until the top of the pancake is no longer wet and the bottom has turned light brown.

Run a spatula around the edge of the pan to loosen then flip and cook for 1 minute or until cooked through.

Transfer to a plate and cover with foil to keep warm. Repeat with remaining batter.

Serve pancakes with cranberry jam.

FLAX CRACKERS

1 cup (150g) flaxseed
3 tbsps chia seeds
1 cup (250ml) water
1 tsp salt
1 tsp dried oregano

Preheat the oven to 95°C. Line two large baking trays with greaseproof paper.

Soak the flax and chia seeds in the water in a large bowl for 15-20 minutes.

After the soaking, add salt and oregano. Mix to combine. Wet your hands and spread the mixture evenly onto one lined baking tray.

Bake for 90 minutes, then flip crackers onto the second lined baking tray. Peel the paper from the top of the cracker dough and bake for an additional 90 minutes.

Allow to cool, then break into pieces.

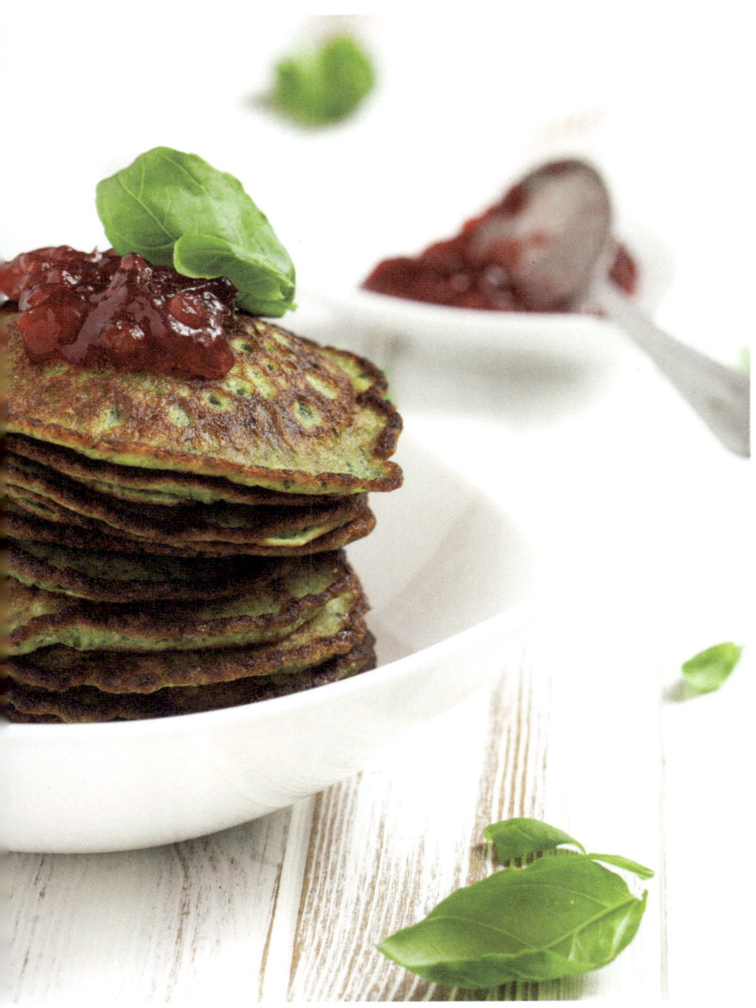

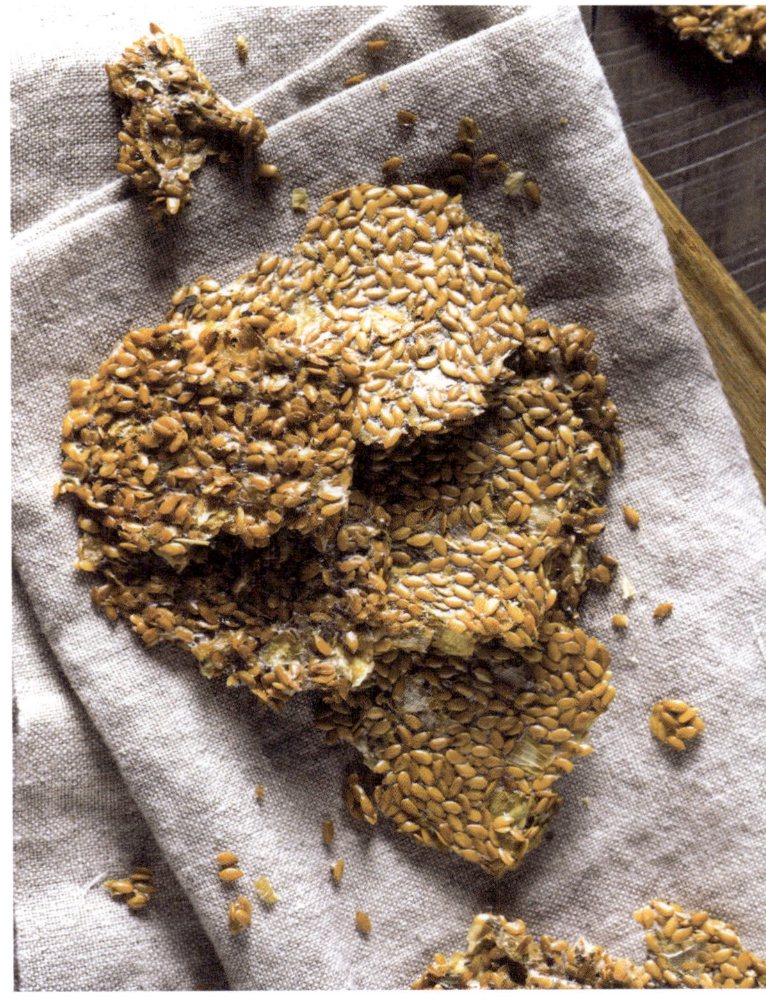

Spinach Pancakes

SERVES 2

PREP + COOK TIME: 30 MINS

VEG • GLUTEN FREE • DAIRY FREE

Flax Crackers

MAKES 25 CRACKERS

PREP + COOK TIME: 3 HOURS 25 MINS

VEG • GLUTEN FREE

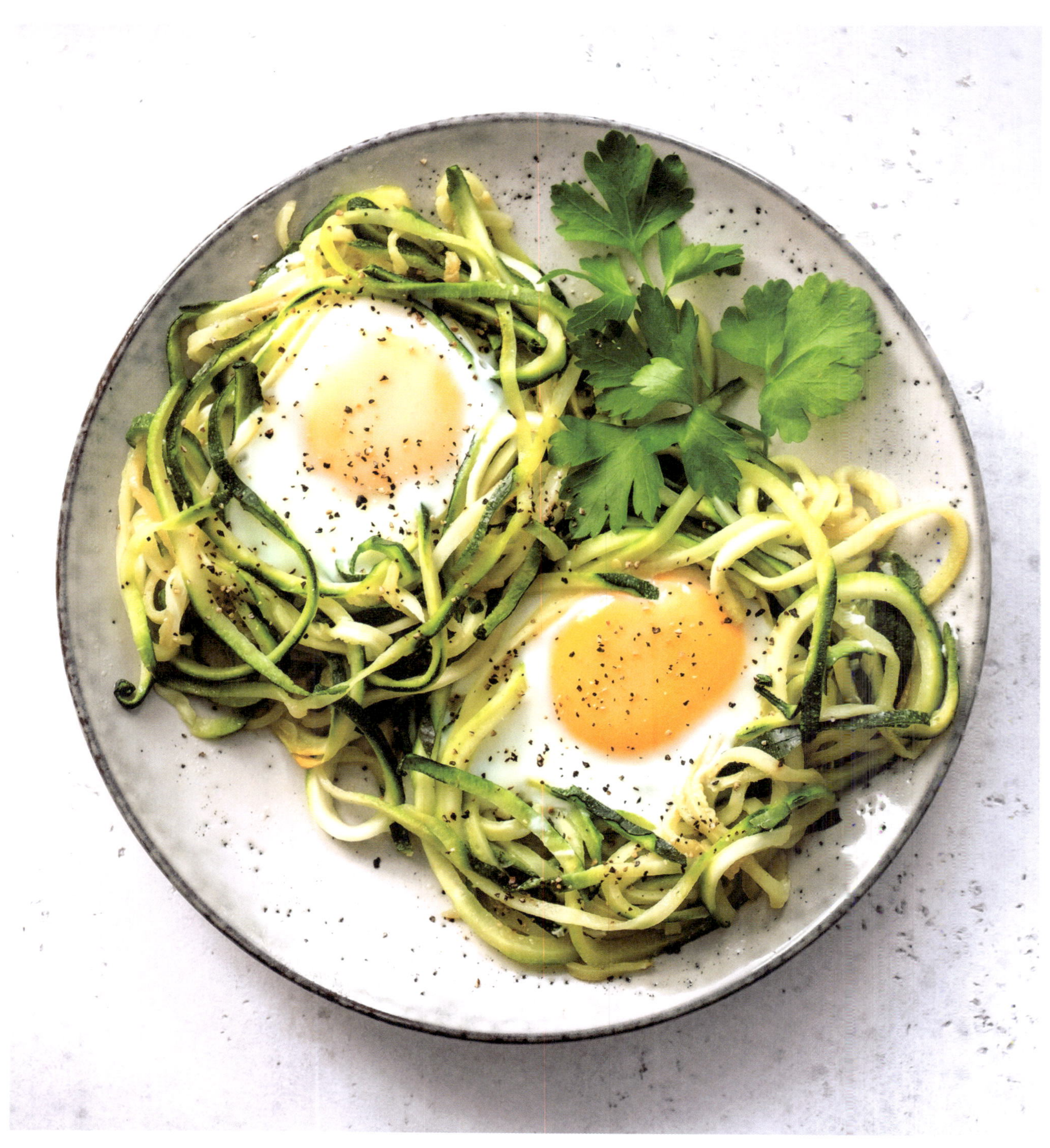

Zucchini Nests

MAKES 6 NESTS

PREP + COOK TIME: 35 MINS

VEG • GLUTEN FREE • DAIRY FREE

ZUCCHINI NESTS

3 large or 4 small zucchinis (enough to yield 6 cups spiralised)

1 tsp salt + more to taste

¼ tsp garlic powder

¼ tsp onion powder

½ cup (20g) chopped fresh basil

Pepper to taste

6 eggs

Use a vegetable peeler or a spiraliser to make zucchini noodles. Place zucchini noodles in a colander over a sink or bowl and toss with salt. Let the zucchini noodles sit for 20 minutes.

Preheat oven to 200°C. Grease and line a large baking tray.

Using your hands, squeeze out the excess moisture from the zucchini noodles. Transfer to a bowl and add garlic powder, onion powder and basil. Season with pepper.

Shape the zucchini noodles into nest shapes with an indent in the centre and carefully slide onto baking tray. Gently crack an egg into the centre of each zucchini nest. Season with more salt and pepper.

Bake for 15-20 minutes until the yolks are cooked to your liking.

Stuffed Spinach Omelette

SERVES 2
PREP + COOK TIME: 15 MINS
VEG • GLUTEN FREE

1 egg
3 egg whites
1 tbsp grated Cheddar cheese
¼ tsp salt
½ tsp chilli flakes (optional)
Pinch of ground nutmeg
Pinch of pepper
Olive oil for frying
1 bunch baby spinach, leaves picked (reserve a few leaves for garnish)
1 tbsp grated Parmesan cheese

Whisk together egg and egg whites in a mixing bowl.

Add Cheddar cheese, salt, chilli flakes, if using, nutmeg and pepper and mix well to combine.

Heat oil in a frying pan over a medium heat. Add egg and stir through, then cook on low for 6-8 minutes or until almost set.

Add spinach and Parmesan and cook until spinach has wilted and cheese melted.

In the last minute of cooking, flip one side of the omelette over the top of the other side.

Serve immediately, garnished with fresh spinach leaves.

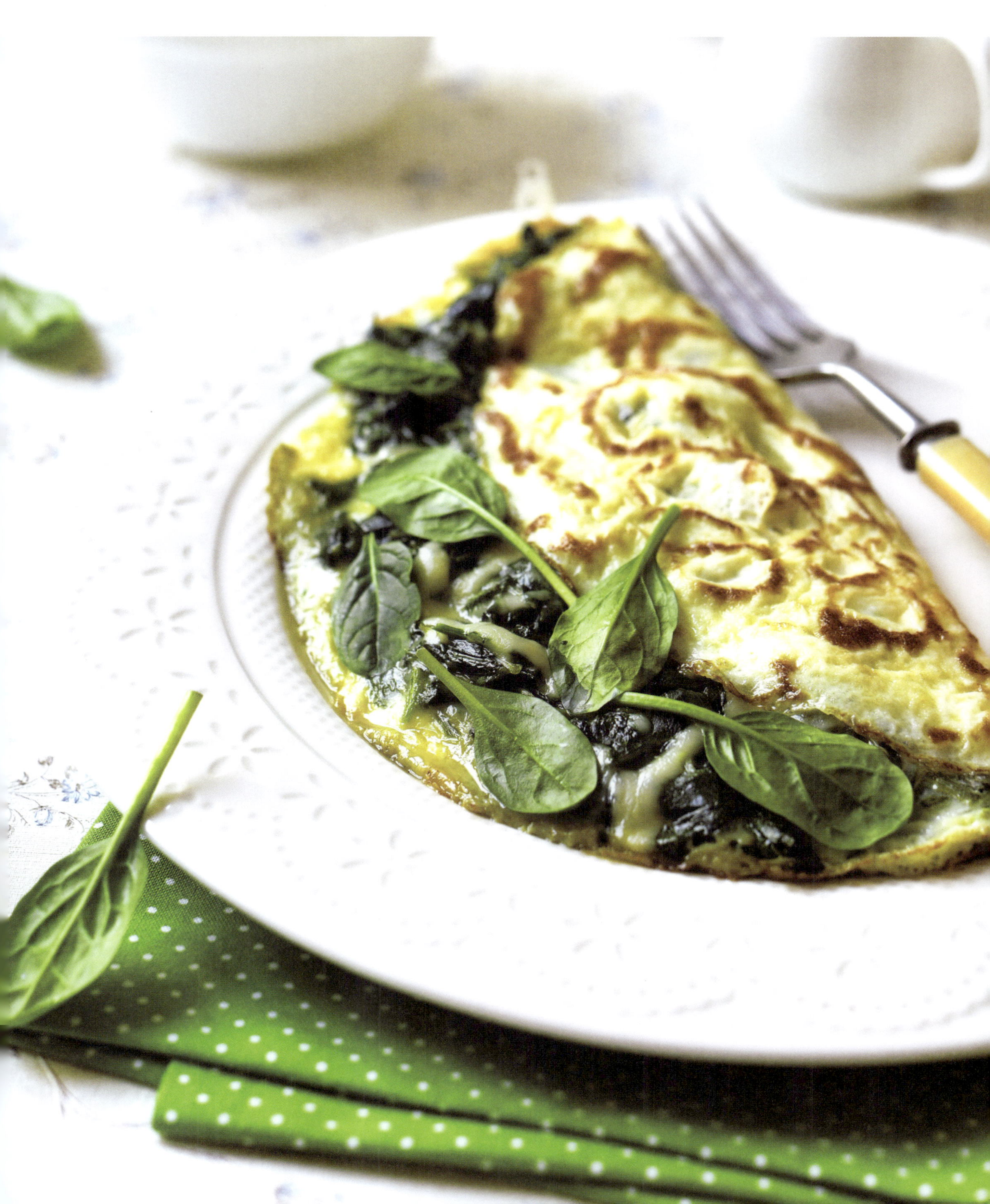

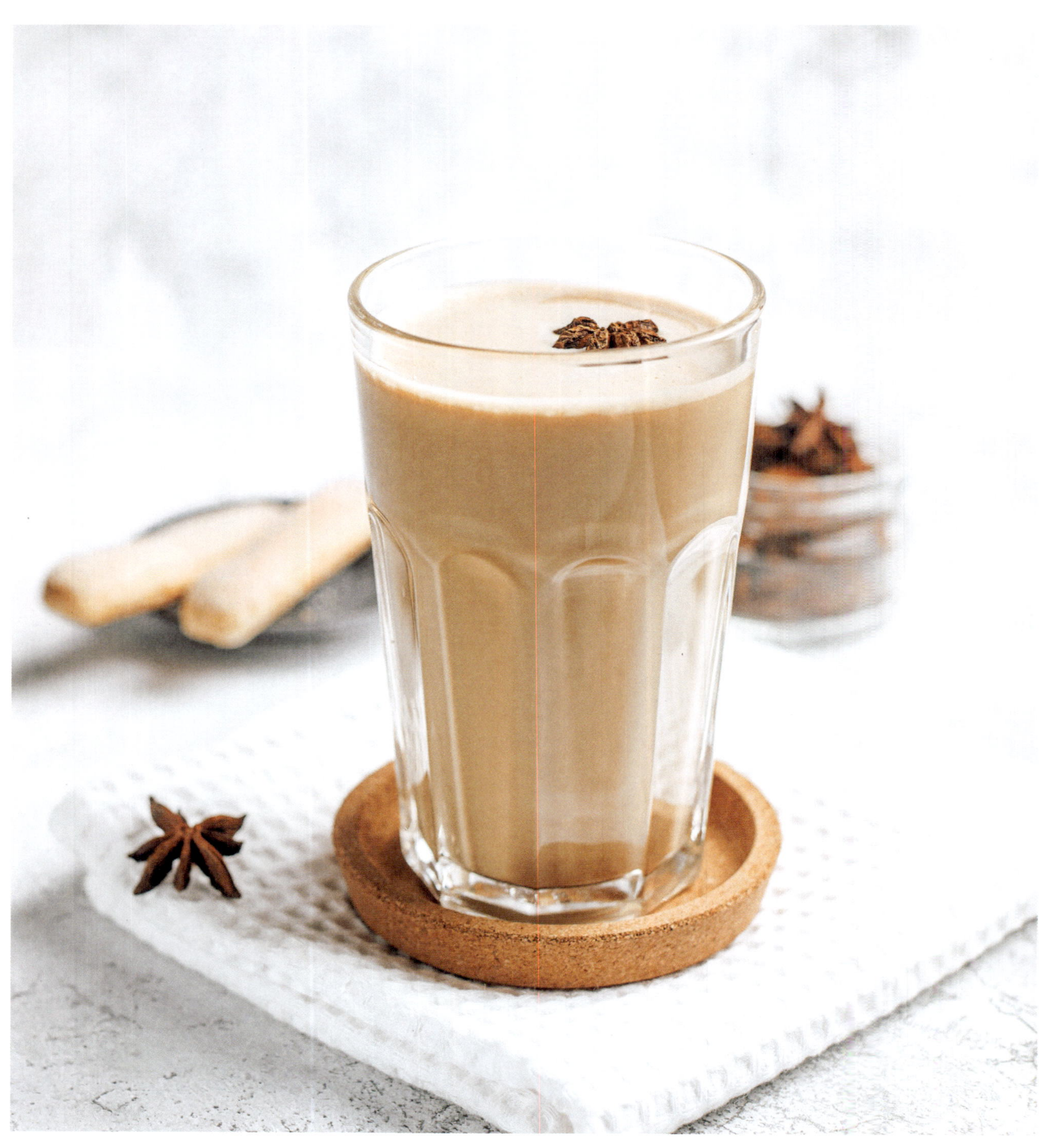

Masala Chai

SERVES 2

PREP + COOK TIME: 10 MINS

VEG • GLUTEN FREE

MASALA CHAI

Small piece ginger, thinly sliced
4 cardamon pods, crushed
2 star anise
1 cinnamon stick
4 black peppercorns
2 cups (500ml) water
2 tbsps black tea leaves
2 tsps keto-friendly granulated sweetener
3 tbsps thickened cream

Place the ginger, cardamon, star anise, cinnamon and peppercorns in a pan with the water.

Place over medium-high heat and bring to a rolling boil.

Add the tea leaves and sweetener and boil for 3 minutes more.

Add in the cream, stir, then turn off the heat and let the tea sit for another 1-2 minutes.

Strain the tea into small cups to serve.

Keto Pancakes

SERVES 6
PREP + COOK TIME: 35 MINS
VEG • GLUTEN FREE

PANCAKES

2½ cups (300g) finely ground almond meal
4 large eggs
¾ cup (185ml) almond milk
¼ cup (60ml) avocado oil
2 tsps vanilla extract
¼ cup (50g) erythritol
2 tsps baking powder
¼ tsp salt
Butter for the pan

TO SERVE

½ cup (60g) flaked almonds
1 cup (125g) fresh raspberries
Mint leaves to serve

Place the almond meal in a blender with the remaining pancake ingredients and blend until smooth. Let the batter rest for 10 minutes.

Grease a large frying pan with butter and place over medium-low heat. Spoon ¼ cup of batter at a time into the pan. Cook each pancake for 3-4 minutes until bubbles begin to appear on the top and the edges are set and dry, then flip and cook for an additional 3-4 minutes. Remove from the pan and keep warm. Repeat with the remaining batter, adding more butter to the pan as needed.

Serve the pancakes topped with flaked almonds, fresh raspberries and mint leaves, if desired.

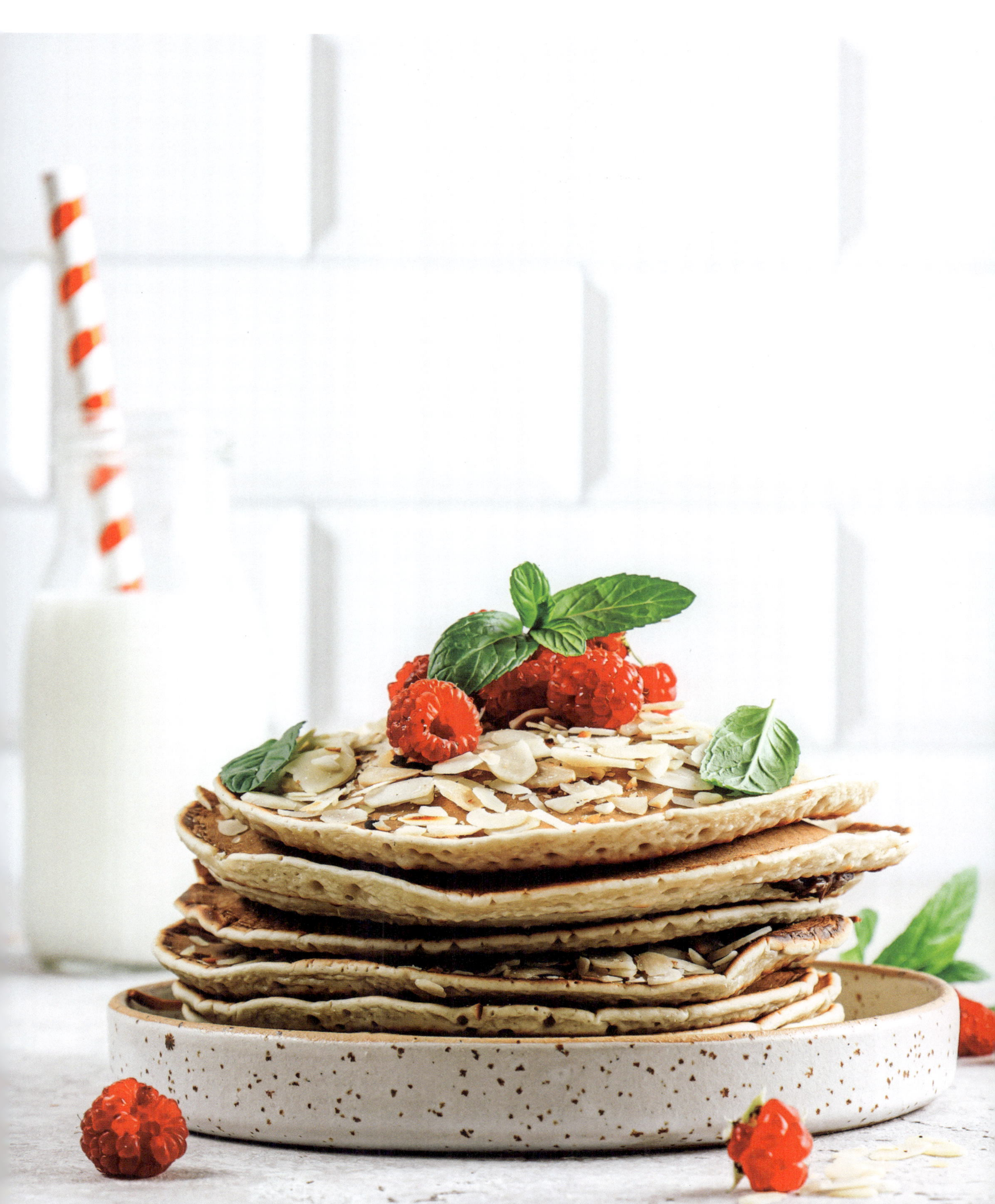

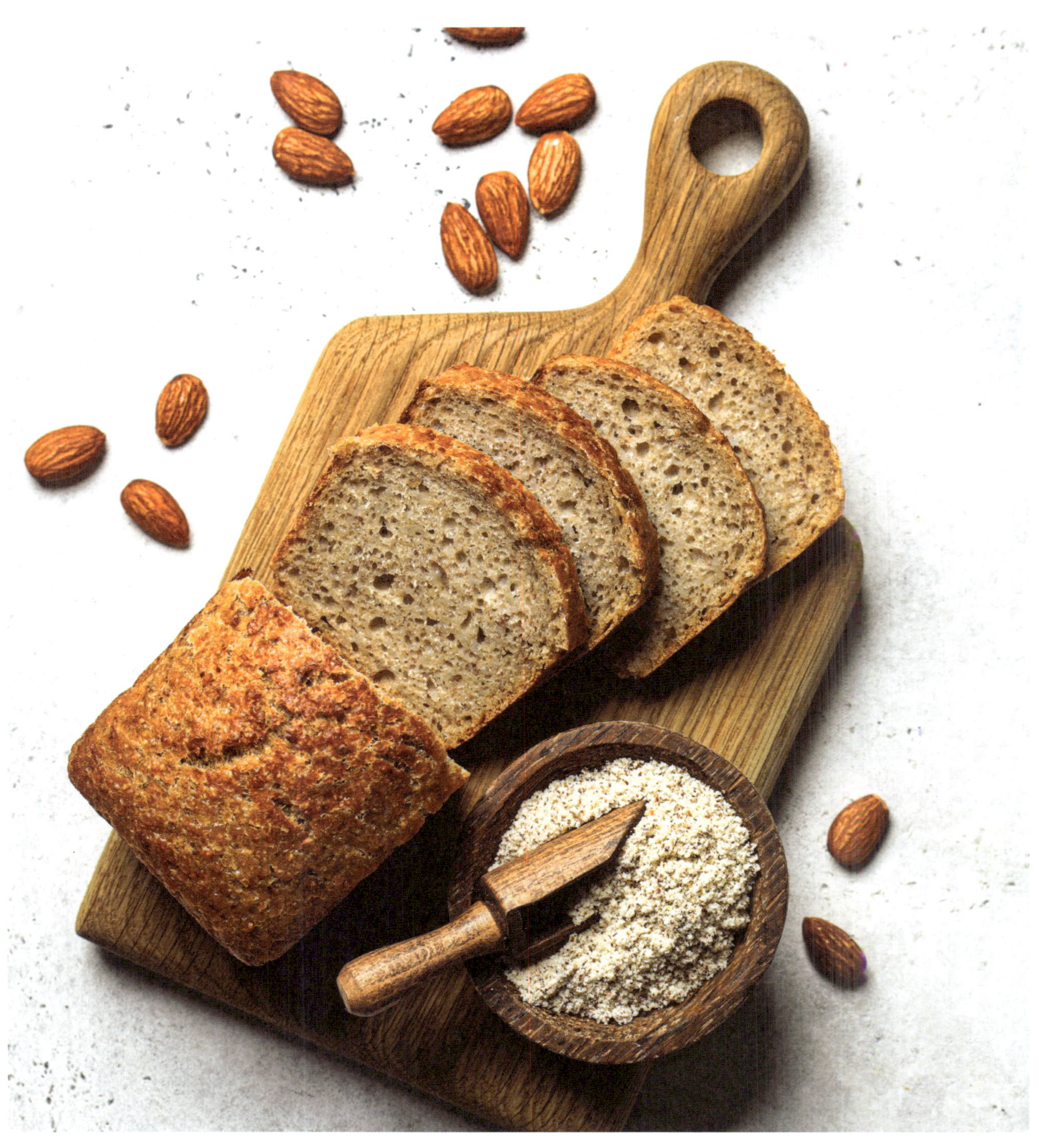

Almond Bread

SERVES 12

PREP + COOK TIME: 1 HOUR

VEG • GLUTEN FREE

ALMOND BREAD

2 eggs, separated + 2 large egg whites, room temperature
2 tbsps butter, melted
½ cup (125ml) warm water
2 cups (240g) almond meal
2 tbsps ground psyllium husks
1½ tsps baking powder
½ tsp xanthan gum
Pinch of salt

Preheat the oven to 180°C. Line a small loaf tin with greaseproof paper.

Beat the four egg whites until stiff peaks form. In another bowl beat the two egg yolks until pale and frothy. Add half of the egg whites to the egg yolks and fold in with a spatula. Set aside the remaining egg whites.

Add melted butter and water to the egg yolk mix and stir gently to combine. Add the almond meal, ground psyllium husks, baking powder, xanthan gum and salt. Blend until you have a smooth batter. Carefully fold in the remaining egg whites with a spatula.

Spoon the batter into a prepared loaf tin and bake for approximately 45 minutes or until a skewer inserted into the centre comes out clean.

Chapter Two

Snacks and Share Plates

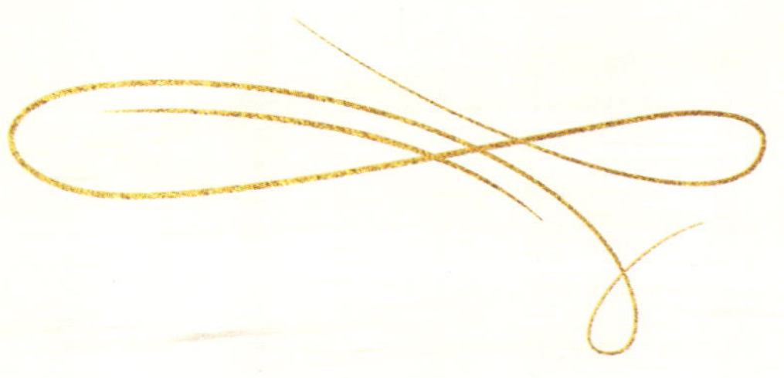

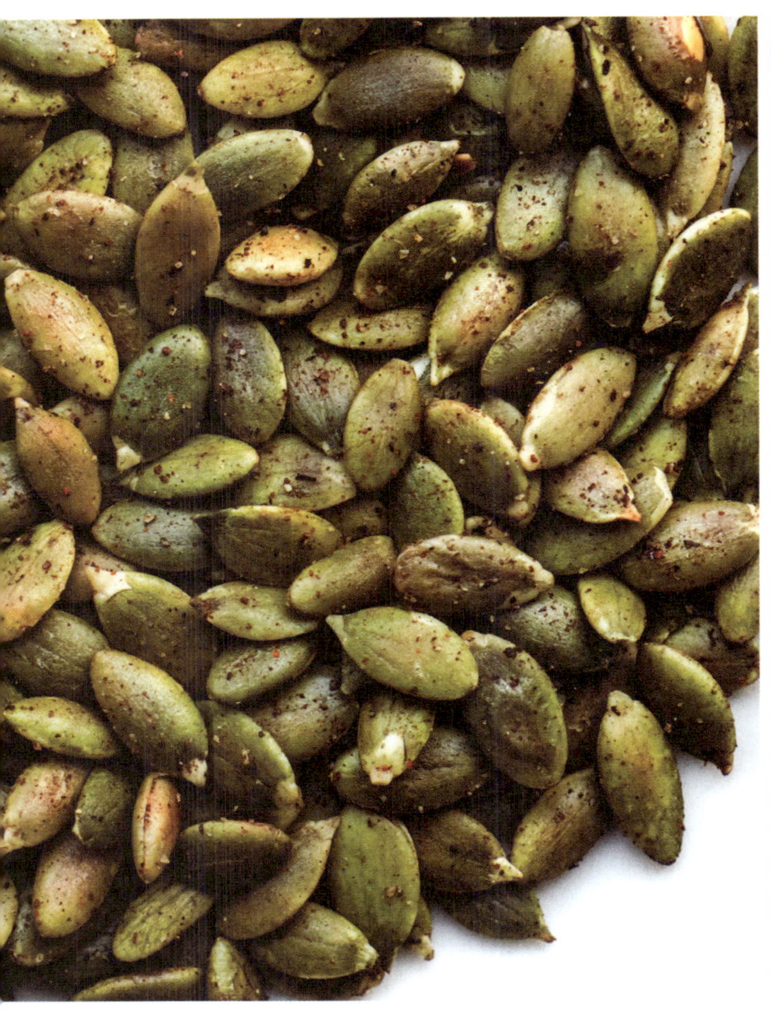

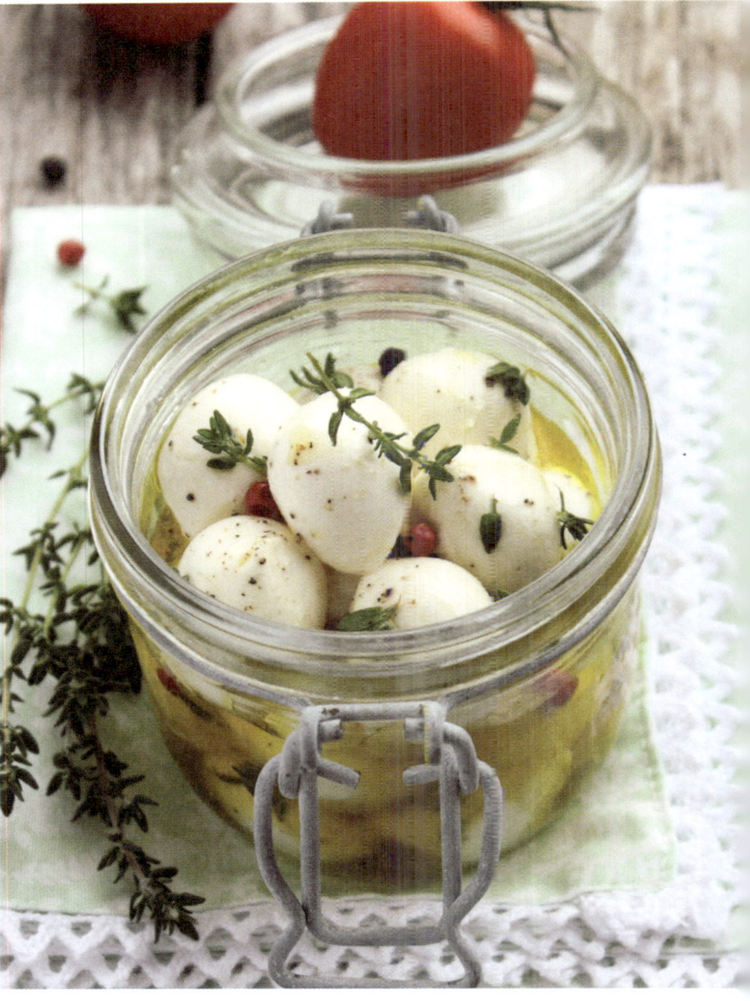

Spiced Roasted Pepitas

MAKES 1 CUP

PREP + COOK TIME: 15 MINS

VEG • GLUTEN FREE • DAIRY FREE

Marinated Mozzarella

SERVES 10

PREP + COOK TIME: 5 MINS + MARINATING

VEG • GLUTEN FREE

SPICED ROASTED PEPITAS

1 cup (130g) pepitas
2 tsps olive oil
1 tsp paprika
½ tsp sweet smoked paprika
Pinch of cayenne pepper
Salt to taste

Preheat oven to 170°C. Line a large baking tray with greaseproof paper.

Add the pepitas to a large bowl along with the olive oil and toss. Add the spices and toss again.

Spread out the pepitas on the baking tray. Transfer to the oven and roast for about 12 minutes until the seeds are lightly toasted.

Season the seed mixture with salt to taste and serve.

MARINATED MOZZARELLA

¾ cup (185ml) olive oil
2 cloves garlic, thinly sliced
1 tbsp fresh thyme, leaves picked
¼ tsp dried chilli flakes
1 tsp pink and black peppercorns
¼ tsp salt
450g bocconcini or ciliegine mozzarella, drained

Mix together the olive oil, garlic, thyme, chilli flakes, peppercorns and salt.

Add the mozzarella balls and stir to fully coat.

Allow to marinate for an hour or longer. The longer they marinate, the better the flavours will be.

Store in an airtight container in the fridge for up to 5 days.

Low-Carb Crackers

MAKES 30

PREP + COOK TIME: 45 MINS

VEG • GLUTEN FREE • DAIRY FREE

- 1 cup (150g) ground flaxseed
- ¼ cup (40g) hulled hemp seeds
- ¼ cup (40g) chia seeds
- 2 tbsps sesame seeds
- 1 tbsp sunflower seeds
- 1 tbsp pumpkin seeds
- 1 tbsp flaxseed
- ½ cup (125ml) warm water

Preheat the oven to 200°C. Line a baking tray with greaseproof paper.

In a medium bowl add the ground flaxseed, hemp seeds, chia seeds, sesame seeds, sunflower seeds, pumpkin seeds and flaxseed. Stir to combine.

Pour in the water and mix into a dough.

Let the mixture sit for 10 minutes.

Roll out the mixture between two layers of greaseproof paper then cut into squares.

Place the squares on the prepared baking tray.

Bake for 15 minutes, remove from the oven and turn over. Return to the oven and bake for a further 10 minutes.

Remove from the oven and allow to cool before eating.

Tip:

Allow your crackers to cool completely and dry out before storing. Store in an airtight container in the pantry for a week.

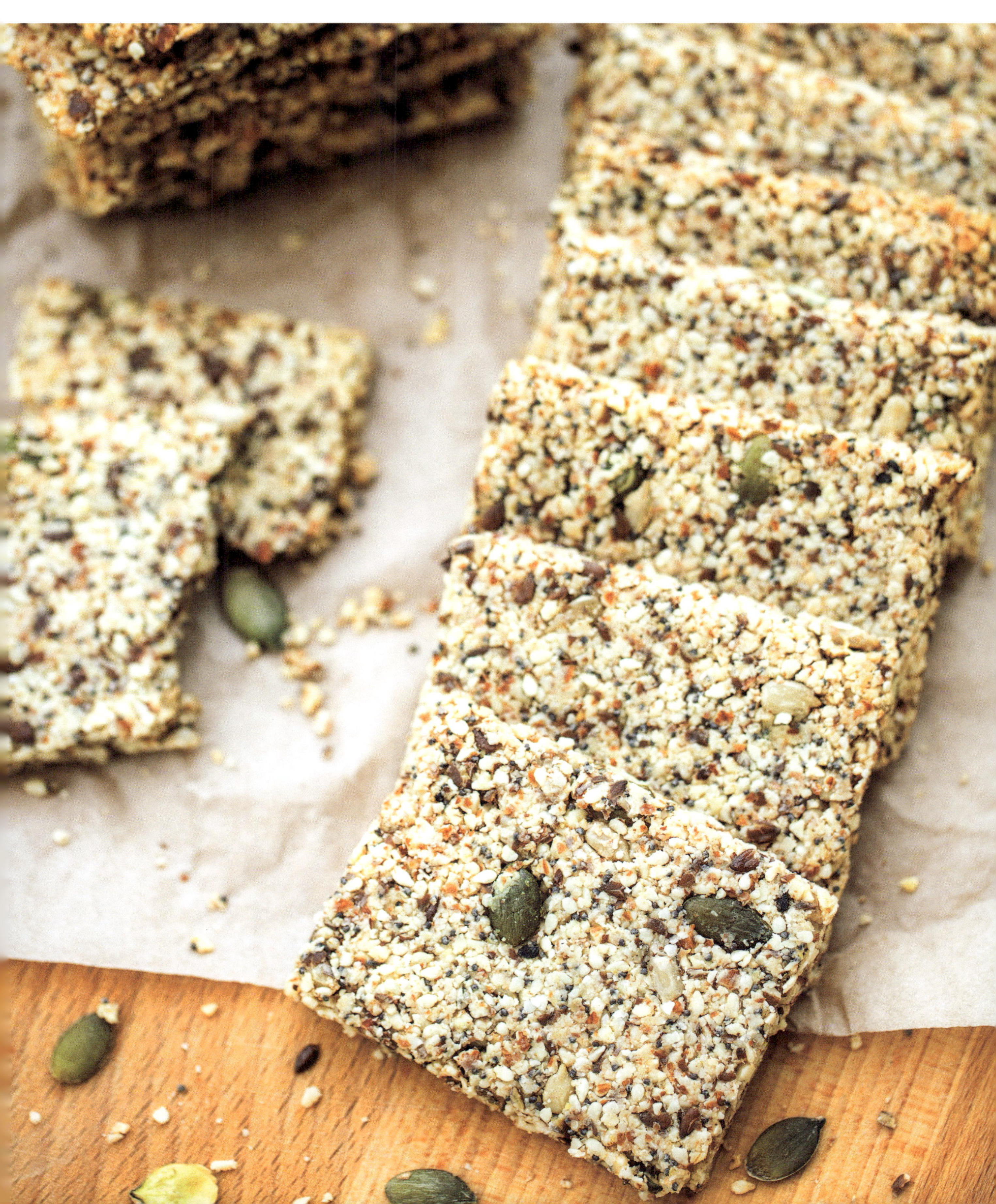

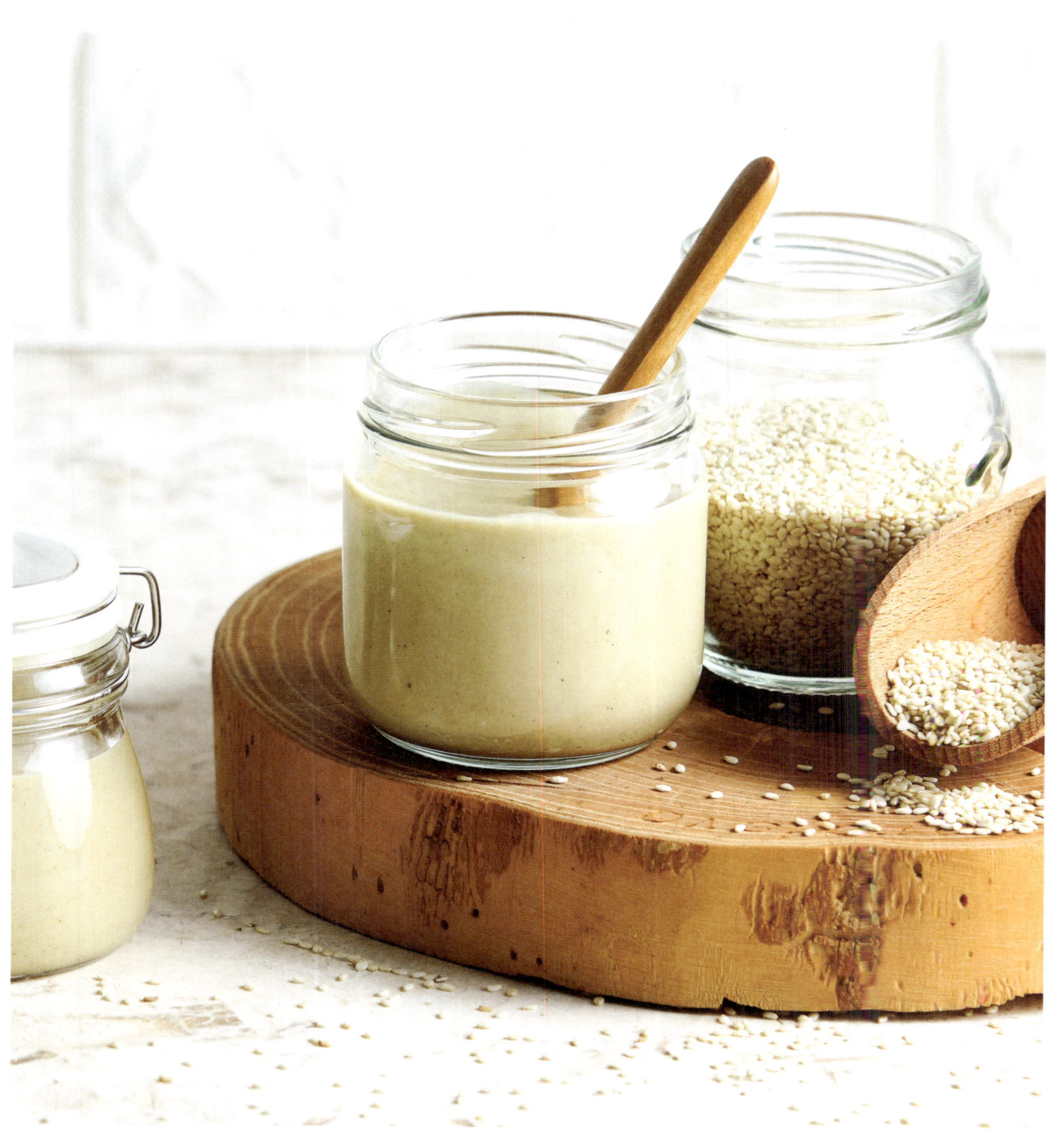

Homemade Tahini

MAKES ½ CUP

PREP + COOK TIME: 15 MINS

VEG • GLUTEN FREE • DAIRY FREE

HOMEMADE TAHINI

1 cup (160g) hulled sesame seeds
4 tbsps light olive oil
Pinch of salt

Add sesame seeds to a wide, dry saucepan over medium-low heat and toast, stirring constantly, for 3-5 minutes, until fragrant and very lightly coloured. Be careful not to let the seeds brown.

Quickly transfer toasted seeds to a plate and cool completely.

Add cooled sesame seeds to the bowl of a food processor and process for 1 minute until a crumbly paste forms.

Add 3 tablespoons of the oil then process for 2-3 minutes more, stopping to scrape down the sides as needed, until the tahini is smooth and pourable. Continue to process or add another spoonful of oil if needed.

Season with salt and pulse to combine.

Serve immediately or store in an airtight container in the fridge for up to 1 month.

Tip:

Tahini may separate over time, so just give it a stir before using.

PICO DE GALLO

3 medium tomatoes, diced
¼ white or red onion, diced
1 jalapeno, chopped
2 tbsps chopped coriander
Juice of ½ lime
Salt to taste

Mix together all the ingredients in a small bowl and season with salt to taste.

HERB BUTTER

100g butter, softened
1 tbsp chopped fresh parsley leaves
1 tbsp chopped fresh basil leaves
1 tsp chopped fresh thyme leaves
1 spring onion, finely diced

Add softened butter, herbs and spring onion to a mixing bowl and whip until thick and creamy using an electric hand mixer or a stand mixer.

Serve with steak or fish or use to flavour vegetables.

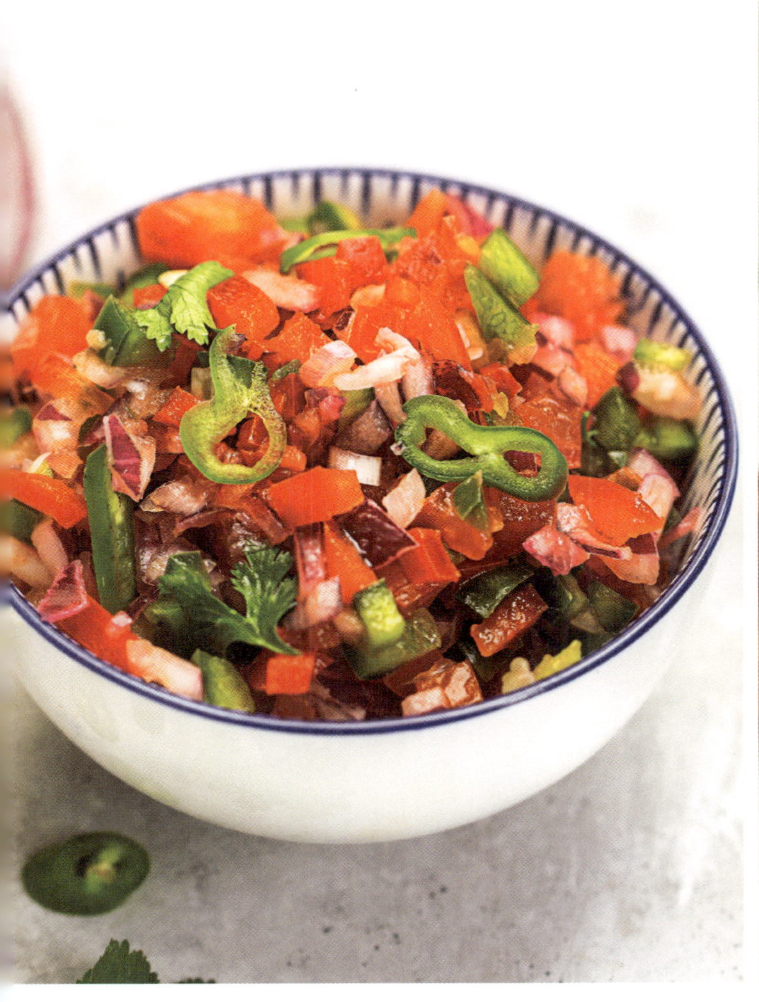

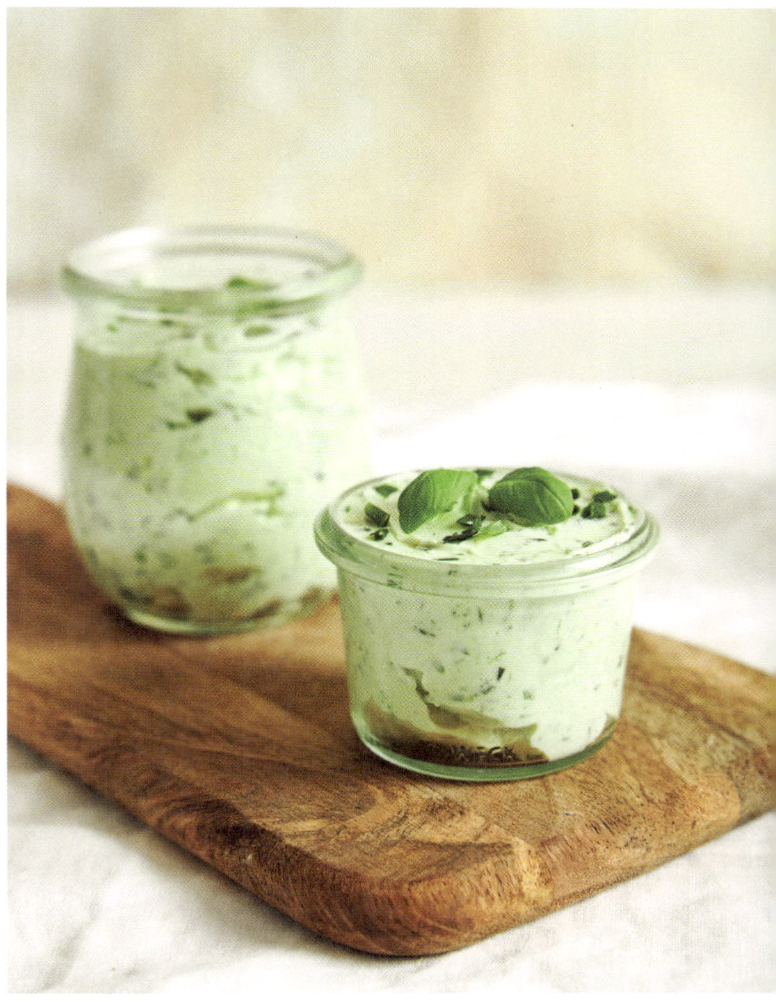

Pico de Gallo

SERVES 4

PREP + COOK TIME: 5 MINS

VEG • GLUTEN FREE • DAIRY FREE

Herb Butter

SERVES 6

PREP + COOK TIME: 10 MINS

VEG • GLUTEN FREE

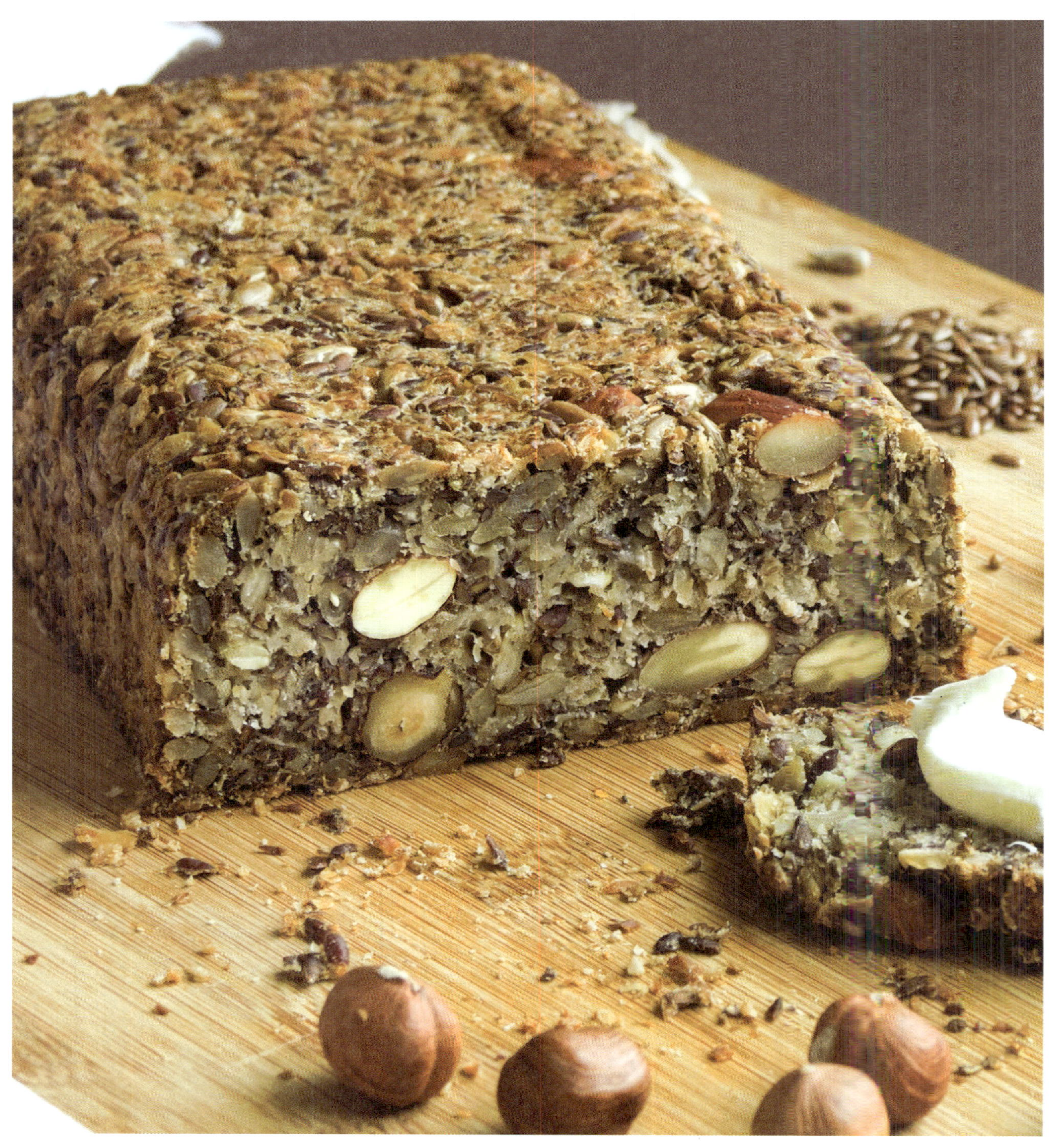

Nut & Seed Loaf

MAKES 1 LOAF

PREP + COOK TIME: 1 HOUR 5 MINS

VEG • GLUTEN FREE • DAIRY FREE

NUT & SEED LOAF

1 cup (125g) almonds
½ cup (75g) flaxseed
½ cup (75g) ground flaxseed
1 cup (125g) hazelnuts
½ cup (75g) Sesame Seeds
½ cup (60g) sunflower seeds
3 eggs
¼ cup (60ml) coconut or avocado oil
⅓ tsp salt

Preheat oven to 160°C. Line a loaf tin with greaseproof paper.

Combine all the ingredients in a large bowl. Mix well until thoroughly combined.

Pour mixture into prepared loaf tin and transfer to the oven. Bake for 50 minutes.

Remove from the oven and leave to cool in the tin for 10 minutes, then transfer to a wire rack to cool completely.

Tip:

Try different combinations of nuts and seeds but be sure not to miss out the ground flaxseed as this works as a binding agent.

CHEESE & HERB CHIPS

2 cups (250g) grated Cheddar cheese
2 tbsps fresh rosemary or thyme leaves, chopped

Preheat oven to 200°C. Line two baking trays with greaseproof paper.

Place the cheese and herbs in a large bowl. Stir to combine.

Arrange cheese mixture in 24 small heaps on the prepared baking trays.

Transfer to the oven and bake for about 7 minutes until melted and golden brown.

Cool for 5-10 minutes before using a spatula to remove from the baking trays.

Serve warm or cold.

ZUCCHINI BALLS

2-3 zucchinis (to make 1½ cups grated zucchini)
3 large eggs, beaten
3 cloves garlic, minced
1 cup (120g) almond meal
2 tbsps whole psyllium husk
2 tbsps flaxseed
½ cup (20g) basil leaves, roughly torn
1 tbsp dried oregano
½ tsp ground cumin
2 tsps paprika
1 tsp salt
1 cup (125g) Cheddar or mozzarella, grated

Preheat oven to 200°C. Line a baking tray with greaseproof paper.

Trim the ends of the zucchini and grate.

Wrap the grated zucchini in a clean tea towel and squeeze to extract the liquid then measure 1½ cups. Place in a large bowl.

Stir in the eggs, garlic, almond meal, psyllium husk, flaxseed, basil, oregano, cumin, paprika, salt and grated cheese.

Combine with a spoon then knead with your hands, squeezing the batter to ensure that all the ingredients come together. It should take 1 minute of squeezing and kneading until it forms a consistent batter.

Form into walnut-sized balls and place onto the baking tray.

Bake for 20-30 minutes or until the outside is golden and crispy.

Serve immediately with dip of your choice.

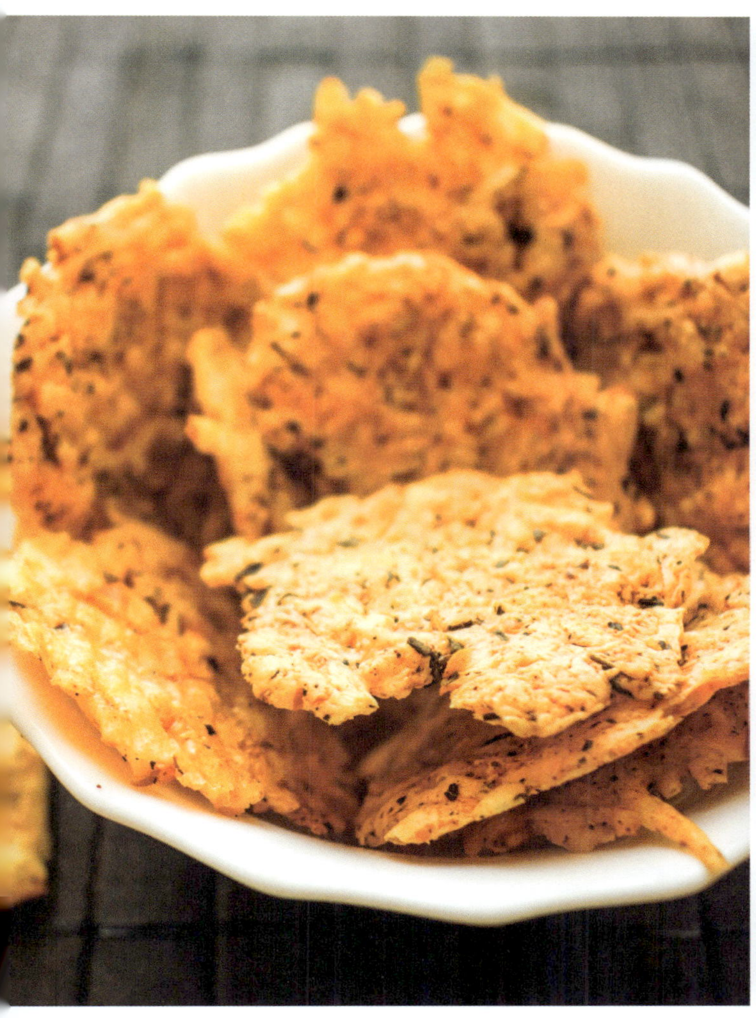

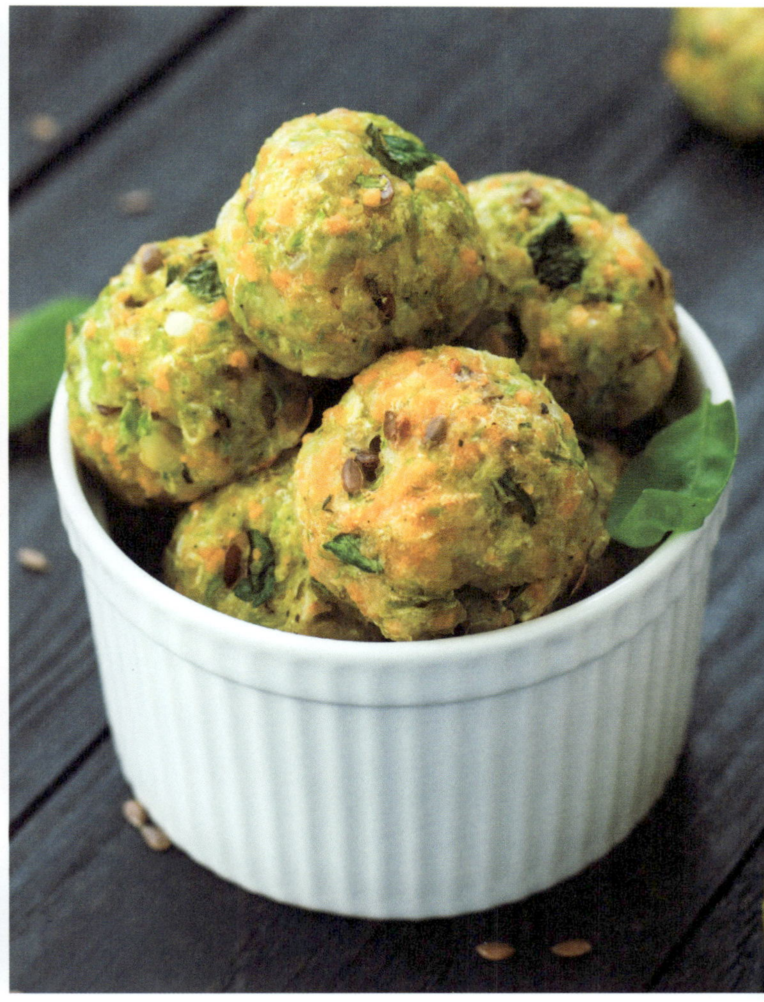

Cheese & Herb Chips

MAKES 24

PREP + COOK TIME: 20 MINS

VEG • GLUTEN FREE

Zucchini Balls

SERVES 4

PREP + COOK TIME: 50 MINS

VEG • GLUTEN FREE

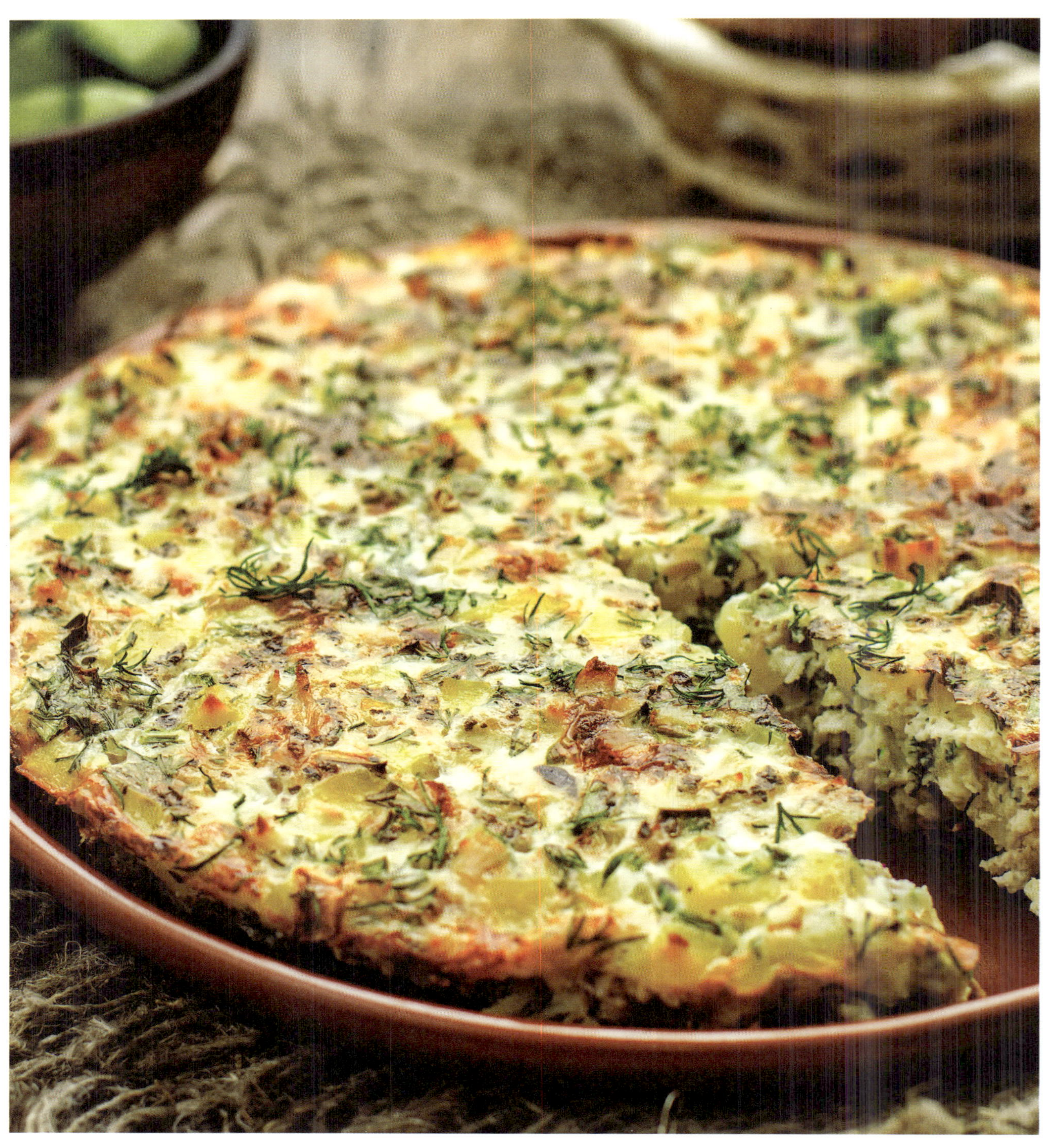

Chicken Frittata

SERVES 4

PREP + COOK TIME: 1 HOUR

GLUTEN FREE

CHICKEN FRITTATA

- 2 tbsps olive oil
- 1 chicken breast, cut into small pieces
- 1 head broccoli, finely chopped
- 1 yellow capsicum, diced
- 3 spring onions, finely chopped
- 2 cloves garlic, minced
- ½ tsp salt
- ¼ tsp pepper
- 8 eggs
- ½ cup (60g) grated Cheddar cheese
- Bunch of dill, finely chopped (reserve some for garnish)

Preheat oven to 180°C. Lightly grease a pie dish.

Heat 1 tablespoon oil in a large frying pan over a medium heat. Fry chicken for 3-4 minutes until lightly golden and cooked through. Remove from heat and set aside.

Heat 1 tablespoon oil in the frying pan over a medium heat. Saute broccoli and capsicum for 5 minutes, until softening.

Add spring onions, garlic, salt and pepper and cook for 1 minute. Remove from heat and set aside.

Whisk eggs in a large bowl. Add cheese, chicken, broccoli, capsicum and dill. Pour egg and chicken mix into pie dish.

Bake for 40 minutes, until set and a skewer inserted into the centre comes out clean.

Let rest for 5 minutes before serving. Garnish with reserved dill to serve.

EGGPLANT ROLLS

1 large eggplant
Salt and pepper to taste
1 cup (250g) ricotta
125g cream cheese, at room temperature
1 tbsp + ¼ cup (60ml) olive oil
½ cup (50g) grated Parmesan cheese
¼ tsp dried chilli flakes
¼ cup (10g) basil, chopped
2 tbsps sour cream

Thinly slice the eggplant lengthways and rub the pieces with salt. Place in a colander and drain for at least 20 minutes to remove moisture and bitterness.

While the eggplant drains, mix together the ricotta, cream cheese, 1 tablespoon olive oil, Parmesan, chilli flakes and chopped basil. Season with salt and pepper to taste.

Rinse and dry the eggplant with paper towels. Brush both sides of slices with olive oil.

Preheat a grill pan and grill the eggplant for 3 minutes on each side until cooked through.

Place a small spoonful of the cheese mixture at the base of each slice. Then roll up and arrange on a platter.

Drizzle with sour cream to serve.

SEED SNAP CRACKERS

2 cups (300g) flaxseed
2 cups (500ml) water, for soaking
⅓ cup (80g) sunflower seeds
½ cup (80g) sesame seeds
1 tsp salt

Place flaxseed in a bowl and cover with water. Cover and set aside to soak overnight.

Preheat the oven to 40°C and line a baking tray with greaseproof paper.

Drain flaxseed and place in a large mixing bowl. Add sunflower seeds, sesame seeds and salt and mix to just combine.

Using a wet spatula spread the mixture in an even layer onto the baking paper.

Score the mixture with a sharp knife into the desired shape and size of crackers.

Transfer to the oven and bake for 1 hour. If the top is dry, turn over and return to the oven for a further 1 hour. If not yet dry, return to the oven and check regularly until dry.

Remove from the oven and set aside to cool. Snap into small crackers down the score lines when cool.

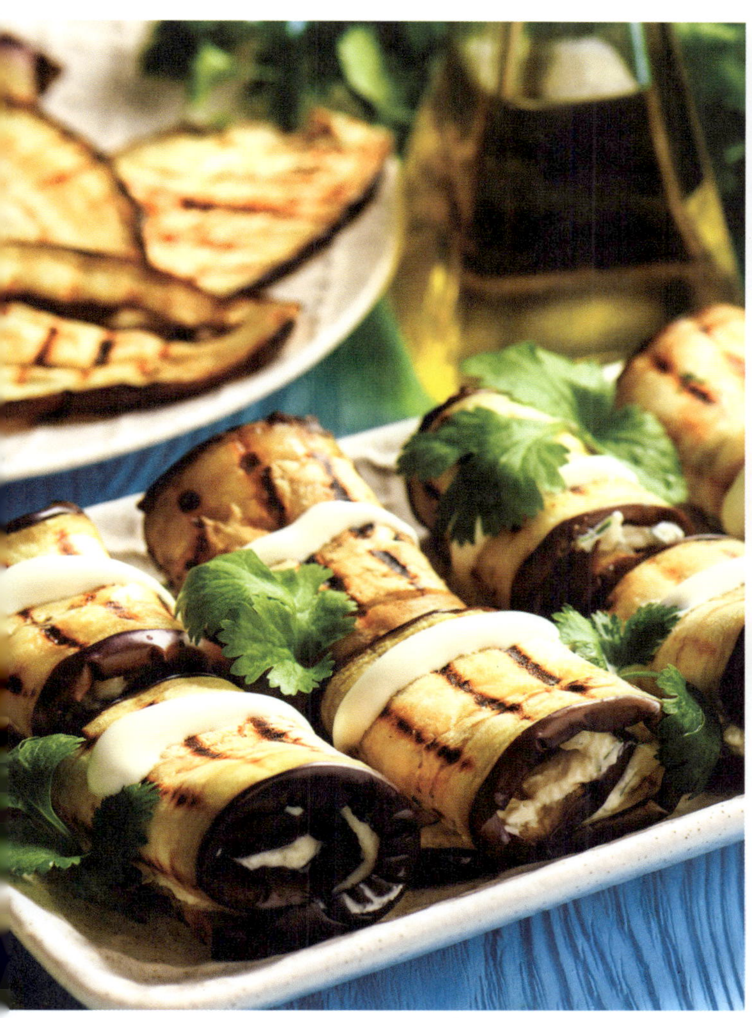

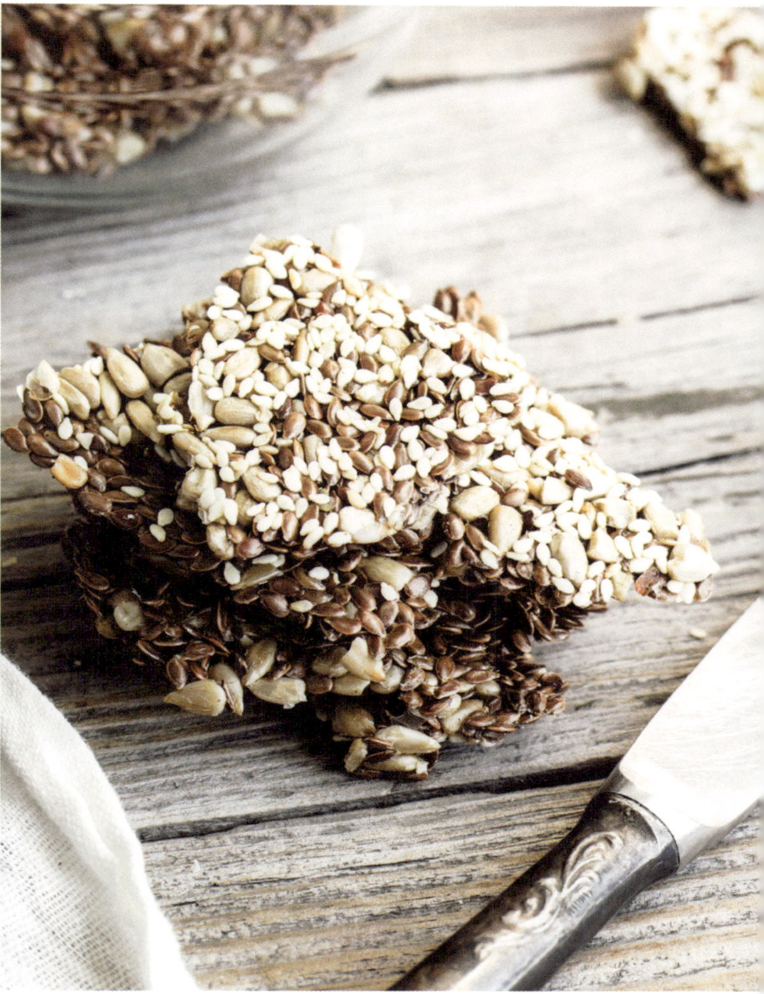

Eggplant Rolls

SERVES 4

PREP + COOK TIME: 1 HOUR

VEG • GLUTEN FREE

Seed Snap Crackers

SERVES 4

PREP + COOK TIME: 30 MINS + SOAKING AND DEHYDRATING

VEG • GLUTEN FREE • DAIRY FREE

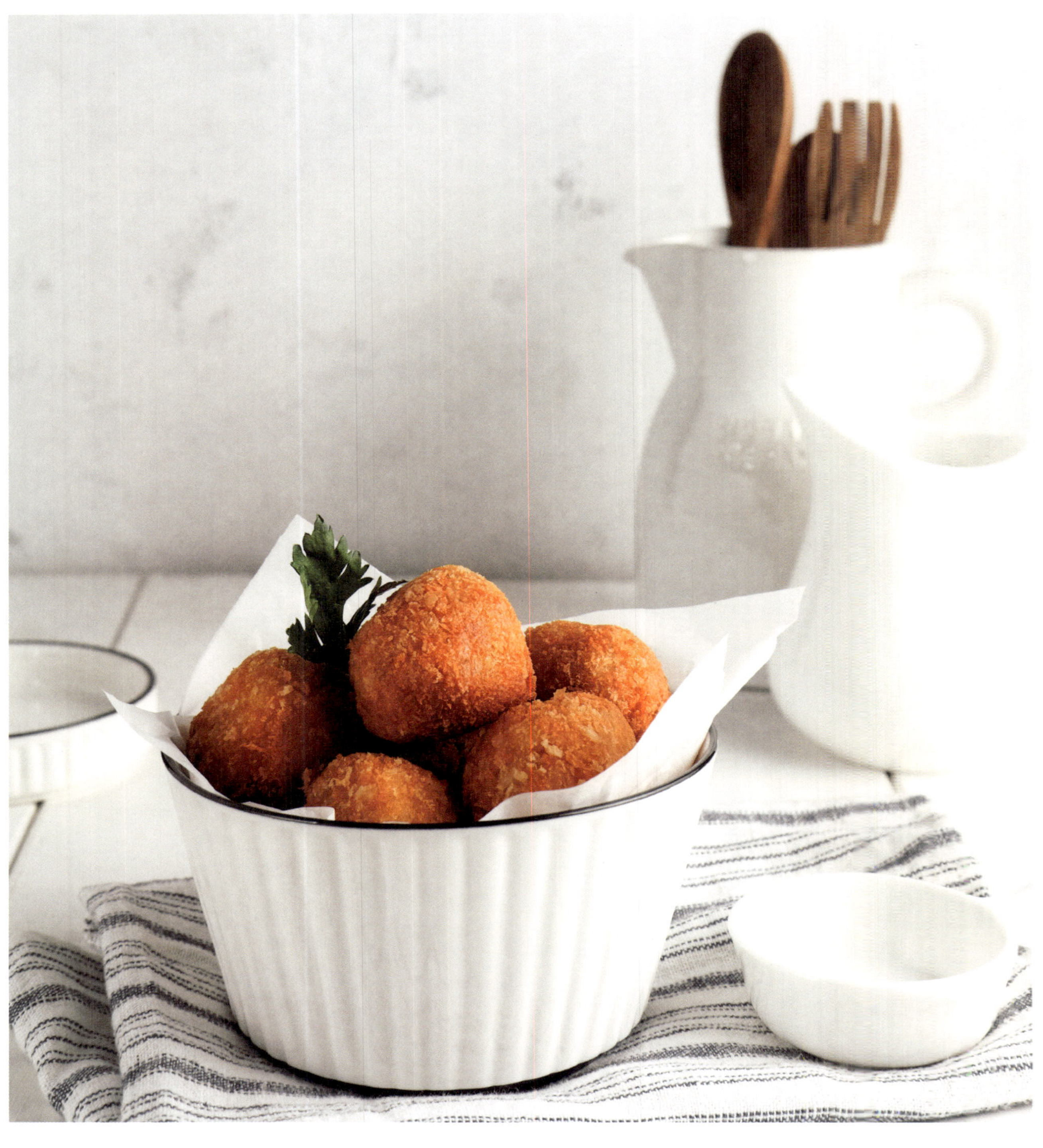

Mozzarella Balls

SERVES 4

PREP + COOK TIME: 15 MINS + FREEZING

GLUTEN FREE

MOZZARELLA BALLS

2 tbsps coconut flour
1 large egg
½ cup (60g) almond meal
½ cup (35g) crushed pork rinds
½ tsp garlic powder
2 tsps Italian seasoning
12 baby bocconcini balls
Avocado oil for frying

Line a baking tray with greaseproof paper.

Place coconut flour in a shallow dish. Beat the egg in a second shallow dish. Mix the almond meal, pork rinds, garlic powder and Italian seasoning in a third shallow dish.

Dredge each bocconcini ball in coconut flour, then dip in the egg, shaking off the excess. Finally roll in the almond meal mixture and coat well. Place the coated bocconcini balls on the prepared baking tray.

Place the baking tray in the freezer for at least 1 hour.

Heat 2 tablespoons oil in a frying pan over medium heat until hot. Working in batches, fry the balls in a single layer for 1-2 minutes per side, until golden brown and soft inside when pressed gently. Add more oil between batches as needed.

Serve hot.

Tip:

You can buy crushed pork rinds online or at health food stores. If you can't find it, you can buy a packet of pork crackle from the supermarket and crush with a rolling pin.

Sesame Chicken

SERVES 4

PREP + COOK TIME: 1 HOUR 10 MINS + MARINATING

GLUTEN FREE • DAIRY FREE

1½ kg chicken wings
4 tbsps tamari
4 tbsps xylitol
1 medium piece of ginger, grated
2 cloves garlic, grated
1 tbsp sesame oil
2 tsps rice wine vinegar
⅛ tsp cayenne pepper
¼ cup (60ml) + 2 tbsps water
½ tsp arrowroot
1 tbsp toasted sesame seeds
1-2 spring onions, finely sliced

Place the chicken in a large shallow dish.

Mix tamari, xylitol, ginger, garlic, sesame oil, vinegar and cayenne pepper in a small bowl. Pour half the marinade over chicken and reserve the rest. Cover and refrigerate for at least two hours.

Preheat oven to 220°C. Line a baking tray with greaseproof paper.

Arrange chicken on baking tray. Roast for 35-40 minutes, until cooked, turning halfway through.

Place reserved marinade in a saucepan with ¼ cup water and simmer for 15-20 minutes. Combine arrowroot with 2 tablespoons water then add to pan. Simmer until just thickened.

Pour glaze over cooked wings. Sprinkle with sesame seeds and spring onions to serve.

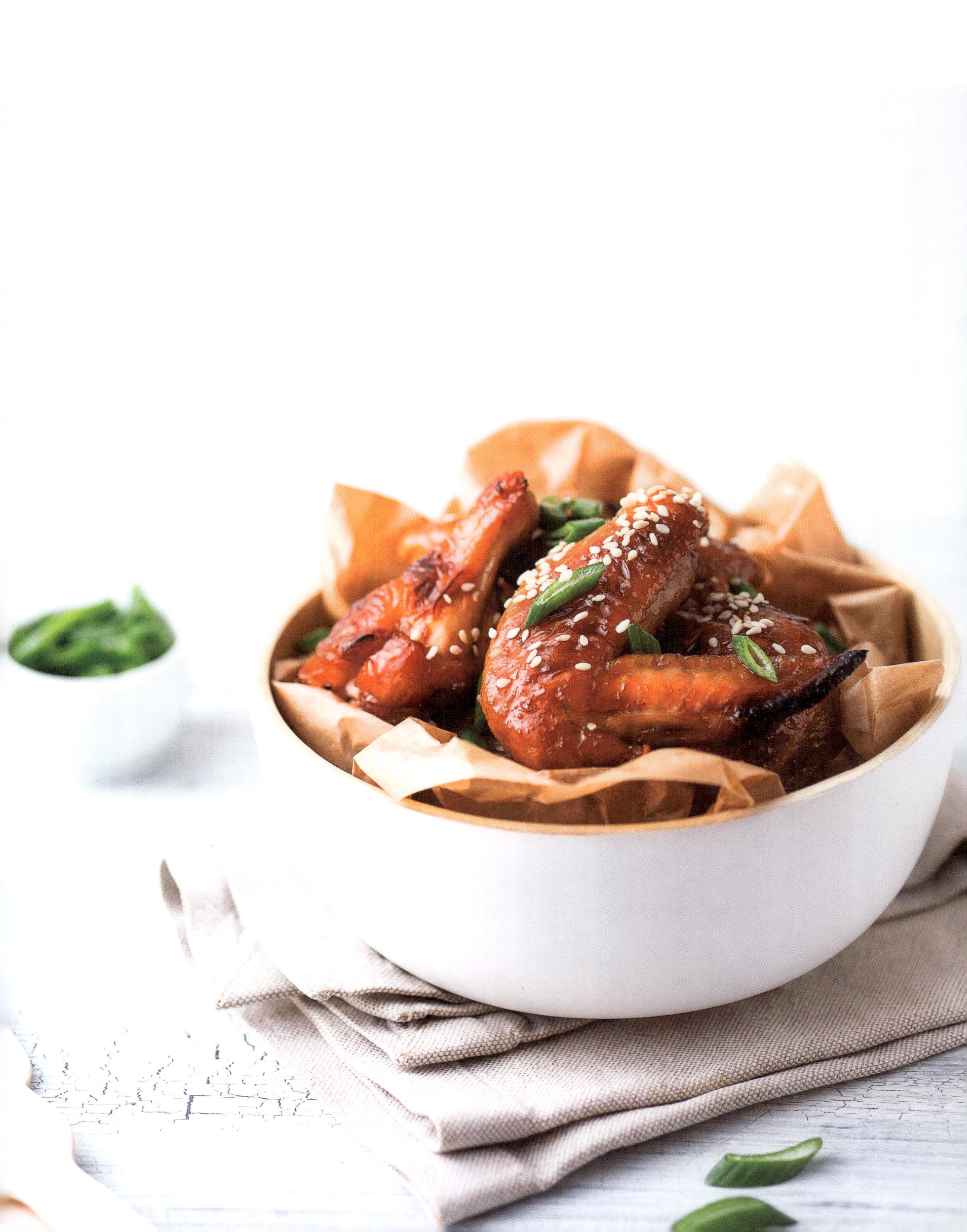

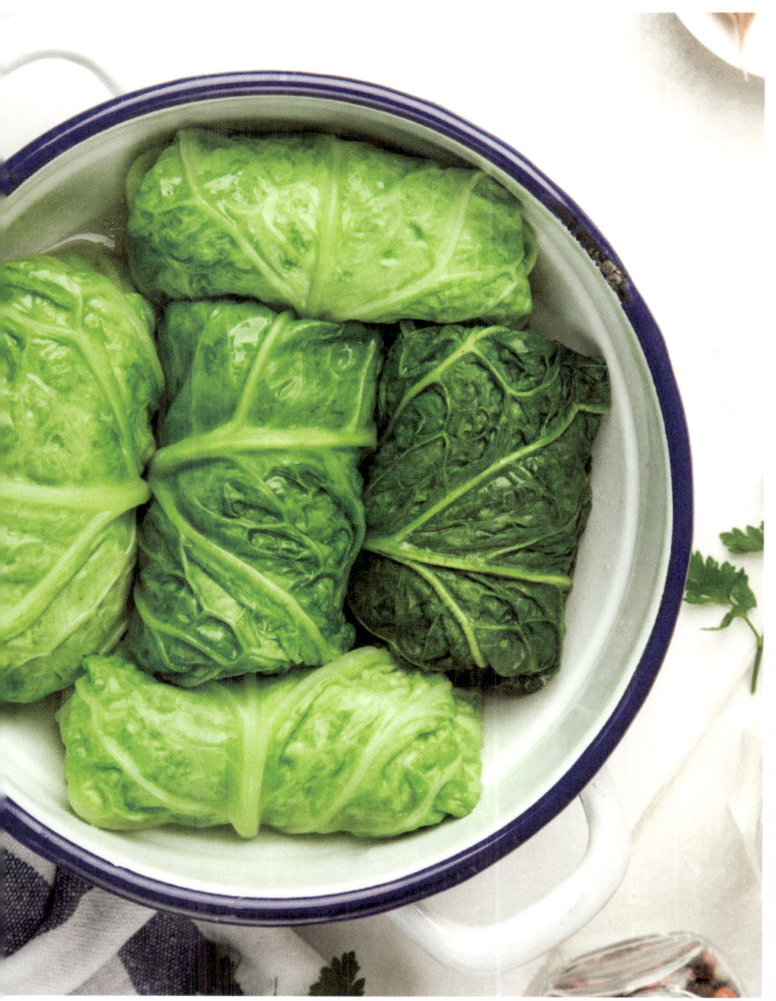

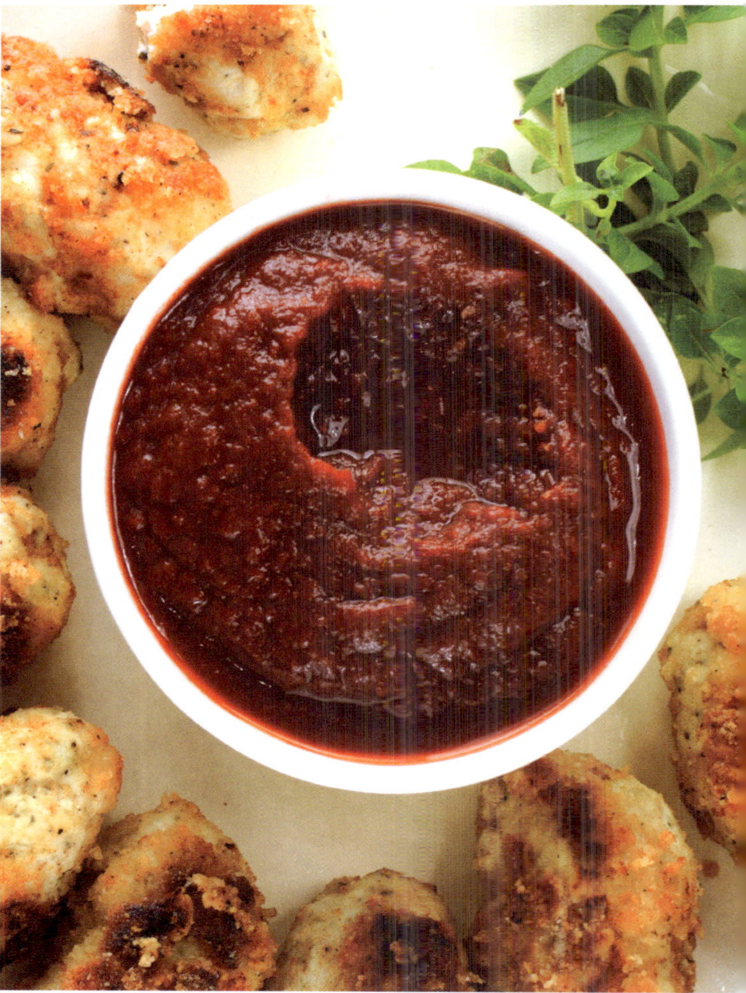

Cabbage Rolls

SERVES 4-6

PREP + COOK TIME: 2 HOURS

GLUTEN FREE • DAIRY FREE

Tomato Sauce

MAKES APPROXIMATELY 1½ CUPS

PREP + COOK TIME: 20 MINS

VEG • GLUTEN FREE • DAIRY FREE

CABBAGE ROLLS

1 tbsp olive oil
1 cup (150g) diced onion
2 cloves garlic, minced
100g mushrooms, finely diced
16 cabbage leaves, core removed
¾ cup (75g) cauliflower florets
250g beef mince
250g pork mince
¼ cup (10g) chopped parsley
1 cup (225g) passata
1½ tsps salt
Pepper to taste
¾ cup (185ml) beef stock

Preheat oven to 180°C.

Heat oil in a frying pan over medium-high heat and saute the onion for 3-5 minutes until soft and translucent. Add garlic and cook for 1 minute until fragrant. Add mushrooms and cook for another 3-4 minutes until soft. Transfer mixture to a large bowl to cool.

In a large pan of boiling water, blanch cabbage leaves for about 1 minute until tender and flexible. Set aside.

To make riced cauliflower, place cauliflower florets into a food processor and pulse until it resembles rice.

In a large bowl, combine the beef and pork mince, cauliflower rice, parsley, passata and cooled onion and mushroom mixture. Season with salt and pepper. Place about ¼ cup of filling into a log shape at one end of each leaf. Fold in the sides, then roll up, and place seam-side down in a large baking dish. Pour stock over rolls.

Cover tightly with foil, and bake for 1½ hours.

Remove from oven and let rest for 10 minutes before serving.

TOMATO SAUCE

¾ cup (170g) tomato paste
2 tbsps apple cider vinegar
2 tbsps white vinegar
¼ cup (40g) keto-friendly brown sugar substitute
1 tsp onion powder
½ tsp garlic powder
1 tsp salt
1 cup (250ml) water

Place all the ingredients into a saucepan over medium heat.

Bring to a simmer then reduce heat to low and cook, stirring, for 5 minutes until the sauce thickens.

Popcorn Chicken

SERVES 4

PREP + COOK TIME: 35 MINS + MARINATING

GLUTEN FREE

- **500g boneless, skinless chicken breasts, cut into bite-size pieces**
- **1 cup (250ml) buttermilk**
- **¼ cup (25g) coconut flour**
- **¼ tsp salt**
- **⅛ tsp pepper**
- **1 large egg**
- **2 cups (150g) crushed pork rinds (see tip)**
- **1 tsp onion powder**
- **½ tsp garlic powder**
- **½ tsp smoked paprika**

Place the chicken in a large bowl. Pour over the buttermilk and toss to coat. Cover and refrigerate for 24 hours.

Preheat the oven to 220°C. Line a baking tray with greaseproof paper.

Prepare three shallow dishes. In the first, combine the coconut flour, salt and pepper. Crack the egg into the second dish and beat lightly with a fork. In the third dish, mix together the pork rinds, onion powder, garlic powder and paprika.

Dredge the chicken first in the coconut flour then dip in egg wash, and finally coat in the pork rind breading.

Place coated chicken pieces on the prepared baking tray.

Transfer to the oven and bake for 20 minutes, until golden brown and crispy.

Tip:

You can buy crushed pork rinds online or at health food stores. If you can't find it, you can buy a packet of pork crackle from the supermarket and crush with a rolling pin. If you buy pork crackle do check the salt content and reduce the amount of salt you add.

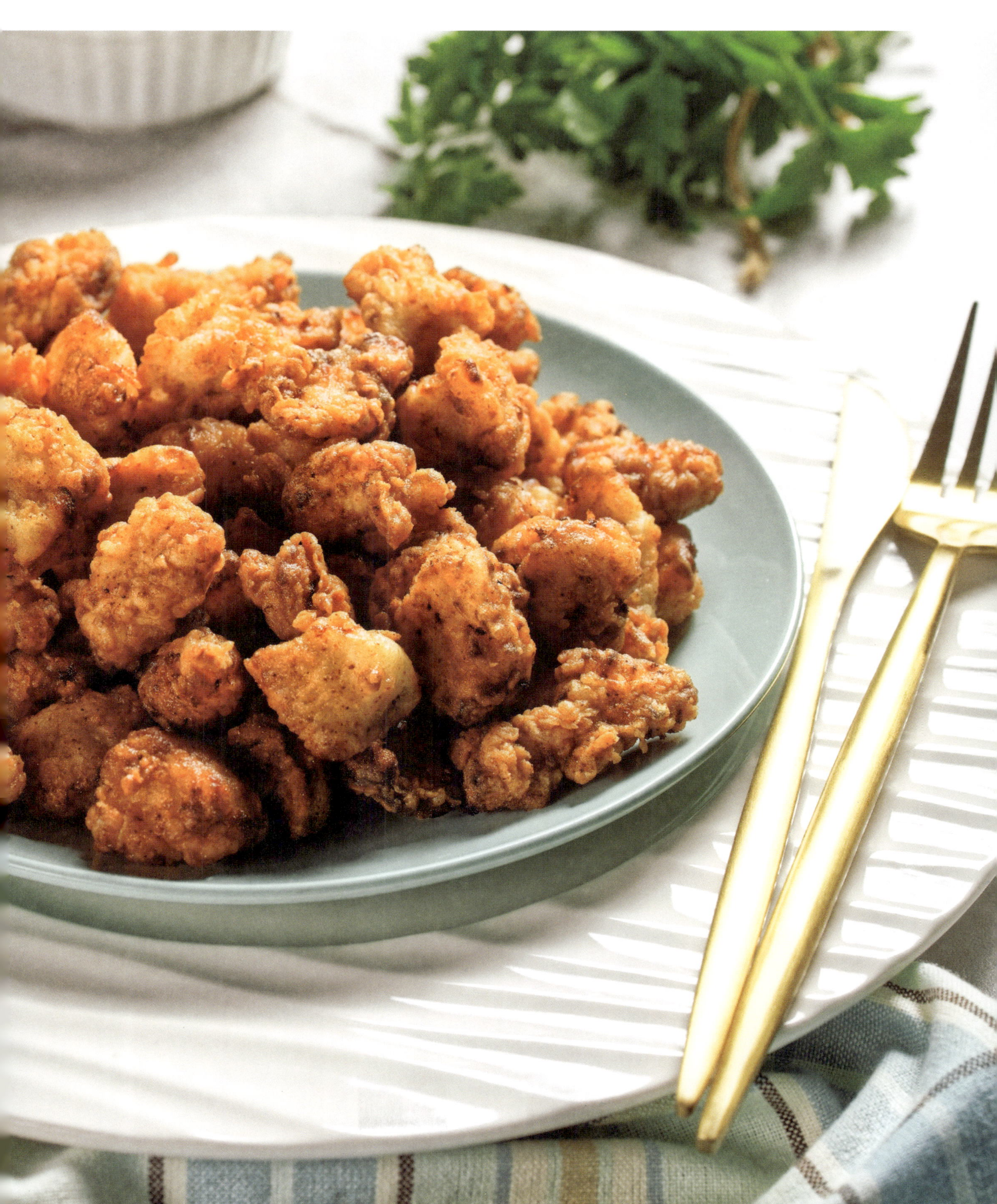

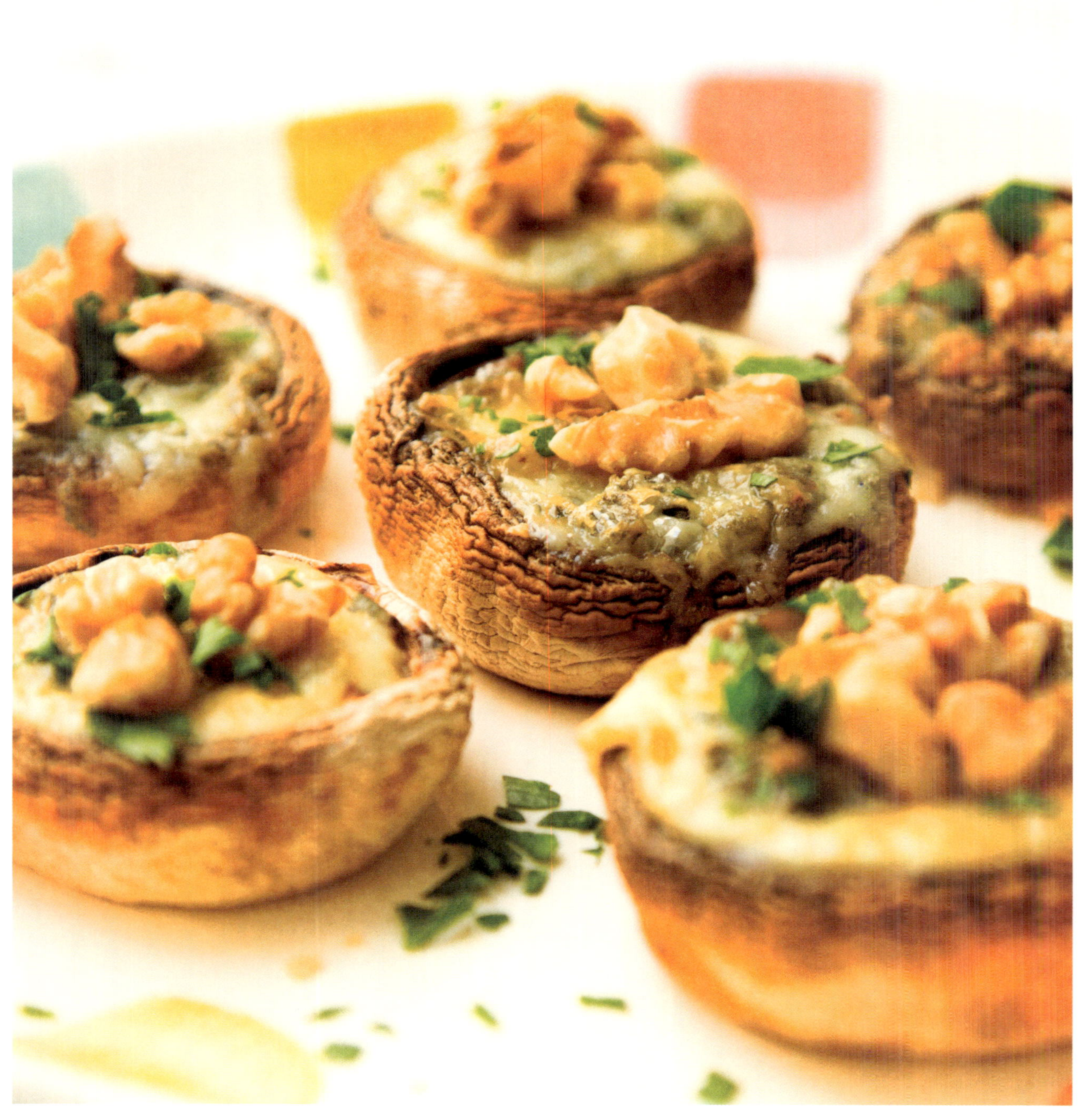

Blue Cheese Mushrooms

SERVES 4

PREP + COOK TIME: 30 MINS

VEG • GLUTEN FREE

BLUE CHEESE MUSHROOMS

500g button mushrooms
Salt and pepper to taste
2 tbsps olive oil
200g blue cheese, crumbled
¼ cup (10g) parsley, chopped + more to serve
½ cup (60g) walnuts, roughly chopped

Preheat oven to 180°C. Line a baking tray with greaseproof paper.

Remove the stems from the mushrooms and set aside.

Arrange the mushrooms stem-side up on the baking tray. Season with salt and pepper.

In a medium frying pan, heat 1 teaspoon olive oil over medium heat.

Chop mushroom stems and add to pan. Season with salt and pepper and saute for 5-7 minutes until soft. Set aside and allow to cool.

In a large mixing bowl combine blue cheese, chopped parsley and mushroom stems. Drizzle filling with remaining olive oil and mix well.

Using your fingers take a portion of the filling and carefully stuff each mushroom cap.

Place into oven and cook for 15 minutes or until golden brown.

Top with chopped walnuts and parsley.

SALMON DEVILLED EGGS

6 hard-boiled eggs
2 ripe avocados
1 tbsp lime juice
½ tsp salt
1 tbsp chopped coriander + extra leaves to garnish
¼ small red capsicum, cut into small pieces
50g smoked salmon, cut into small pieces

Cut the eggs in half lengthwise and remove the yolks.

In a mixing bowl, mash the yolks together with the avocado flesh, lime juice and salt. Gently stir through the chopped coriander, capsicum and smoked salmon.

Fill the egg white halves with the mixture. Sprinkle with coriander leaves to serve.

AVOCADO YOGHURT DRESSING

1 avocado
⅔ cup (160ml) Greek yoghurt
Juice of 1 lime
¼ cup (5g) fresh coriander, loosely packed
Pinch of salt

In a food processor or blender, add the avocado flesh, yoghurt, lime juice and coriander.

Blend until smooth, then add salt to taste.

Use as a dressing for salads or serve with chicken or fish.

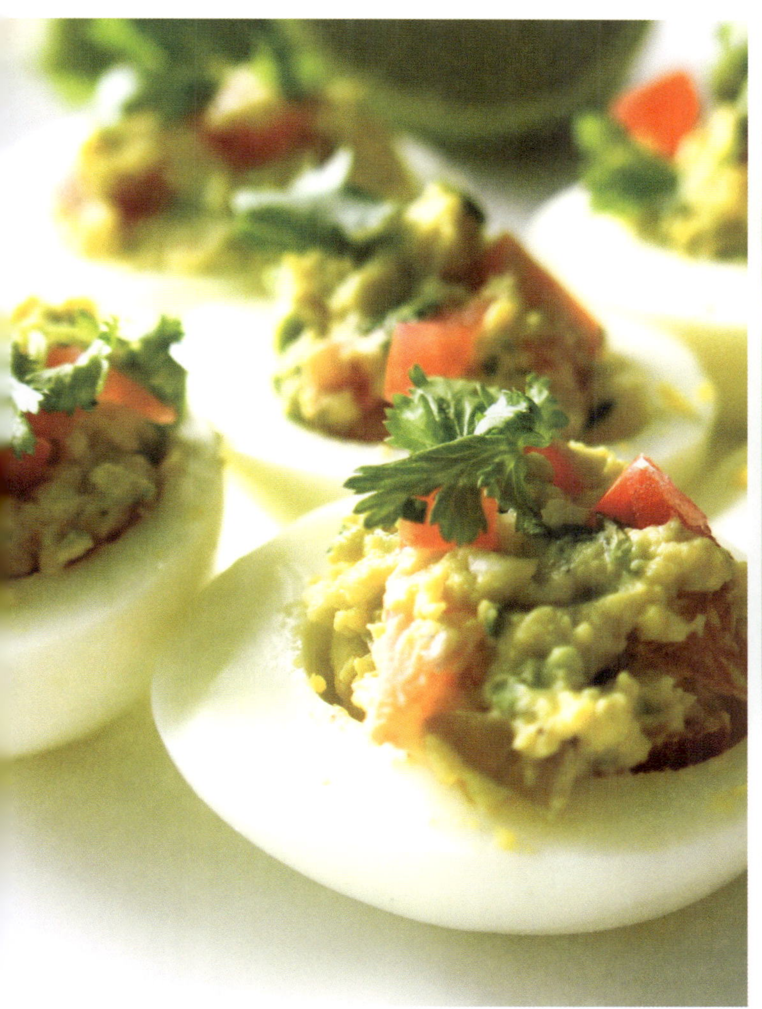

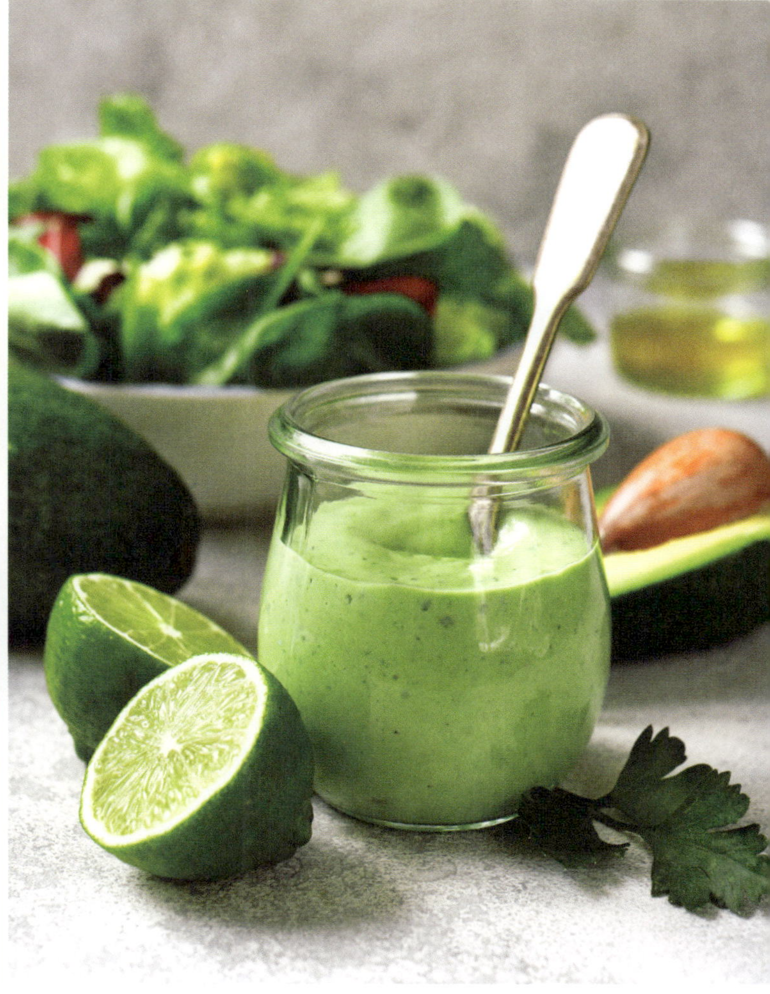

Salmon Devilled Eggs

MAKES 12

PREP + COOK TIME: 10 MINS

GLUTEN FREE • DAIRY FREE

Avocado Yoghurt Dressing

SERVES 8

PREP + COOK TIME: 5 MINS

VEG • GLUTEN FREE

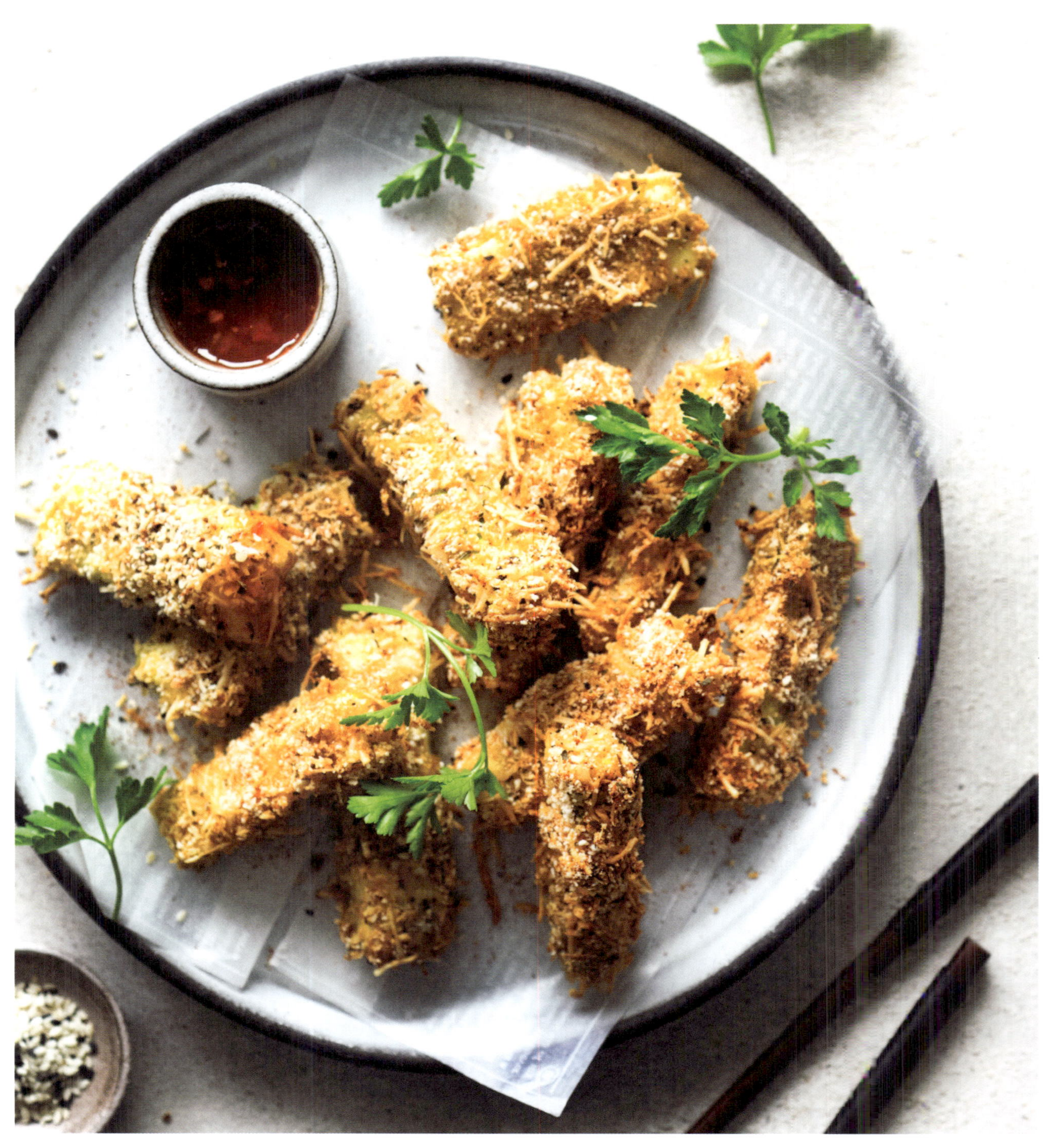

Zucchini Fries

SERVES 4

PREP + COOK TIME: 40 MINS

VEG • GLUTEN FREE

ZUCCHINI FRIES

2 large zucchinis
½ cup (50g) coconut flour
2 eggs, lightly beaten
1 tbsp mayonnaise
½ cup (60g) almond meal
¾ cup (75g) shredded Parmesan cheese
½ tsp paprika
¼ tsp Italian seasoning
¼ tsp garlic powder
⅛ tsp salt
1 tbsp olive oil
Pepper to taste

Preheat oven to 200°C.

Slice zucchinis into 6cm-long batons. Pat the zucchini dry.

Place the coconut flour in one shallow dish, whisk together the egg and the mayonnaise in another dish and combine the almond meal, Parmesan, paprika, Italian seasoning, garlic powder and salt in a third shallow dish.

Dredge the zucchini first in the coconut flour then the egg mixture, then the almond meal and Parmesan mixture. Place the coated zucchini on the baking tray. Drizzle with olive oil.

Bake for 15 minutes, turn carefully with a fork and bake for 10 minutes more until golden brown and crisp. Season with pepper to serve.

SPINACH & FETA MUFFINS

4 eggs
¼ cup (60ml) melted butter
¼ cup (60ml) water
Salt and pepper, to taste
⅓ cup (30g) coconut flour
½ tsp baking powder
4 spring onions, chopped
1 zucchini, grated
½ cup (115g) cooked spinach
4 tbsps fresh parsley, chopped
½ tsp ground nutmeg
¼ cup (25g) Parmesan, grated
150g feta cheese, diced

Preheat oven to 200°C. Fill a muffin tin with eight paper liners.

Combine eggs, butter, water, salt and pepper in a large bowl. Whisk thoroughly.

Add coconut flour and baking powder and mix well.

Add in spring onions, zucchini, spinach, parsley and nutmeg. Mix thoroughly.

Stir through Parmesan and half the feta cheese. Add more water if the mixture is too stiff.

Spoon the mixture into the muffin tin, filling each cup two-thirds full. Top the muffins with the remaining feta cubes.

Bake for 20-25 minutes until firm and golden.

STRAWBERRY AVOCADO SMOOTHIE

2½ cups (500g) fresh or frozen strawberries
1½ cups (375ml) unsweetened almond milk
1 large avocado, pitted and peeled
1 cup (30g) baby spinach
1 tbsp monkfruit sweetener or to taste
½ cup (75g) ice (if using fresh fruit)

Combine all ingredients in a high-speed blender.

Add ice, if using. Blend until smooth.

Adjust sweetener to taste as needed.

Pour into glasses to serve.

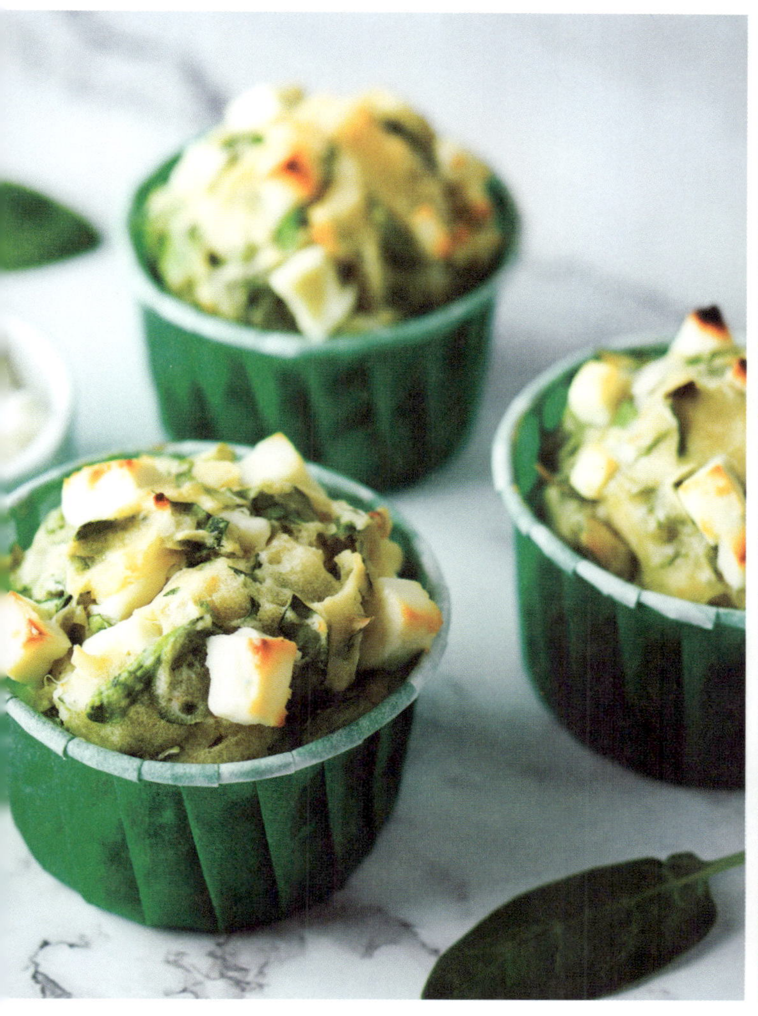

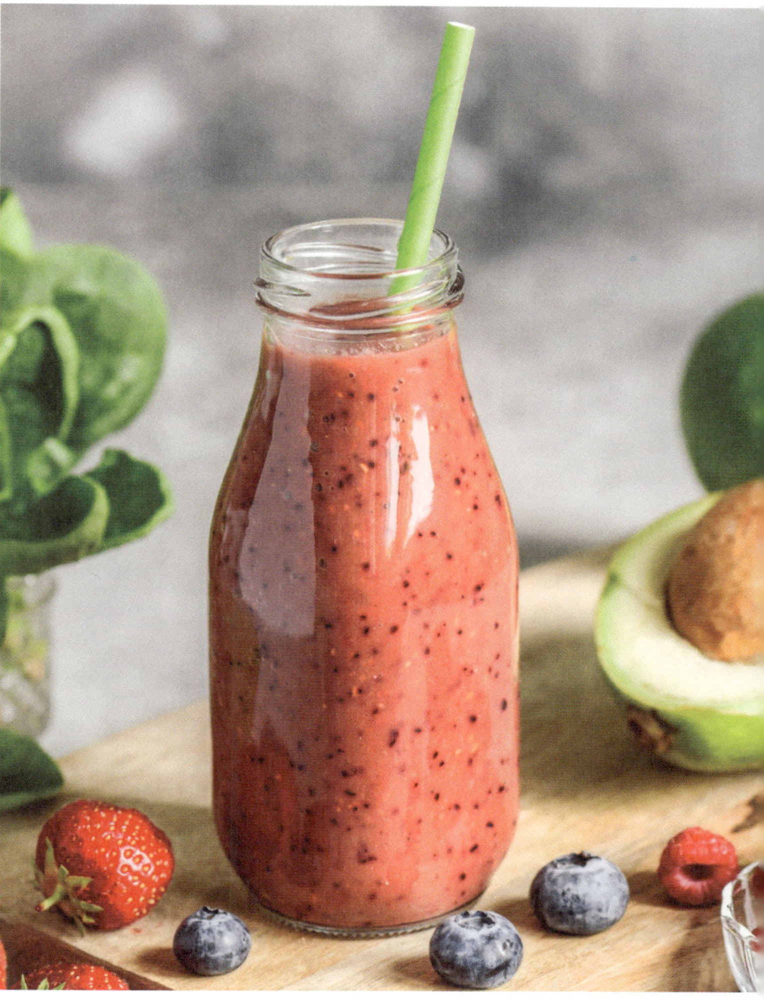

Spinach & Feta Muffins

MAKES 8

PREP + COOK TIME: 40 MINS

VEG • GLUTEN FREE

Strawberry Avocado Smoothie

SERVES 5

PREP + COOK TIME: 5 MINS

VEG • GLUTEN FREE • DAIRY FREE

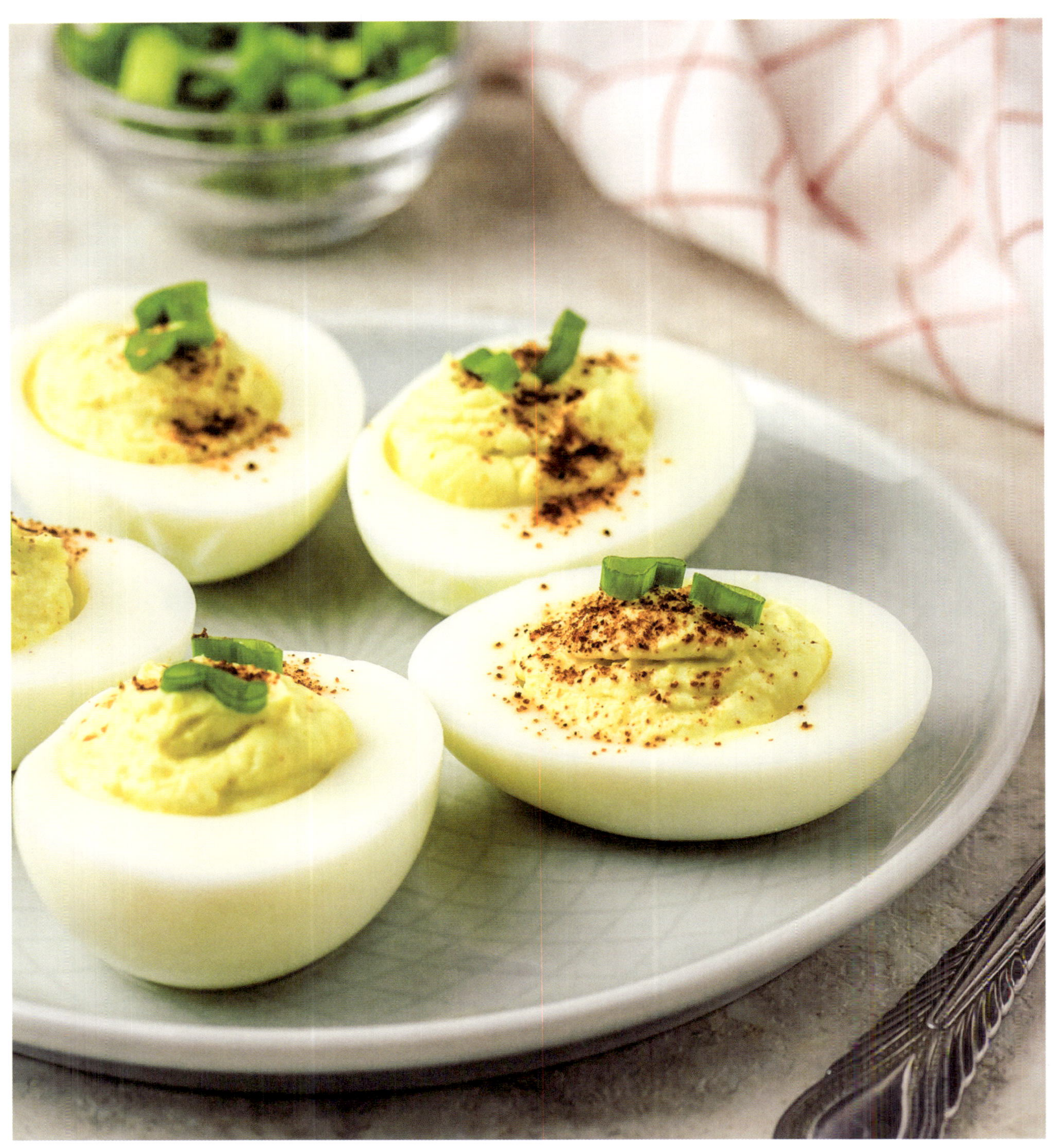

Avo Devilled Eggs with Smoked Paprika

MAKES 8

PREP + COOK TIME: 20 MINS

VEG • GLUTEN FREE

AVO DEVILLED EGGS WITH SMOKED PAPRIKA

4 eggs
1 large avocado
1 tbsp lime juice
1 tbsp sour cream
Pinch of salt
⅛ tsp smoked paprika
1 tbsp chopped spring onions, (green part only) to serve

Place eggs in a medium pan and cover with cold water. Bring to a boil, then cover the pan and turn the heat off. Let the eggs stand in the hot water for 10-12 minutes.

Transfer the eggs to a bowl of ice water or run under cold water.

Peel the hard-boiled eggs and cut them in half lengthways.

Remove the cooked yolk and add to a mixing bowl along with the avocado flesh, lime juice and sour cream.

Mash with a fork, then beat with a wooden spoon until smooth and creamy. Season with a pinch of salt. Stir to combine.

Either spoon the mixture back into the eggs or use a piping bag to pipe in the mixture.

Sprinkle with smoked paprika and scatter with chopped spring onion to serve.

ZUCCHINI BITES

2 zucchinis, sliced into rounds
1 tsp coconut flour
1 egg
1 tbsp fish sauce
1 tbsp avocado oil

In a medium bowl, toss the zucchini and coconut flour, ensuring each piece is lightly coated.

In a separate bowl, whisk the egg and fish sauce.

Heat the oil in a large frying pan over medium-high heat.

Working in batches, dip and coat the floured zucchini rounds in the egg mixture, then add to the pan and cook for 3 minutes each side, until lightly browned.

Use a spatula to transfer finished zucchini rounds to a wire rack lined with paper towels.

Serve with sesame soy dipping sauce (see next recipe).

SESAME SOY DIPPING SAUCE

2 tbsps tamari
2 tbsps rice wine vinegar
½ tsp maple syrup
¼ tsp sesame seeds
1 spring onion, thinly sliced

Whisk all ingredients together in a bowl.

Store in the refrigerator in a covered container for up to 1 week.

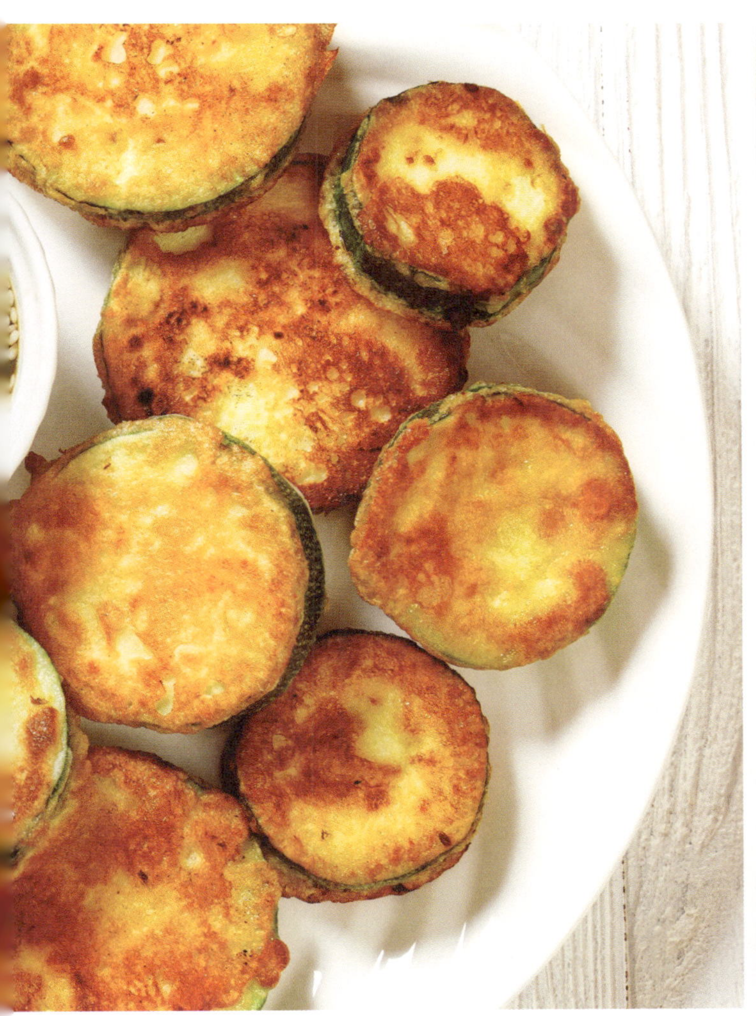

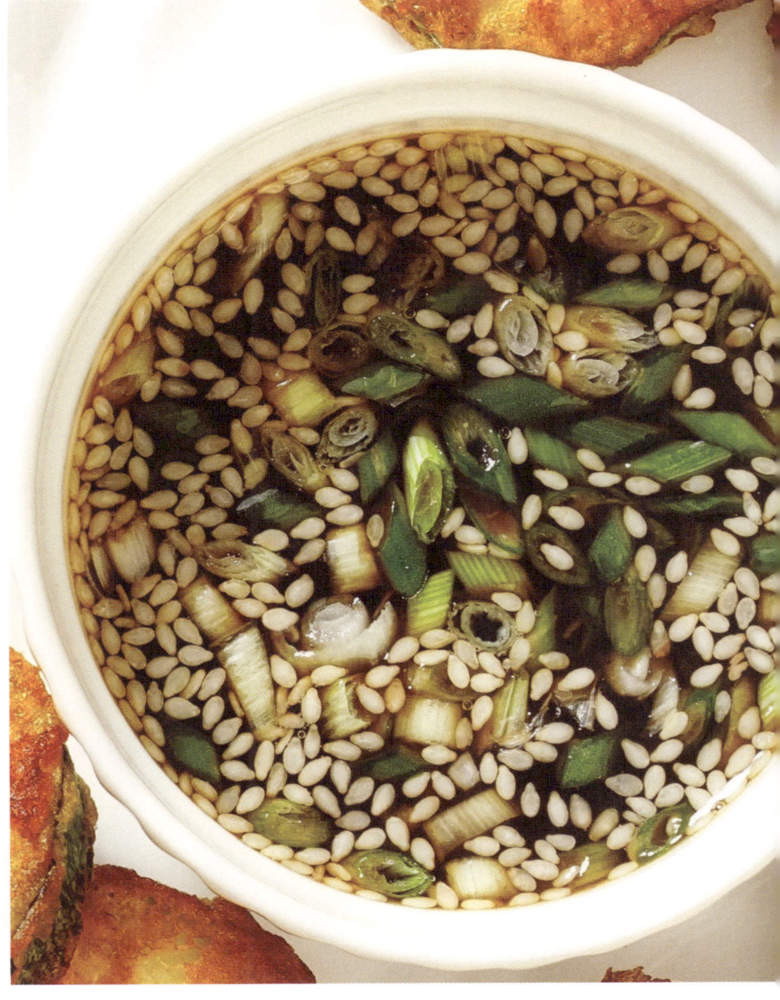

Zucchini Bites

SERVES 4

PREP + COOK TIME: 20 MINS

VEG • GLUTEN FREE • DAIRY FREE

Sesame Soy Dipping Sauce

SERVES 4

PREP + COOK TIME: 20 MINS

VEG • GLUTEN FREE • DAIRY FREE

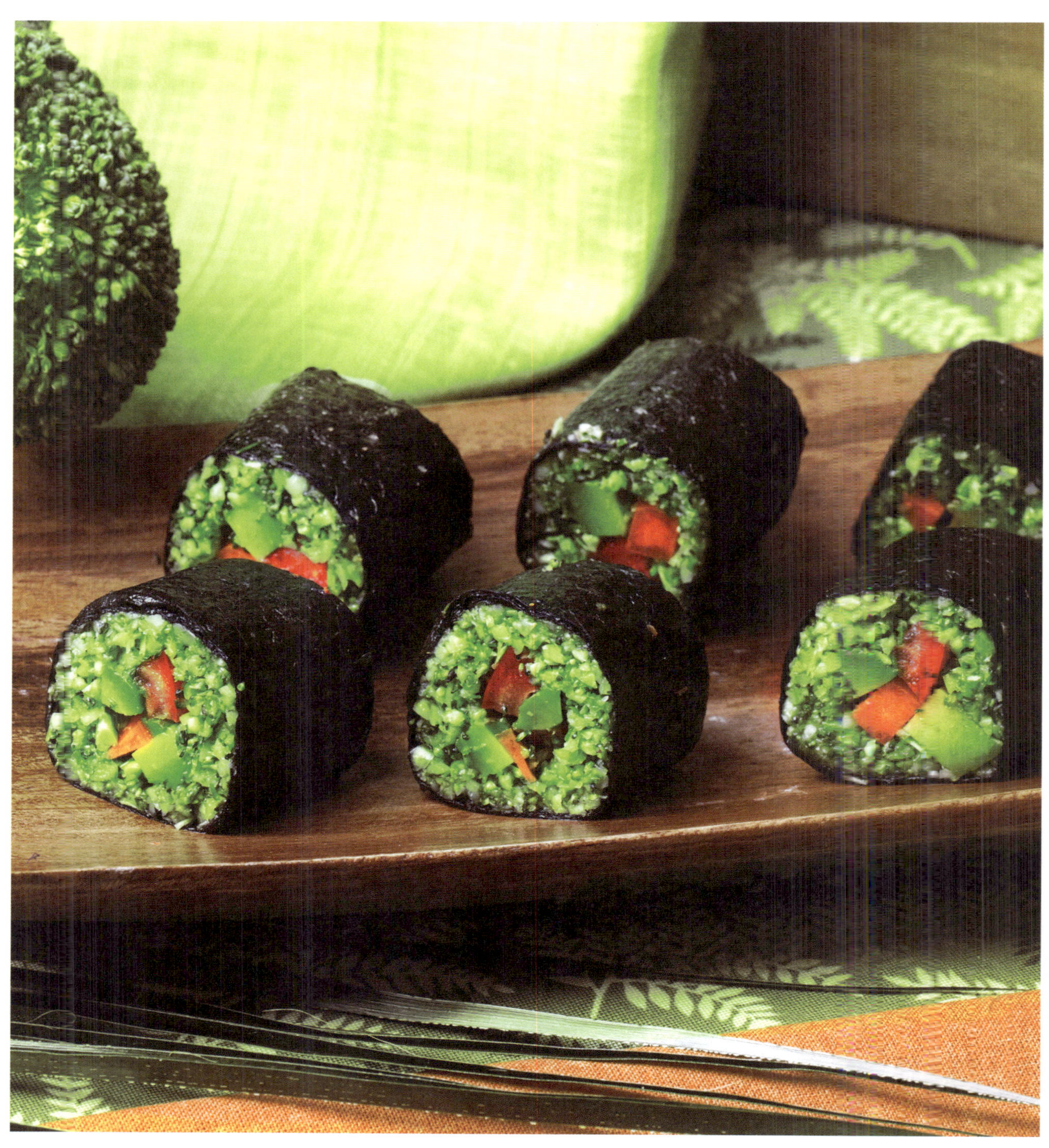

Raw Green Sushi Rolls

SERVES 4

PREP + COOK TIME: 30 MINS

VEG • GLUTEN FREE • DAIRY FREE

RAW GREEN SUSHI ROLLS

4 sheets of nori

RICE

½ head cauliflower, cut into florets
1 head broccoli, cut into florets
½ cup (20g) parsley
1 tbsp grated fresh ginger
¼ cup (40g) hemp seeds
1 tbsp ground flaxseed
2 tsps apple cider vinegar

FILLING

1 avocado, cut into strips
1 carrot, julienned
1 red capsicum, sliced into strips

Place the cauliflower, broccoli and parsley in a food processor and process until a rice-like consistency forms.

Add the grated ginger, hemp seeds, flaxseed and apple cider vinegar to the food processor and pulse until combined.

Lay the nori sheets shiny-side down on a clean surface and spread the rice mixture onto each sheet until it reaches the edges, but leave a border at the top and bottom.

Place the filling vegetables at the bottom of the sheet on top of the rice.

Roll from the bottom, using thumbs to roll and fingers to keep the vegetables intact. Apply even and firm pressure.

Dab water or lemon juice at the top of the nori roll to create a seal at one end.

Cut into slices using a very sharp knife.

Tip:

Use a bamboo mat to roll the sushi if you have one.

BAKED AVOCADO CHIPS

1 large avocado
¾ cup (75g) grated Parmesan cheese
1 tsp lemon juice
½ tsp garlic powder
¼ tsp onion powder
⅛ tsp pepper

Preheat oven to 165°C. Line two baking trays with greaseproof paper.

Scoop avocado flesh into a medium bowl. Mash with a fork until smooth. Add in cheese, lemon juice, garlic powder, onion powder and pepper. Stir well to combine.

Add heaped teaspoons of batter to the prepared baking trays, spacing each one about 7cm apart.

Press into thin rounds using a spatula or the back of a spoon.

Bake chips for 15 minutes or until the cheese is golden brown. Gently flip the chips with a spatula. Cook for an additional 2-3 minutes on the other side.

Transfer to a wire rack to cool. Chips will crisp up further as they cool.

Let chips cool completely before eating.

RICOTTA PANCAKES

4 large eggs
1 cup (250g) ricotta cheese
¼ cup (60ml) milk
1 tbsp vanilla extract
½ tsp stevia glycerite
6 tbsps coconut flour
½ tsp bicarbonate of soda
¼ cup (40g) dried blueberries
Butter for frying
1 cup (250ml) sour cream to serve

In a large bowl, whisk together the eggs, ricotta, milk, vanilla extract and stevia.

Add the coconut flour and bicarb and whisk to combine. Stir in the dried blueberries.

Heat 1 tablespoon butter in a large nonstick frying pan over medium-low heat.

Scoop 2 tablespoonfuls of batter at a time into mounds in the pan. Gently flatten the tops with a spatula.

Cook the pancakes for 3-4 minutes until the bottoms are golden brown and set.

Carefully flip the pancakes and cook for 2-3 more minutes until golden and set. Transfer to a plate and keep warm.

Repeat with the remaining batter, adding more butter between each batch if needed.

Serve the pancakes with a dollop of sour cream.

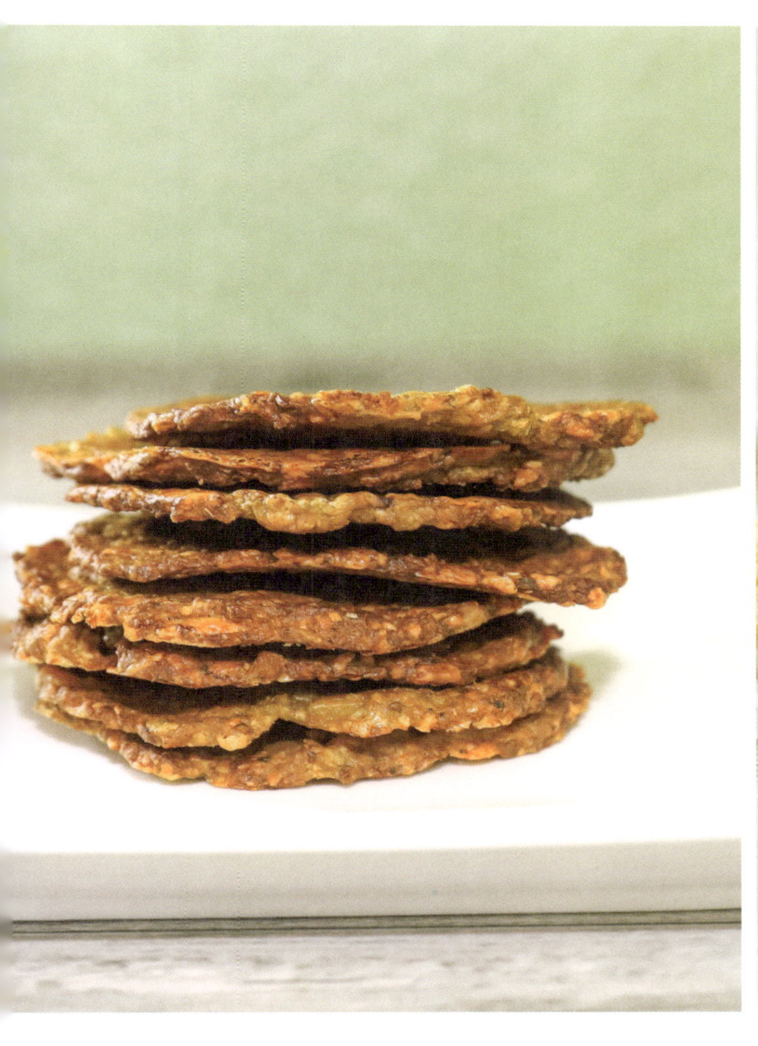

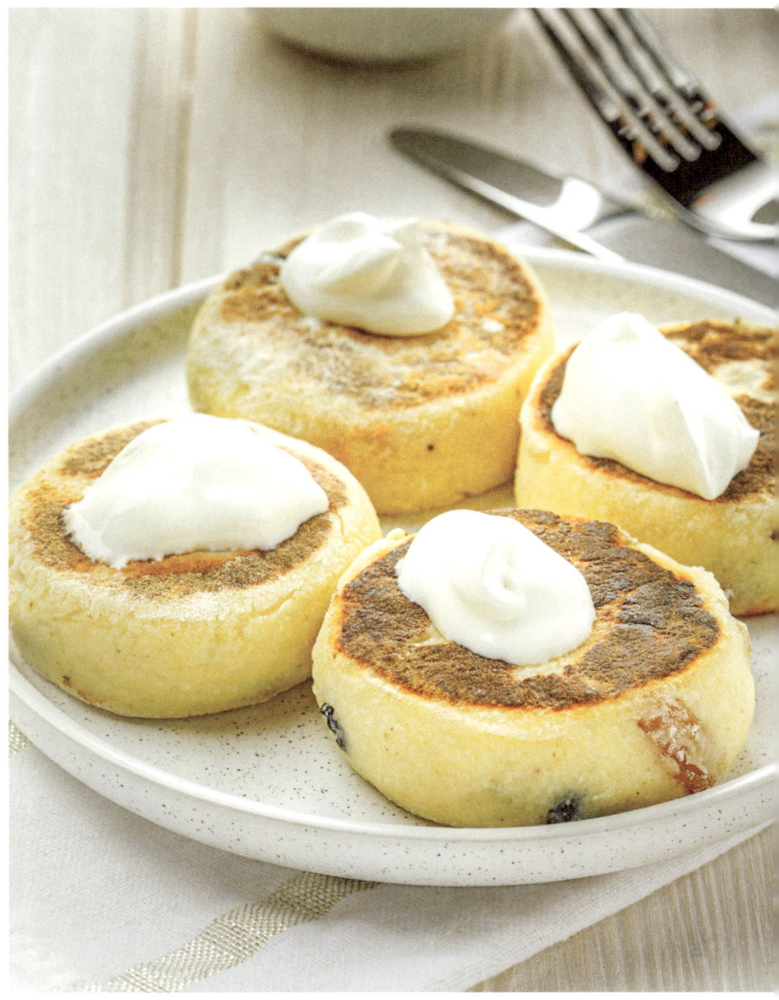

Baked Avocado Chips

MAKES 24

PREP + COOK TIME: 35 MINS

VEG • GLUTEN FREE

Ricotta Pancakes

SERVES 4

PREP + COOK TIME: 30 MINS

VEG • GLUTEN FREE

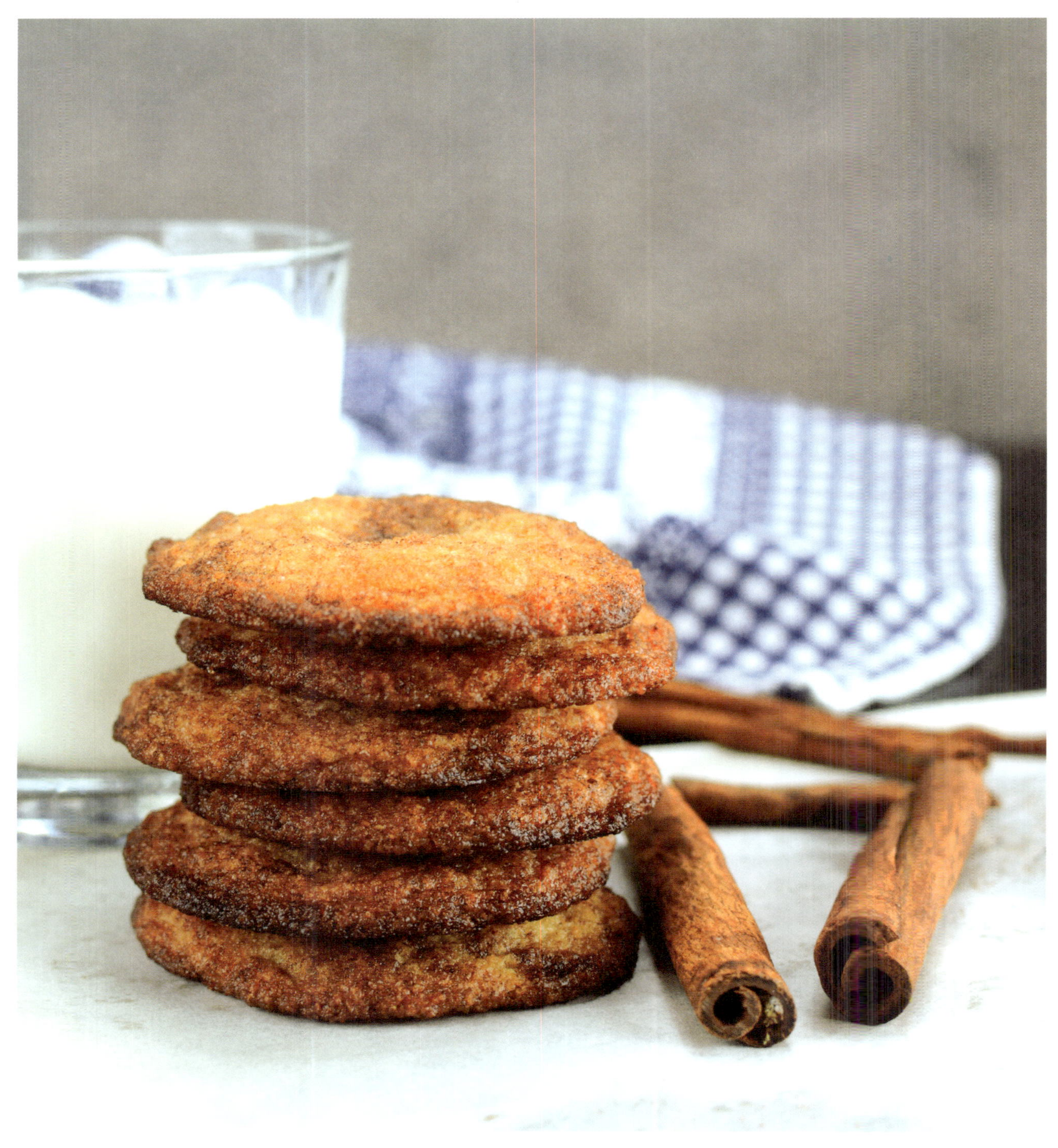

Snickerdoodle Cookies

MAKES 24

PREP + COOK TIME: 30 MINS

VEG • GLUTEN FREE

SNICKERDOODLE COOKIES

1¼ cups (150g) almond meal
2 tbsps coconut flour
½ tsp xanthan gum
½ tsp bicarbonate of soda
½ tsp cream of tartar
Pinch of salt
125g butter at room temperature
⅓ cup (60g) to ¾ cup (150g) erythritol or xylitol, to taste
1½ tsps vanilla extract
1 egg

CINNAMON SUGAR

2-3 tbsps erythritol or xylitol
2 tsps cinnamon

Preheat oven to 190°C and line a baking tray with greaseproof paper.

Add almond meal, coconut flour, xanthan gum, bicarb, cream of tartar and salt to a medium bowl. Stir to combine and set aside.

Cream butter in a large bowl with an electric mixer until soft. Add in sweetener to taste and continue to cream for 6-8 minutes until light and fluffy. Add vanilla extract and egg, mixing until just incorporated. With your mixer on low, add in the flour mixture until combined.

To make the cinnamon sugar, combine the sweetener and cinnamon in a shallow dish.

Using a tablespoon, scoop out small balls of the cookie mixture. Roll in cinnamon sugar then place on the baking tray and flatten slightly.

Transfer to oven and bake for 6-8 minutes, until golden brown. Allow to cool for 10 minutes before removing from the tray and serving.

Almond Butter Pumpkin Bread

MAKES 1 LOAF
PREP + COOK TIME: 1 HOUR, 15 MINS
VEG • GLUTEN FREE

- 1 cup (250g) smooth almond butter
- 2 large eggs
- ⅔ cup (120g) erythritol
- ⅔ cup (150g) mashed cooked pumpkin
- 1 tsp baking powder
- ½ tsp ground cinnamon
- ½ tsp ground nutmeg
- ⅛ tsp ground ginger
- ⅛ tsp ground cloves

ICING

- 125g cream cheese, softened
- 2 tbsps butter, softened
- ½ cup (80g) powdered erythritol
- 1 tsp vanilla extract
- 1 tbsp cream
- 1-2 tsps cinnamon

Preheat oven to 180°C. Line a 20cm loaf tin with greaseproof paper.

Add almond butter and eggs to a large mixing bowl. Whisk until smooth. Add erythritol and whisk to combine. Add pumpkin and baking powder, cinnamon, nutmeg, ginger and cloves and whisk to incorporate.

Pour batter into prepared loaf tin. Bake for 45-55 minutes or until golden brown and springy to touch and a toothpick inserted in the centre has only a few moist crumbs attached.

Allow to cool in the tin for 10 minutes then transfer to a wire rack to cool completely.

Meanwhile use an electric hand mixer to beat together the cream cheese and butter until light and fluffy. Add the sweetener, vanilla and cream and beat until smooth and creamy.

When the bread is completely cool, spread with the icing.

Dust with cinnamon, slice and serve.

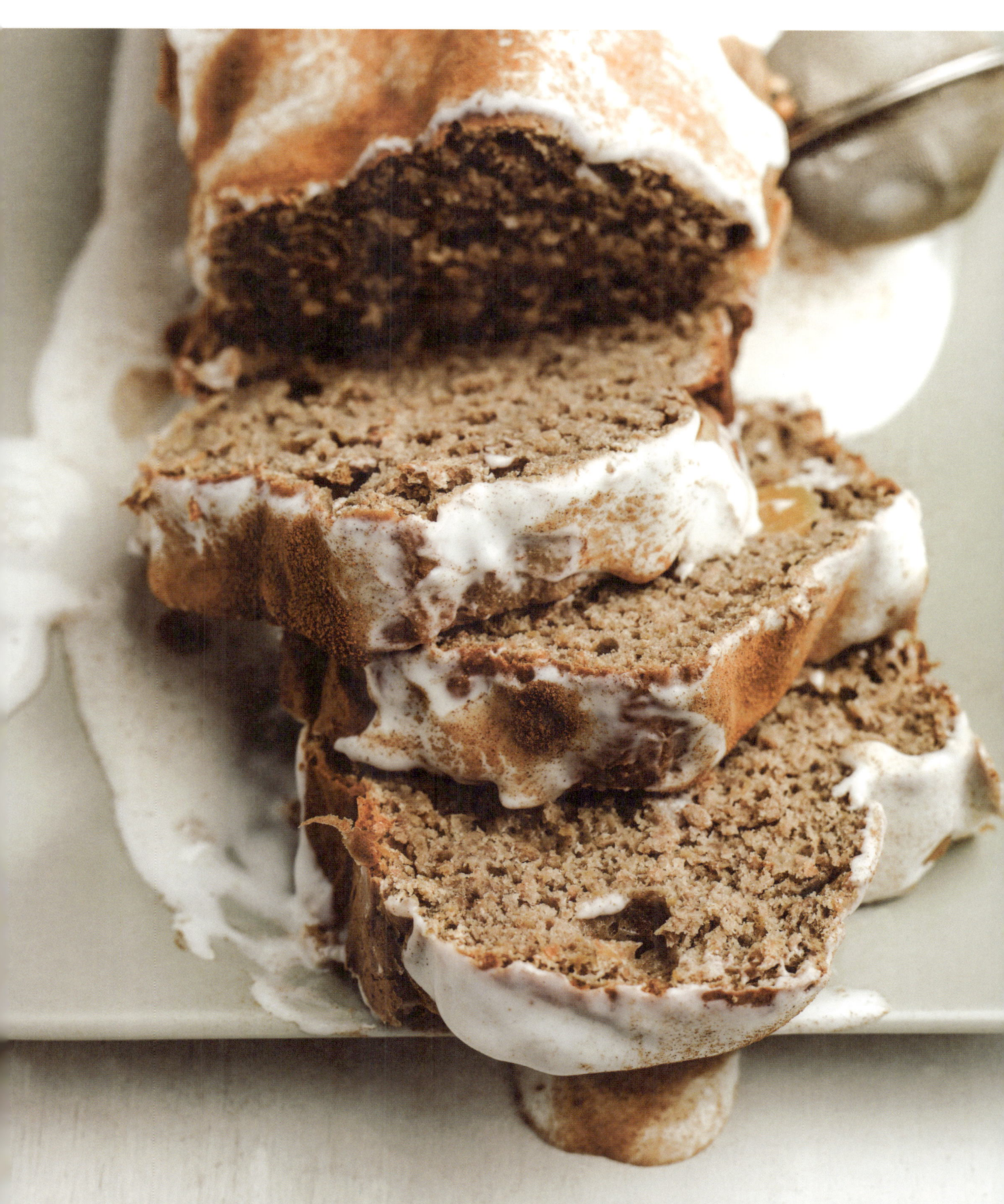

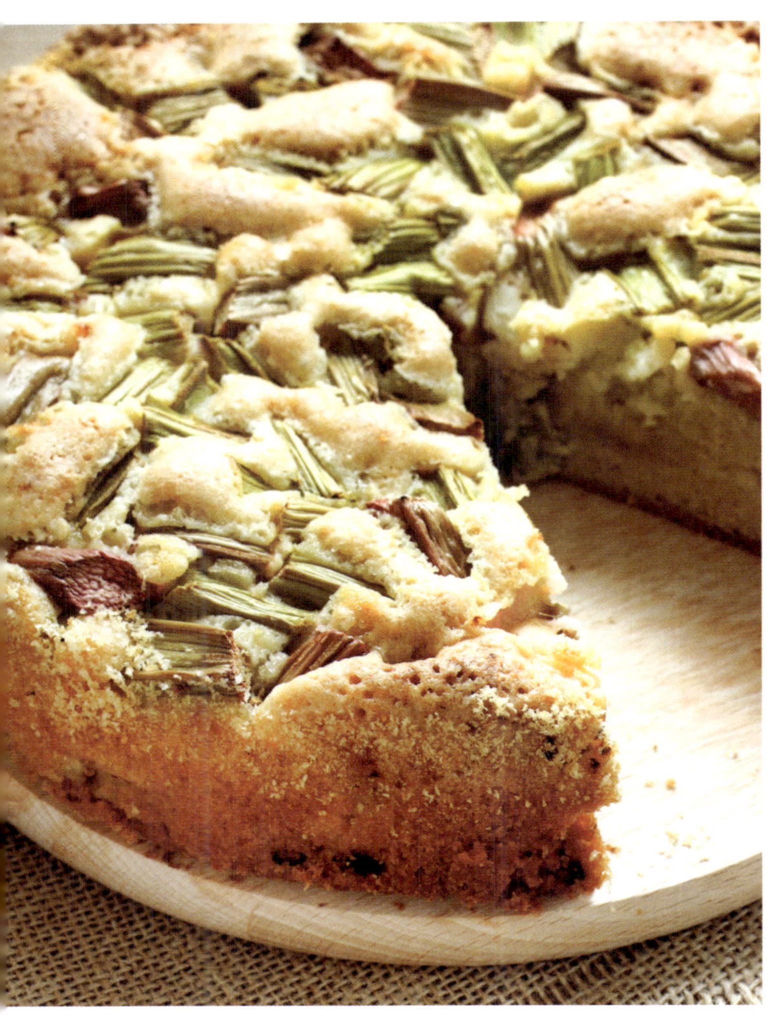

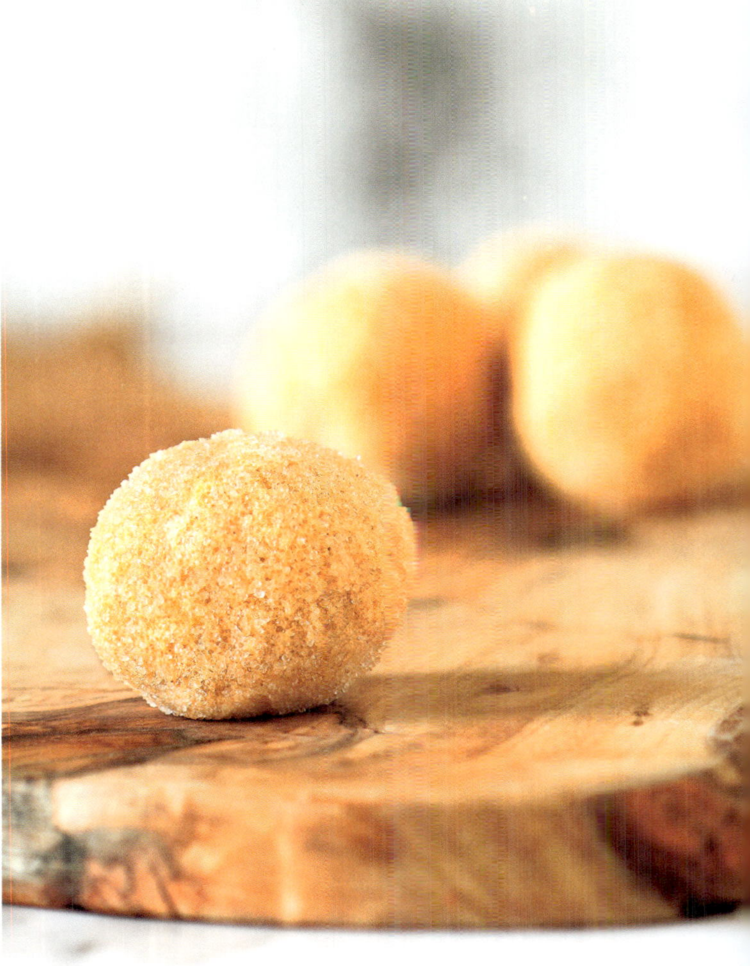

Rhubarb Cake

SERVES 8-10

PREP + COOK TIME: 1 HOUR

VEG • GLUTEN FREE • DAIRY FREE

Cream Cheese Fat Bombs

MAKES 24

PREP + COOK TIME: 20 MINS + CHILLING

VEG • GLUTEN FREE

RHUBARB CAKE

1¾ cups (150g) shredded coconut
½ cup (100g) granulated erythritol
½ cup (60g) almond meal
1 tsp baking powder
1 tsp bicarbonate of soda
3 large eggs
¾ cup (185ml) almond milk
¼ cup (60ml) melted coconut oil
2 cups (200g) roughly chopped rhubarb
½ cup (100g) strawberries, halved

Preheat oven to 170°C. Grease and line a 22cm springform tin.

Add coconut to a food processor and process until finely ground. Reserve about 2 tablespoons of the granulated sweetener for topping. Add all of the remaining dry ingredients to the coconut and pulse once or twice to combine. Add eggs, almond milk and coconut oil and process for a few seconds to mix.

Allow the mixture to sit for about 5 minutes then pour into the prepared tin. Scatter the chopped rhubarb evenly over the top, and then top with the reserved 2 tablespoons of sweetener.

Bake for 40-45 minutes until golden brown and the edges are starting to come away from the sides. A skewer inserted in the centre should come out mostly clean.

Store the cake in an airtight container in the fridge for up to a week.

CREAM CHEESE FAT BOMBS

250g cream cheese at room temperature
125g butter or coconut oil
½ cup (125ml) double cream
2-3 tbsps erythritol
2 tsps vanilla extract
3 tbsps granulated erythritol

Place the cream cheese, butter or coconut oil, cream, erythritol and vanilla in medium mixing bowl. Beat with an electric mixer for 1-2 minutes or until smooth and creamy.

Scoop batter using an ice-cream scoop into a mini cupcake tin. Place in the fridge to set for 1-2 hours or in the freezer for up to 30 minutes.

Place the granulated erythritol in a shallow dish.

Remove the batter from cupcake tin. Gently shape into balls if needed, then roll in the granulated erythritol.

Eat immediately or transfer to an air-tight container and refrigerate for up to 2 weeks.

Keto Chocolate Cookies

MAKES 9

PREP + COOK TIME: 20 MINS

VEG • GLUTEN FREE

½ cup (60g) almond meal
½ tsp baking powder
3 tbsps cocoa powder
4 tbsps granulated erythritol
1 egg
4 tbsps butter, softened
¼ cup (65g) almond butter
¼ cup (30g) sugar-free chocolate chips or chopped dark chocolate (minimum 85% cocoa solids)

Preheat the oven to 175°C. Line a baking tray with greaseproof paper.

Mix the almond meal, baking powder, cocoa powder and granulated erythritol in a bowl.

Add the egg, softened butter and almond butter and mix with a fork until you have a smooth dough.

Add half the chocolate chips and mix.

Form into nine cookies and place on prepared baking tray. Top with the remaining chocolate chips and press gently into the dough.

Bake for 12 minutes.

Allow to cool completely on the baking tray.

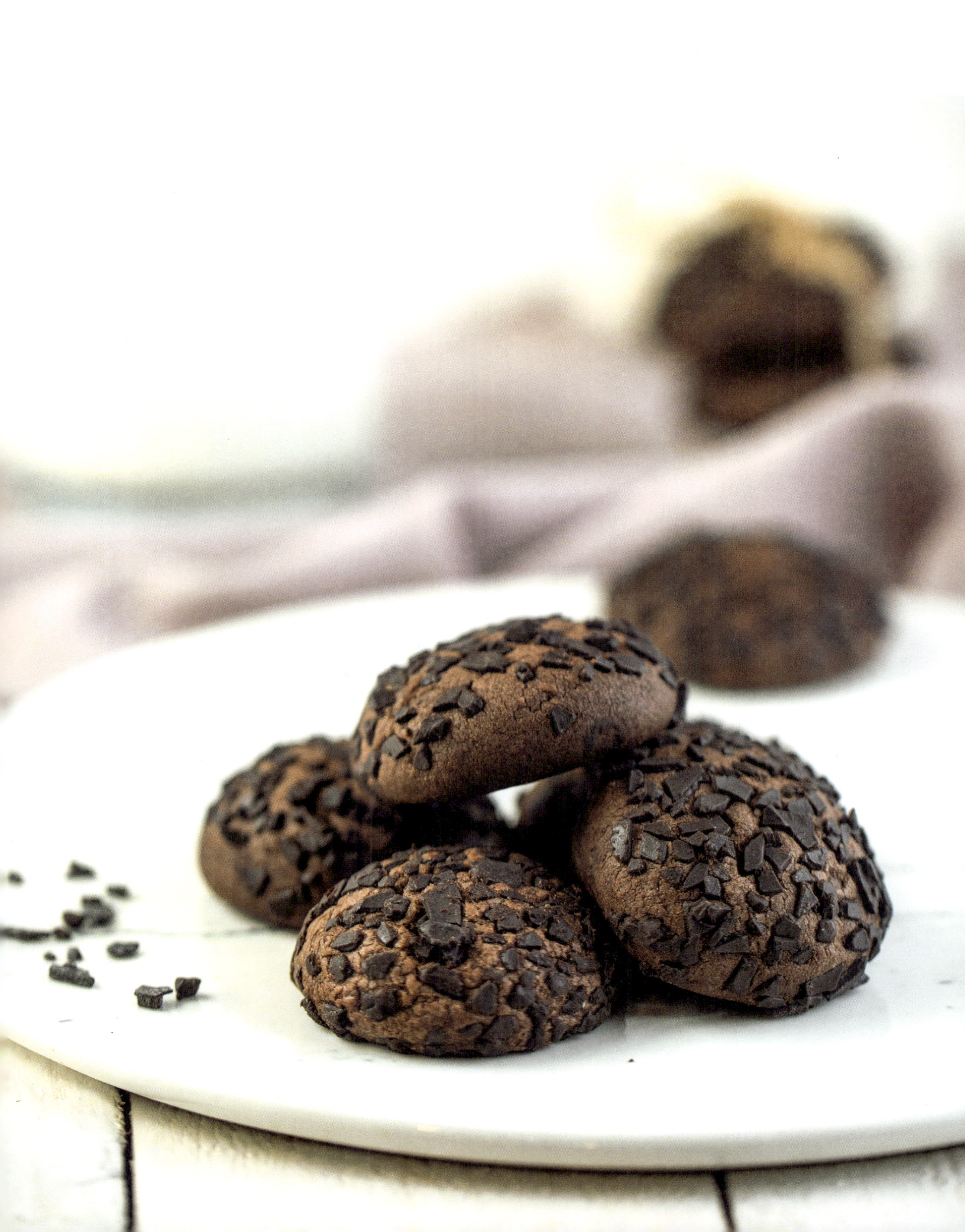

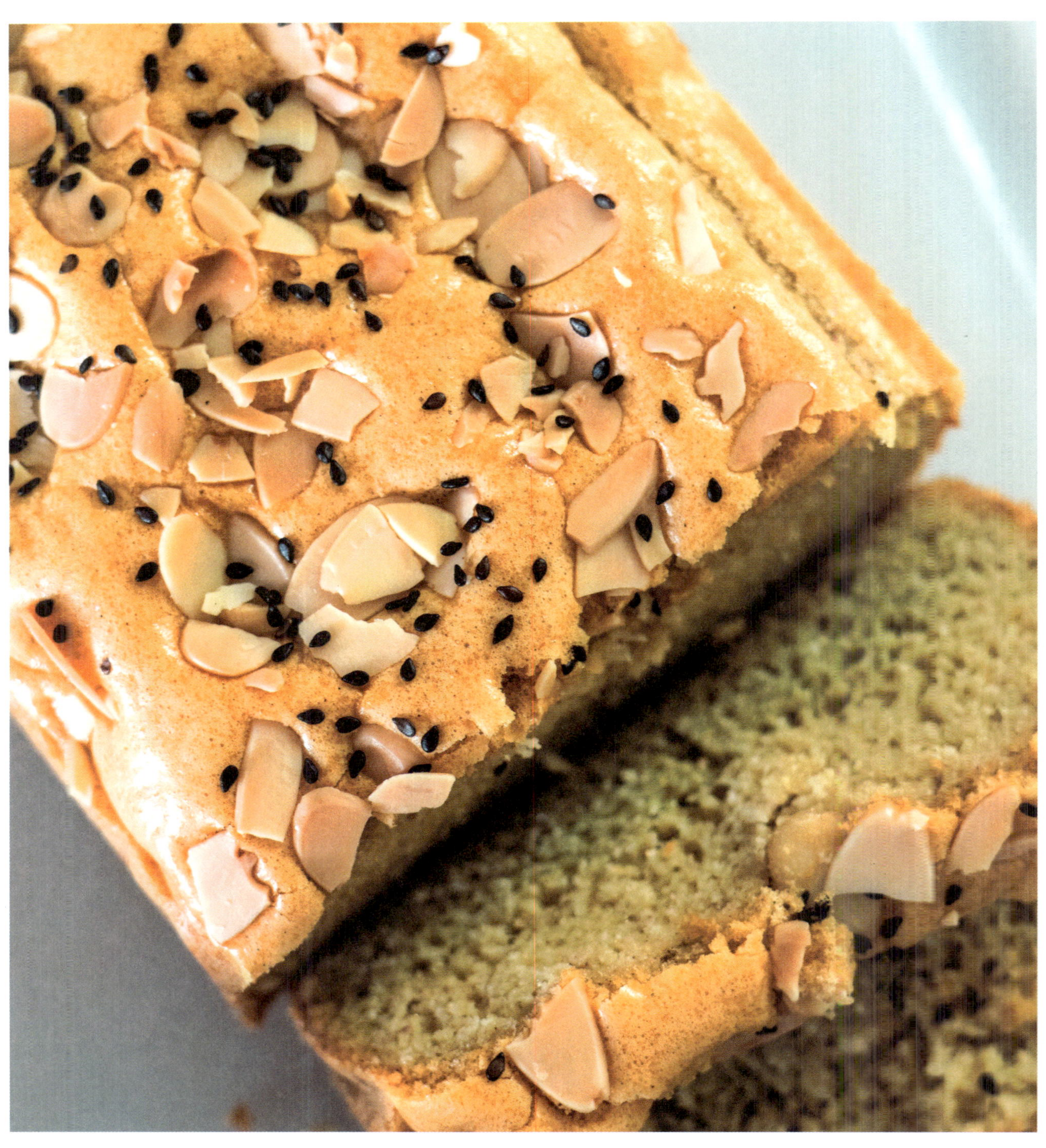

Low-Carb Bread

SERVES 6

PREP + COOK TIME: 55 MINS

VEG • GLUTEN FREE • DAIRY FREE

LOW-CARB BREAD

2 tbsps coconut oil
½ cup (125ml) olive oil
½ cup (50g) coconut flour
1½ cups (150g) almond flour
1 tsp baking powder
½ tsp xanthan gum
Pinch of salt
7 large eggs, room temperature
¼ cup (30g) flaked almonds
½ tbsp black sesame seeds

Preheat oven to 180°C and grease and line a 23 x 13cm loaf tin.

Gently heat the coconut oil to a liquid if needed and mix it together with the olive oil.

Sift together the flours, baking powder, xanthan gum and salt and set aside.

In a standing mixer bowl, whisk the eggs together for 1 minute until light and aerated. Drizzle the oil in while whisking to mix through thoroughly.

Change to a paddle attachment and stir in the flours, ½ cup at a time, until everything is fully incorporated.

Pour the mix into the loaf tin and smooth the top. Scatter the almonds over the top and gently press into the loaf.

Bake for 40 minutes or until it starts to turn golden and a skewer inserted into the middle comes out clean. Let sit for 10 minutes before removing to a wire rack to cool. Sprinkle with the sesame seeds.

COCONUT BALLS

⅓ cup (50g) ground flaxseed

4 tbsps almond butter, peanut butter or tahini

2 scoops (60g) sugar-free chocolate protein powder

2 tbsps refined coconut oil

⅓ cup (30g) shredded coconut + more to coat the balls

2-3 tbsps cacao nibs

Place flaxseed and nut butter or tahini in a food processor or high-powered blender. Blend until combined.

Next add protein powder, coconut oil and shredded coconut. Blend until a smooth batter is formed. Scrape down the sides as needed.

Transfer batter into a large mixing bowl and stir in cacao nibs. Roll the batter into one large ball, cover with plastic wrap and place in the fridge to firm up for about 20 minutes.

Remove batter from fridge and then roll the dough into walnut-sized balls.

Place the additional shredded coconut in a shallow dish.

Roll each ball in the shredded coconut, pressing gently to coat.

Eat immediately or store in an airtight container in the freezer.

BLUEBERRY MUFFINS

2½ cups (300g) finely ground almond meal

½ cup (80g) erythritol or low-carb sweetener of choice

1½ tsps baking powder

¼ tsp salt

85g butter, melted

⅓ cup (80ml) unsweetened almond milk, room temperature

3 large eggs, room temperature

½ tsp vanilla extract

¾ cup (75g) blueberries

Preheat the oven to 175°C. Line a 12-hole muffin tin with paper liners.

In a large bowl, stir together the almond meal, sweetener, baking powder and salt. Mix in the melted butter, almond milk, eggs and vanilla extract. Fold in the blueberries.

Divide the batter evenly between the muffin cups.

Bake for 20-25 minutes, until the tops are golden and an inserted toothpick comes out clean.

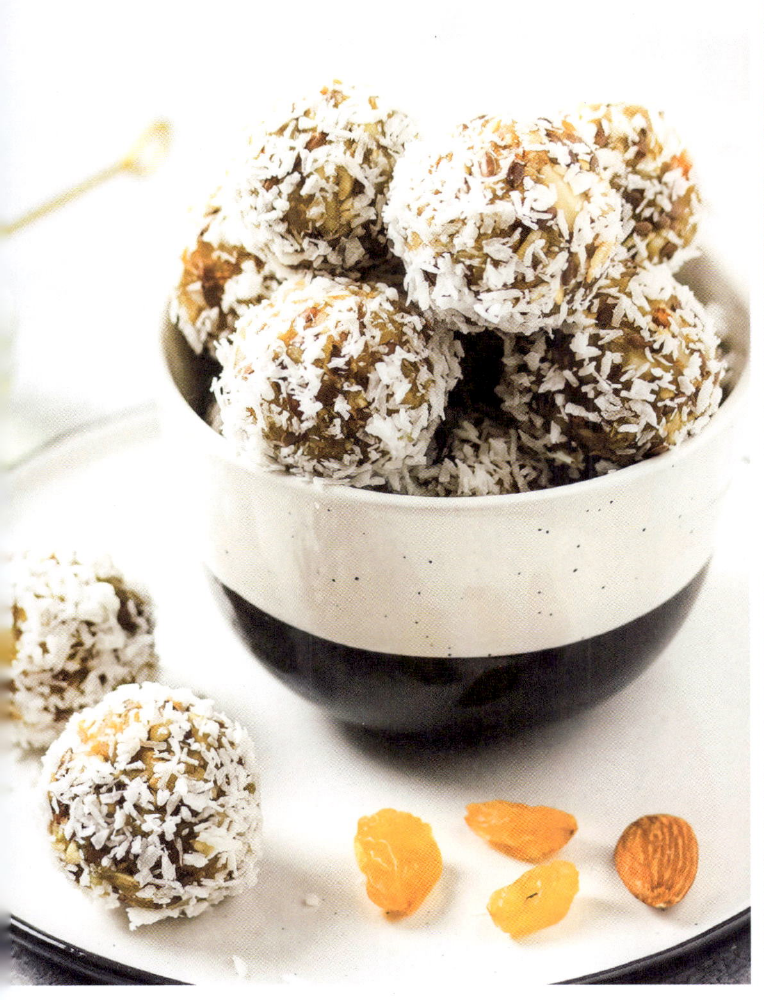

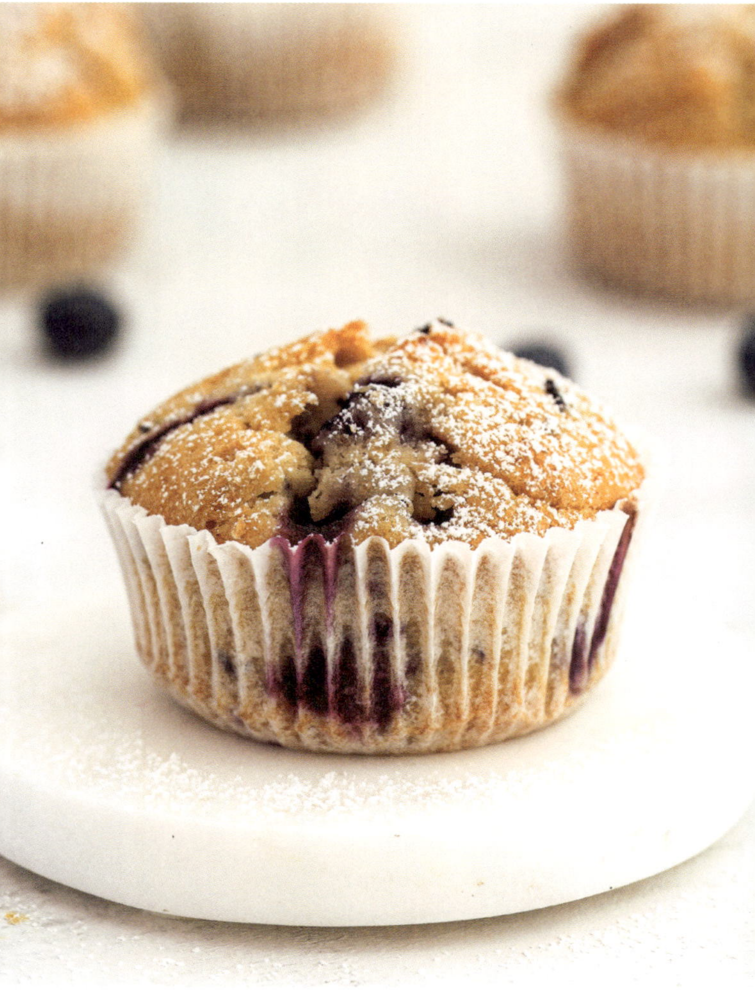

Coconut Balls

MAKES 8

PREP + COOK TIME: 15 MINS + CHILLING

VEG • GLUTEN FREE

Blueberry Muffins

MAKES 12

PREP + COOK TIME: 30 MINS

VEG • GLUTEN FREE

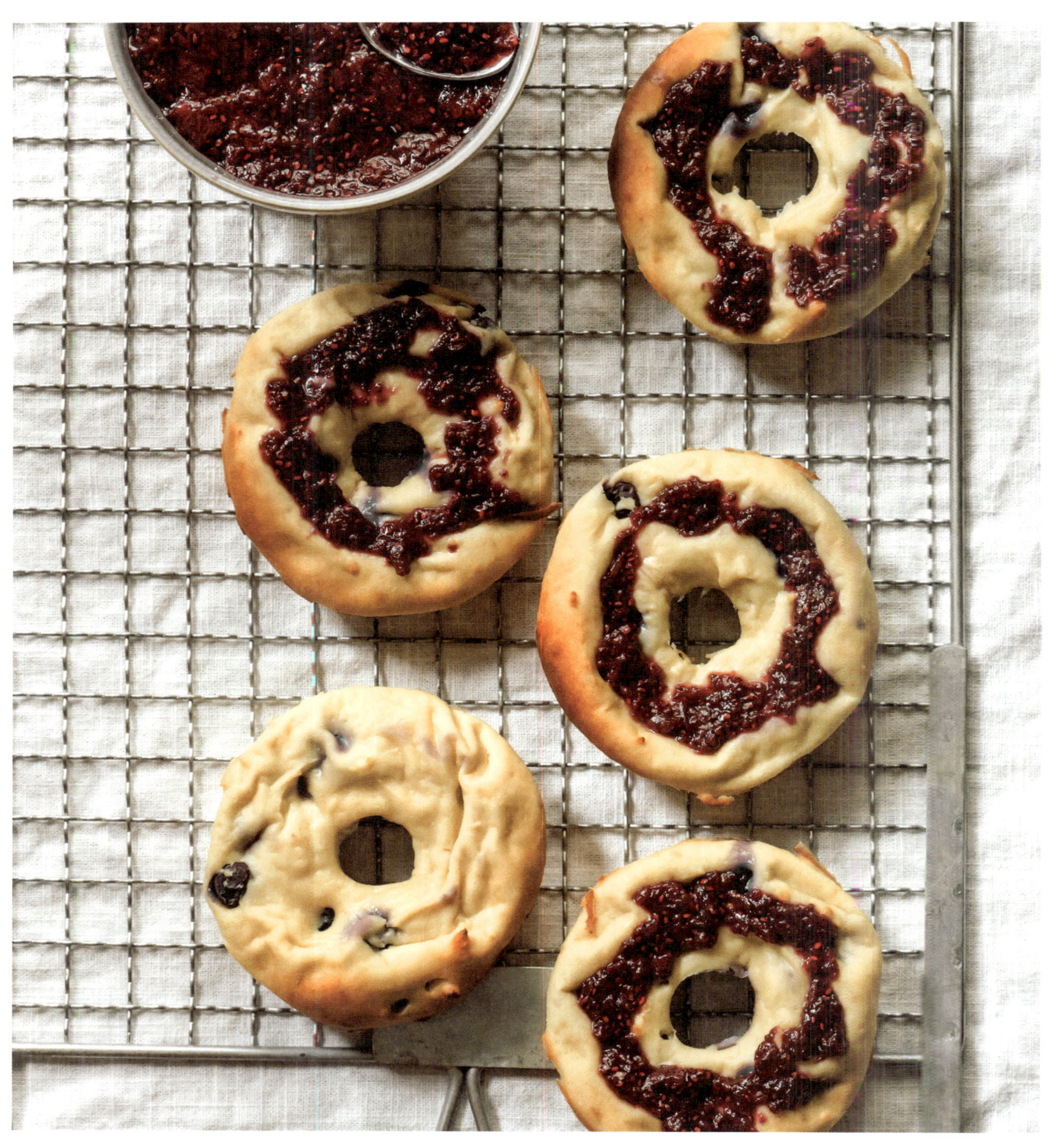

Mascarpone Doughnuts with Raspberry Jam

MAKES 12

PREP + COOK TIME: 40 MINS

VEG • GLUTEN FREE

MASCARPONE DOUGHNUTS WITH RASPBERRY JAM

FRUIT JAM

2 cups (250g) mixed berries, fresh or frozen

2 tbsps chia seeds

1 tbsp lemon juice

¼ tsp stevia (optional)

SOUR CREAM DOUGHNUTS

1½ cups (150g) almond flour

½ cup (50g) coconut flour

2 tsps baking powder

¼ tsp salt

⅓ cup (60g) low-carb powdered sweetener

¾ cup (185ml) mascarpone cheese

3 eggs

60g unsalted butter, melted and cooled

1 tsp vanilla extract

1 cup (100g) fresh blueberries

Place the fruit in a small saucepan over a medium heat. Bring it to the boil, then reduce to a simmer. Stir until berries have reached a desirable consistency. Add the chia seeds, lemon juice and stevia, if using, and stir. Simmer for a further 5 minutes. Remove the jam from the heat and allow to cool. Transfer to a glass jar and store in the fridge until needed.

Preheat the oven to 180°C. Grease two six-hole doughnut pans.

Place the almond flour, coconut flour, baking powder, salt, sweetener, mascarpone, eggs, melted butter and vanilla extract into the mixing bowl of a food processor. Beat on high until a smooth batter is formed.

Gently stir through the fresh berries.

Fill the cavities of a doughnut baking pan almost to the top (they won't rise much), and transfer to the oven. Bake for 15-20 minutes until browned and cooked through.

Allow the doughnuts to cool completely before serving with jam.

Tip:

Look out for keto-friendly low-sugar jams at your local health-food store or supermarket, and skip the jam-making part of this recipe.

Raspberry Chia Smoothie Pot

SERVES 4

PREP + COOK TIME: 15 MINS + CHILLING

VEG • GLUTEN FREE • DAIRY FREE

COCONUT PUDDING

2 tbsps chia seeds

¾ cup (185ml) coconut milk

2 tsps powdered erythritol (optional)

½ tsp vanilla extract

RASPBERRY SMOOTHIE

1 cup (125g) frozen raspberries

1 tbsp powdered erythritol (optional)

¾ cup (185ml) coconut milk

¼ cup (40g) chia seeds

¼ tsp vanilla extract

ADDITIONAL LAYERS

¾ cup (185ml) Greek yoghurt or coconut yoghurt for dairy free

2 tsps chia seeds

½ cup (60g) frozen raspberries

Place all the ingredients for the coconut pudding in a medium bowl. Whisk to combine. Cover and place in the fridge overnight.

For the raspberry smoothie add the raspberries and erythritol (if using) to a food processor or high-speed blender and pulse into a puree. Add the coconut milk and the chia seeds and pulse just enough to combine.

Pour into a medium bowl, cover and place in the fridge overnight.

To serve, spoon a layer of the coconut pudding into the base of each serving bowl or glass, next add a layer of raspberry smoothie, then a layer of yoghurt and finish with another layer of raspberry smoothie.

Sprinkle with chia seeds and scatter with raspberries to serve.

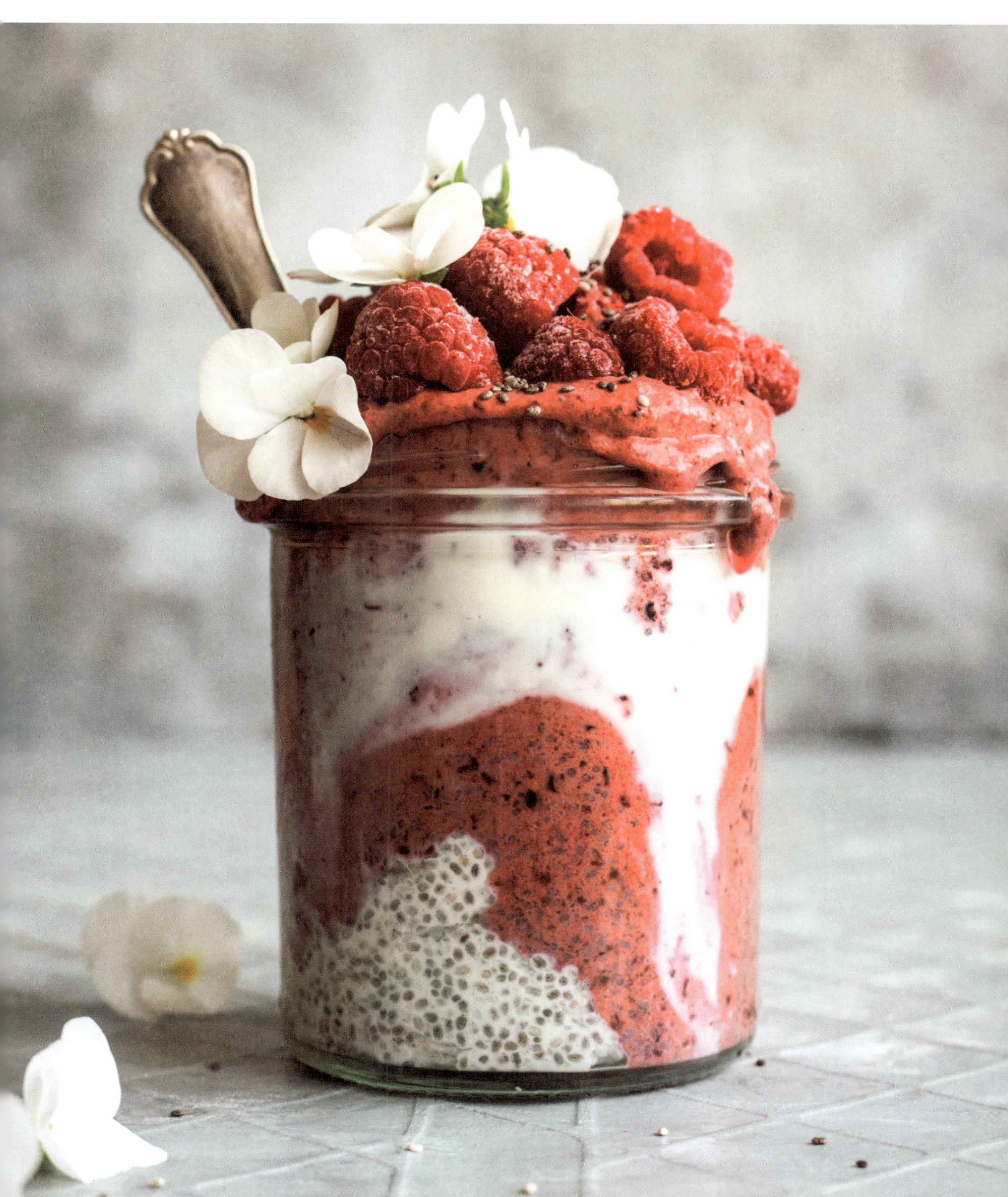

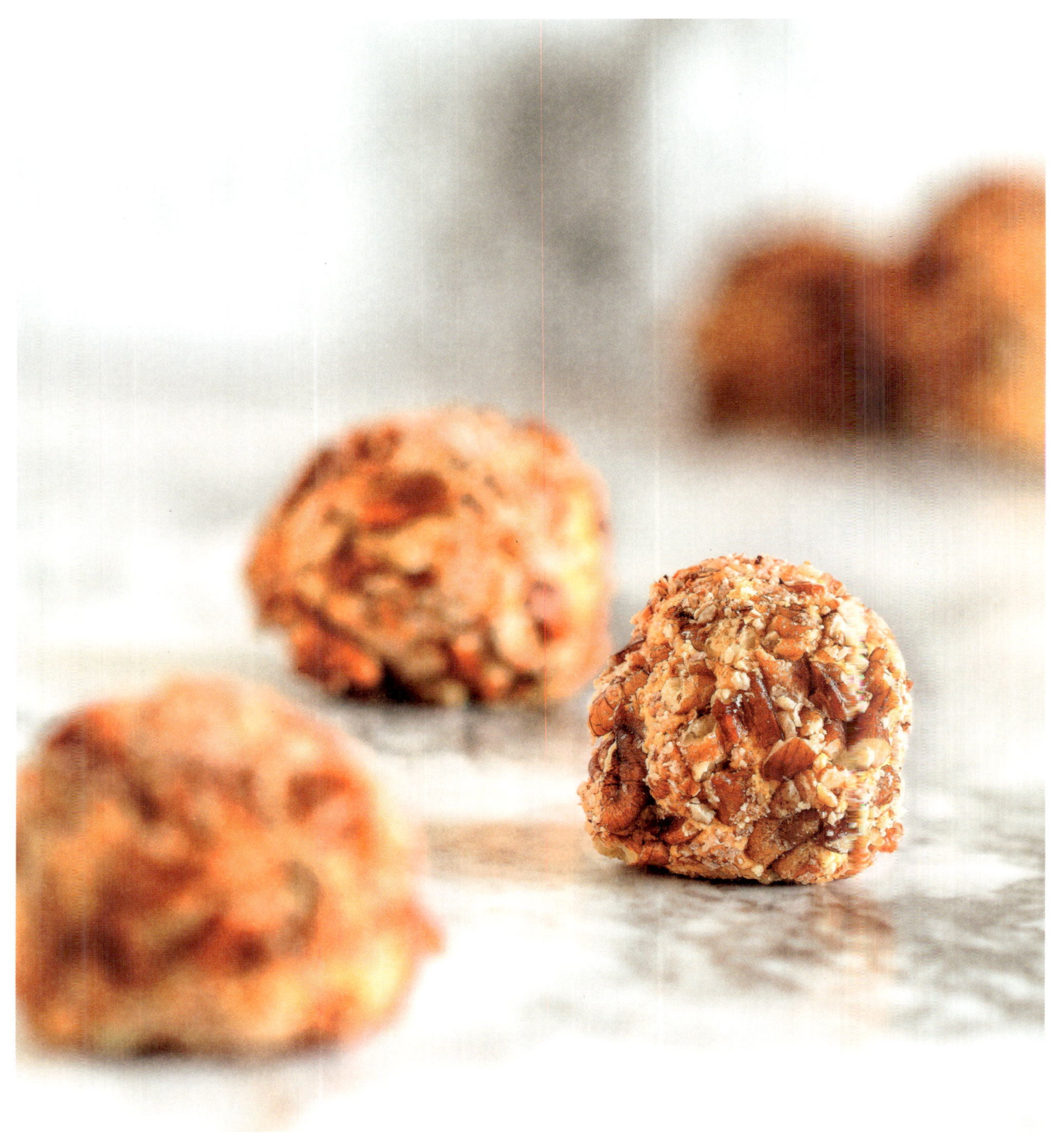

Pumpkin & Pecan Fat Bombs

MAKES 10

PREP + COOK TIME: 10 MINS + CHILLING

VEG • GLUTEN FREE

PUMPKIN & PECAN FAT BOMBS

4 tbsps almond meal
3 tbsps (45g) melted butter or coconut oil
2 tbsps (30g) cooked and mashed pumpkin
1½ tbsps erythritol
1 tbsp coconut flour
½ tsp vanilla powder
¼ tsp cinnamon
⅛ tsp ground ginger
½ cup (60g) pecans, chopped

Place the almond meal, butter or oil, pumpkin, erythritol, coconut flour, vanilla, cinnamon and ginger in a large bowl.

Stir until well combined.

Place in freezer to chill for 10-15 minutes.

Remove the bowl from the freezer and use your hands to form the mixture into walnut-sized balls.

Spread the pecans on a large plate. Roll the finished balls in the pecans.

Chill the finished fat bombs in the fridge for at least 30 minutes, then serve.

Cinnamon Cheesecake Slice

MAKES 14

PREP + COOK TIME: 1 HOUR 20 MINS

VEG • GLUTEN FREE

BASE

60g cream cheese

⅓ cup (30g) almond flour

⅓ cup (30g) coconut flour

1 tsp baking powder

½ tsp salt

½ tsp xanthan gum

½ tsp ground cinnamon

2 tbsps granulated erythritol

1 tsp vanilla extract

1¾ cups (225g) shredded mozzarella cheese

1 egg

CHEESECAKE FILLING

450g cream cheese

2 eggs

½ cup (95g) granulated erythritol

1 tsp vanilla extract

LEMON CINNAMON TOPPING

2 tbsps butter, melted

2 tsps lemon juice

2 tbsps granulated erythritol

1 tbsp cinnamon

Preheat the oven to 180°C. Grease and line a square baking dish with greaseproof paper.

Soften the cream cheese by heating it in the microwave in 30-second increments until just melted. Pour into the bowl of a food processor and add the remaining ingredients for the base. Process until a smooth and uniform dough forms. Divide dough into two equal portions and set aside while you make the filling.

Add the filling ingredients to the food processor and process until smooth.

Roll the dough into two squares just larger than the size of your baking dish. Press one portion into the prepared baking dish. Pour the cheesecake batter over the dough base and use a spatula to create a smooth even surface. Gently place the other portion of dough over the top of the filling.

Whisk together the melted butter and lemon juice.

Sprinkle the top of the slice with sweetener and cinnamon, and drizzle over the melted lemon butter. Transfer to the oven to bake for 50-60 minutes until golden brown.

Tip:

If the top browns too much cover with foil and continue cooking.

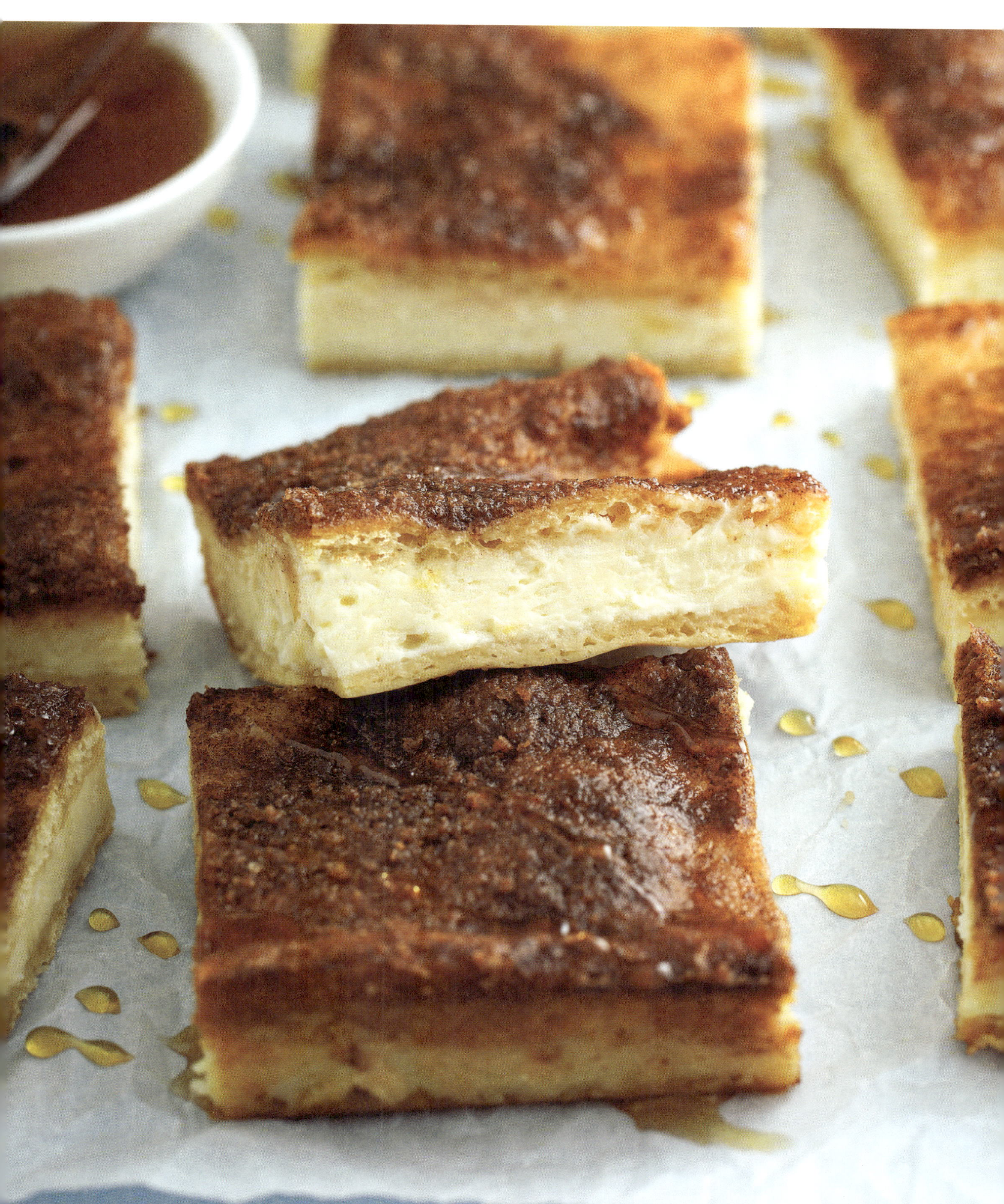

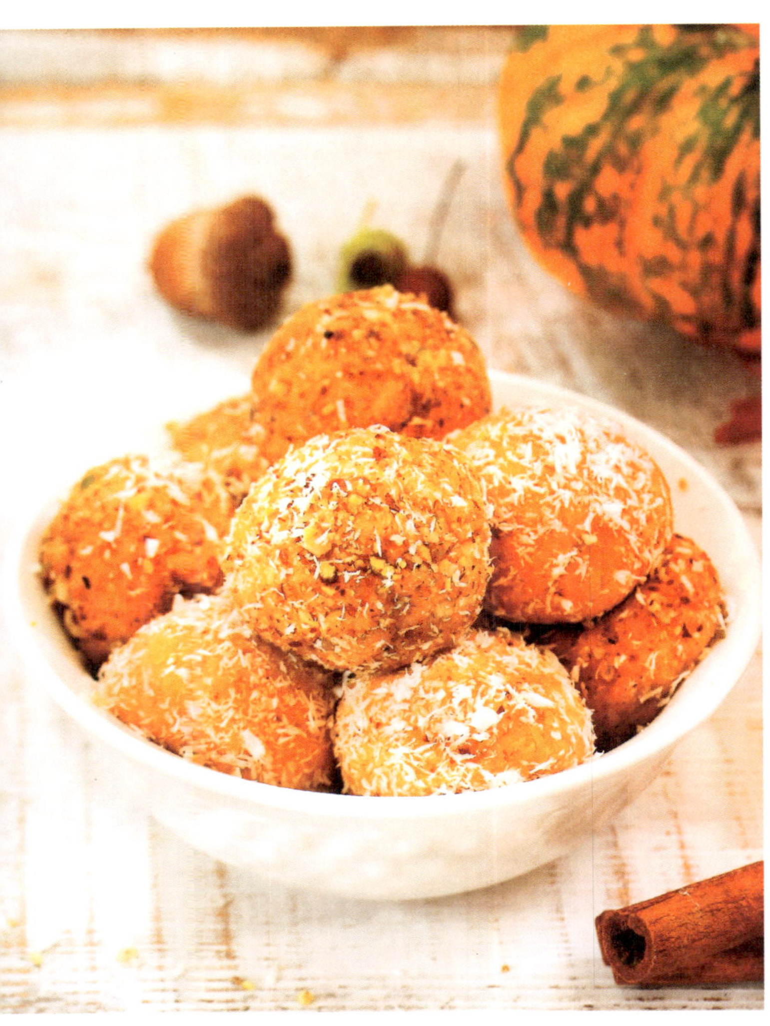

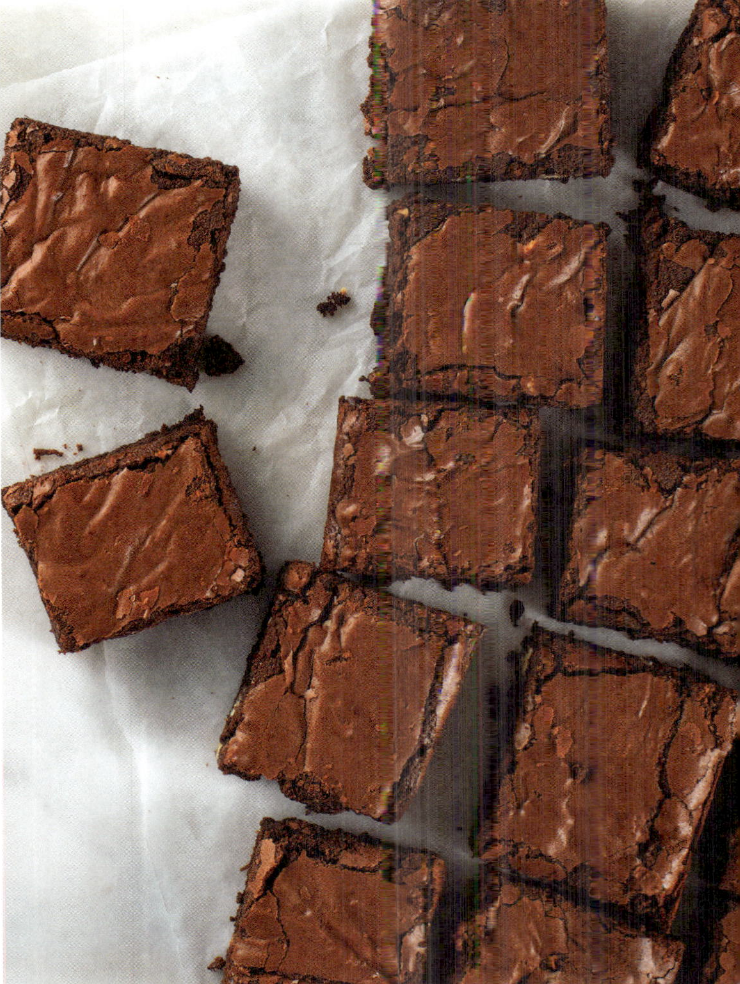

Pumpkin Pie Protein Balls

MAKES 10

PREP + COOK TIME: 20 MINS + CHILLING

VEG • GLUTEN FREE • DAIRY FREE

Chocolate Brownies

MAKES 16

PREP + COOK TIME: 45 MINS

VEG • GLUTEN FREE

PUMPKIN PIE PROTEIN BALLS

⅓ cup (85g) almond butter
¼ cup (50g) cooked and mashed pumpkin
2 tbsps erythritol
1 tbsp coconut flour
¼ tsp ground cinnamon
⅛ tsp ground ginger
⅛ tsp ground nutmeg
2 tbsps desiccated coconut
2 tbsps pistachios, chopped

Line a baking tray with greaseproof paper.

Place the almond butter, pumpkin, erythritol, coconut flour and spices into a bowl. Mix until well incorporated. Place bowl in the freezer for about 20 minutes so batter is firm but not frozen.

Place the coconut and pistachios on two shallow dishes.

Scoop 1 tablespoon of batter and roll between your hands to form a ball.

Roll ball in coconut and pistachios and place onto prepared baking tray. Place baking tray back into the freezer for 10 minutes until firm.

Once firm eat immediately or store in an airtight container in the freezer and allow to defrost for a few minutes before eating.

CHOCOLATE BROWNIES

⅔ cup (80g) almond meal
¼ cup (30g) cocoa powder
1 tsp baking powder
½ tsp guar gum
1 tsp instant coffee powder
½ tsp salt
100g unsweetened cooking chocolate, chopped
100g butter
3 eggs
½ cup (95g) granulated erythritol
½ tsp vanilla extract

Preheat oven to 180°C. Line a 20 x 20cm cake tin with greaseproof paper.

In a large bowl mix together almond meal, cocoa powder, baking powder, guar gum, coffee and salt.

Place chocolate and butter in a small heatproof bowl over a pan of simmering water. Heat for 3-5 minutes, stirring regularly, until chocolate and butter melt. Remove from heat and set aside.

In a large bowl whisk together eggs, erythritol and vanilla extract. Add the dry ingredients and mix well. Add melted butter and chocolate and stir to combine.

Pour into the prepared tin. Transfer to the oven. Bake for 25-30 minutes or until an inserted skewer comes out clean.

Avocado Lime Popsicles

SERVES 8

PREP TIME: 20 MINS + FREEZING

VEG • GLUTEN FREE • DAIRY FREE

3 medium ripe avocados, flesh roughly chopped

1 lime, to make 1 tbsp lime zest + 2 tbsps lime juice

½ tsp ground cardamom

2 cups (500ml) coconut milk

½ tsp stevia, more to taste

Place all the ingredients in a food processor and blend until smooth. Taste and adjust for sweetness.

Pour the mixture into eight large popsicle moulds or 12 small popsicle moulds and insert the popsicle sticks.

Freeze for at least 4 hours, preferably overnight.

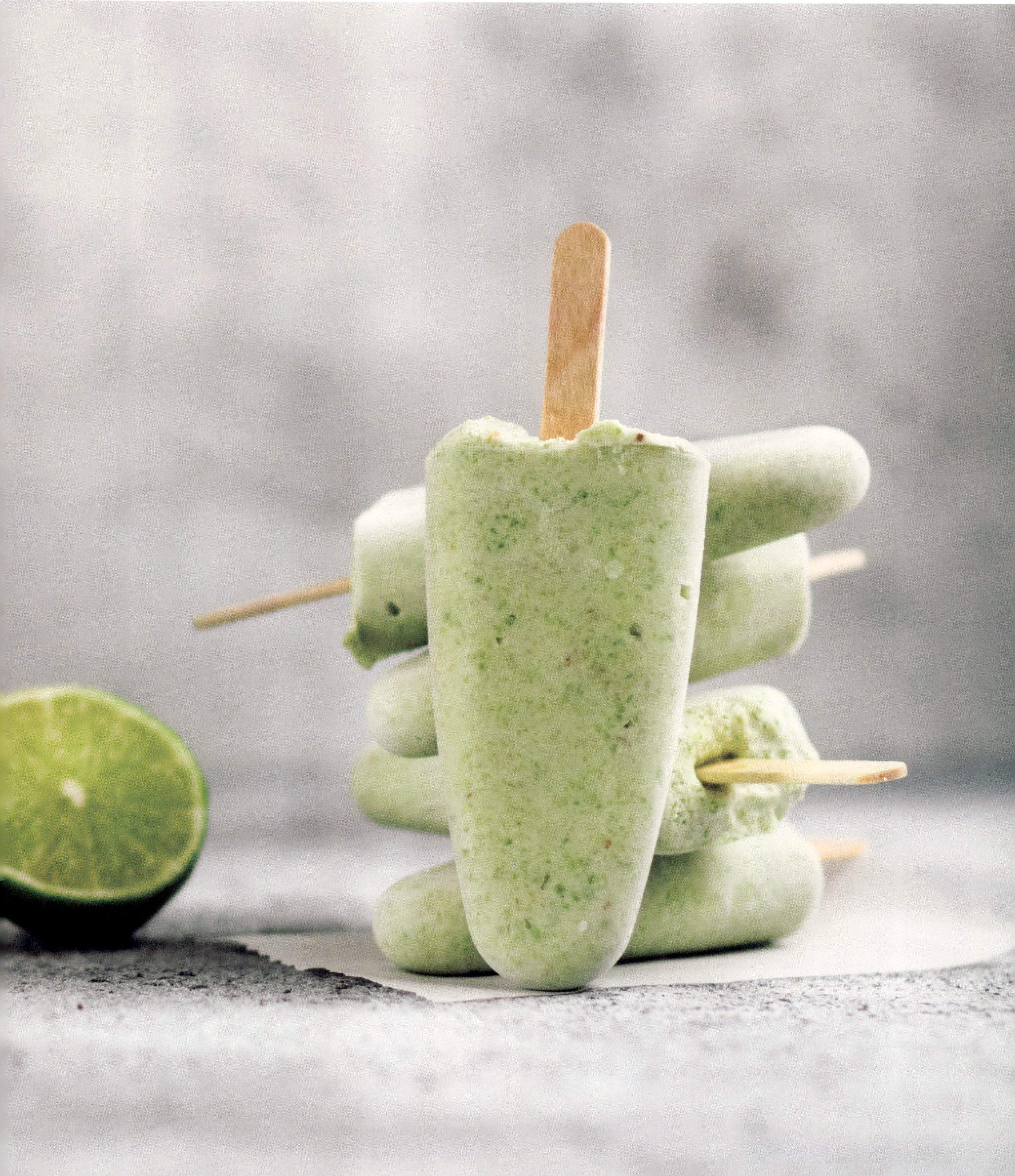

Chapter Three

Light Meals

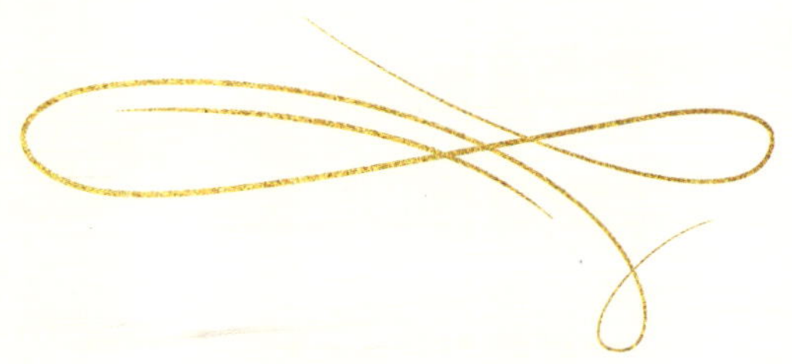

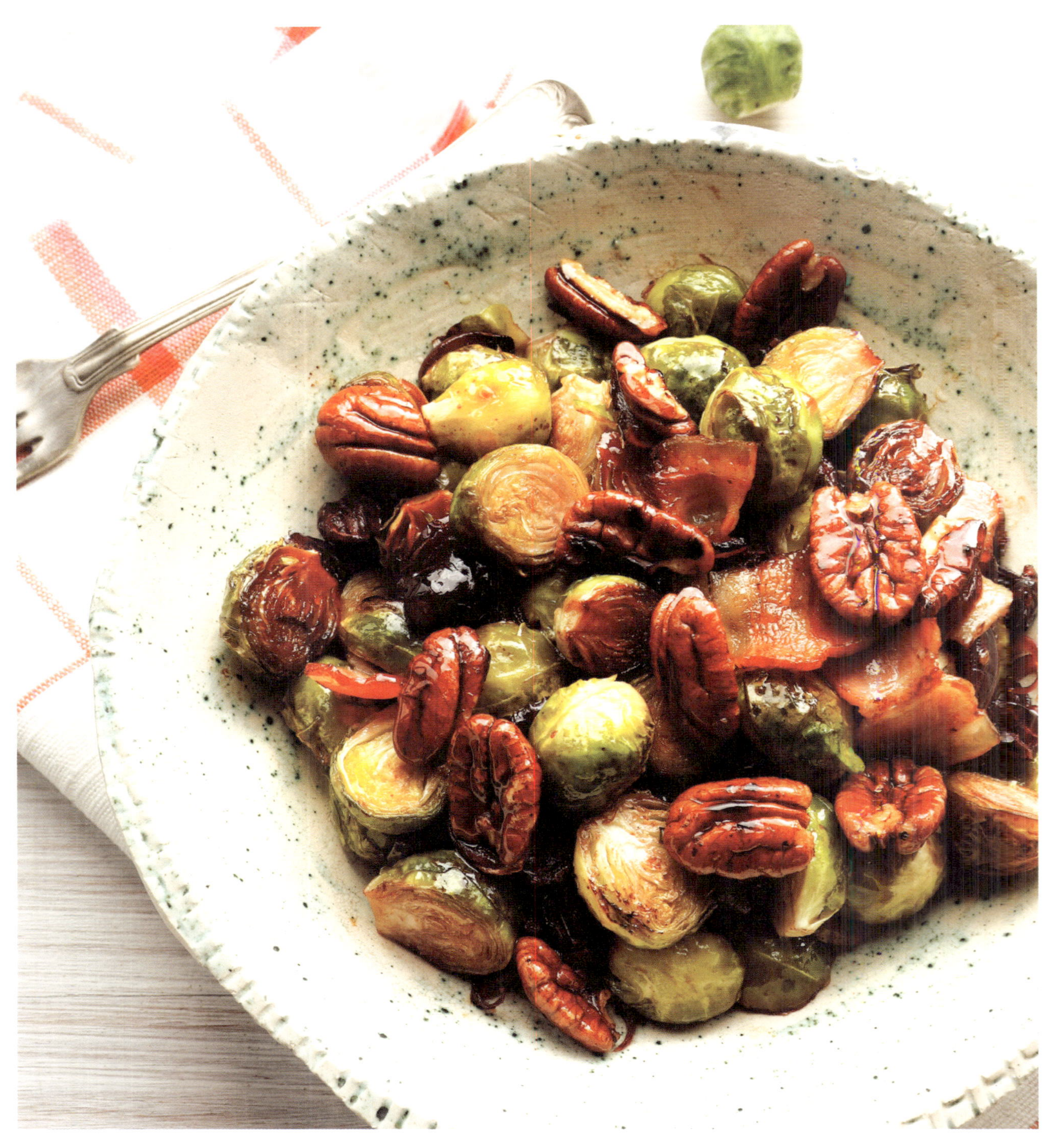

Brussels Sprout Salad

SERVES 4

PREP + COOK TIME: 1 HOUR

GLUTEN FREE • DAIRY FREE

BRUSSELS SPROUT SALAD

350g Brussels sprouts, trimmed and halved

2 tbsps olive oil

¼ tsp salt

4 rashers bacon

1 cup (125g) pecans

2 tbsps dried cranberries (optional, only add if following a targeted or cyclical ketogenic diet)

Preheat oven to 200°C. Line two baking trays with greaseproof paper.

In a medium bowl, combine Brussels sprouts, olive oil and salt. Toss to combine.

Place Brussels sprouts on one baking tray, cut-side down.

Arrange bacon on other tray.

Roast Brussels for 25 minutes, flipping over for last 10 minutes of roasting. They should be partially charred but not blackened.

Roast bacon for 20 minutes or until crisp. Remove from oven then cut into 3cm-wide strips.

Place pecans on the bacon baking tray. Reduce oven to 170°C. Bake for 5 minutes until darker in colour.

Place Brussels sprouts, bacon and pecans in a large bowl. Add the cranberries if using and toss together. Serve warm.

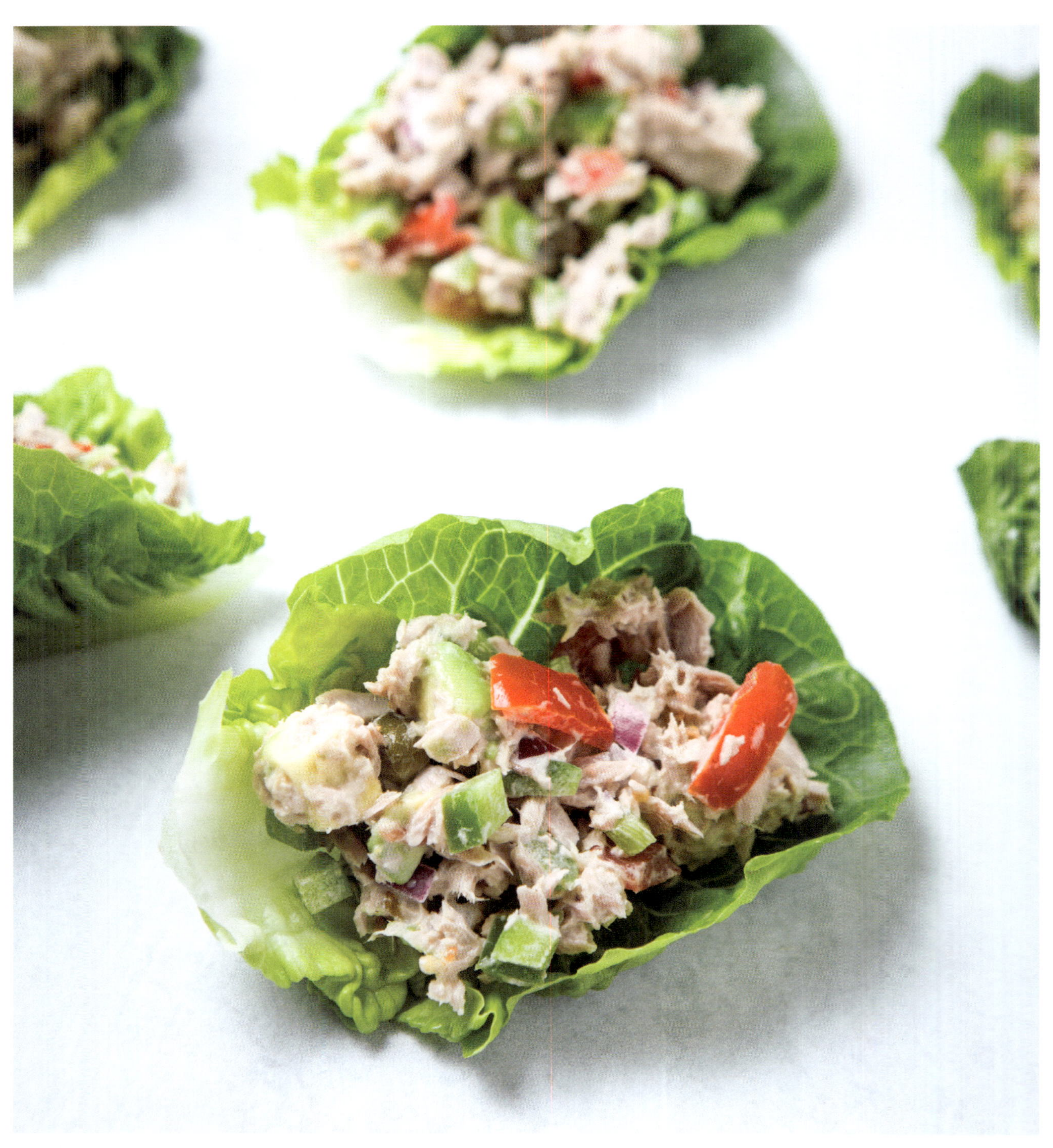

Tuna Lettuce Wraps

SERVES 4

PREP + COOK TIME: 10 MINS

GLUTEN FREE • DAIRY FREE

TUNA LETTUCE WRAPS

1 x 185g can tuna, drained
¼ red capsicum, diced
¼ green capsicum, diced
¼ red onion, diced
3-4 gherkins, sliced
½ avocado, diced
¼ cup (60g) mayonnaise
1 tbsp lemon juice
1 tbsp Dijon mustard
Salt and pepper to taste
1 head baby cos lettuce or butter lettuce, washed and cut into cups

Place the tuna in a large mixing bowl and break it up using the back of a fork.

Add the capsicums, onion, gherkins and avocado and mix to combine.

Add the mayonnaise, lemon juice and seasonings and stir gently to combine.

Spoon the mixture into lettuce leaf cups before serving.

Tip:

To make your own mayo see the recipe on page 22. If using a store-bought mayo, check the label carefully and avoid 'light' versions which often contain less fat and more sugar.

Satay Chicken Skewers

SERVES 4

PREP + COOK TIME: 15 MINS + MARINATING

GLUTEN FREE • DAIRY FREE

500g boneless, skinless chicken breasts, cut into 3cm-wide strips

Lime wedges to serve

MARINADE

2 tbsps tamari

2 tbsps coconut milk

2 tsps fish sauce

2 tbsps lime juice

1 tbsp Sriracha sauce

2 tsps ground ginger

2 tsps ground turmeric

1 tbsp monkfruit sweetener

2 cloves garlic, minced

PEANUT SAUCE

1 cup (250ml) chicken stock

5 tbsps smooth peanut butter

1 tbsp monkfruit sweetener

1 tbsp tamari

2 tsps fish sauce

2 tsps Sriracha sauce

1 tsp ground ginger

2 cloves garlic, minced

1 tbsp lime juice

In a large mixing bowl, whisk together all of the marinade ingredients. Add the chicken, toss to coat, then cover and place in the fridge to marinate for 2 hours or overnight. Let stand at room temperature for 30 minutes prior to grilling. If using wooden skewers, soak the skewers in water for 30 minutes prior to grilling.

Meanwhile, prepare the peanut sauce. In a medium saucepan, combine all the sauce ingredients except the lime juice. Bring to a simmer over medium heat, then cook, stirring often, for 5-6 minutes until the sauce is smooth and thick. Stir in the lime juice and set aside.

Preheat a grill pan or barbecue to medium-high heat. Thread the chicken onto skewers. Grill chicken for 2-3 minutes per side until cooked through.

Serve with lime wedges and peanut sauce.

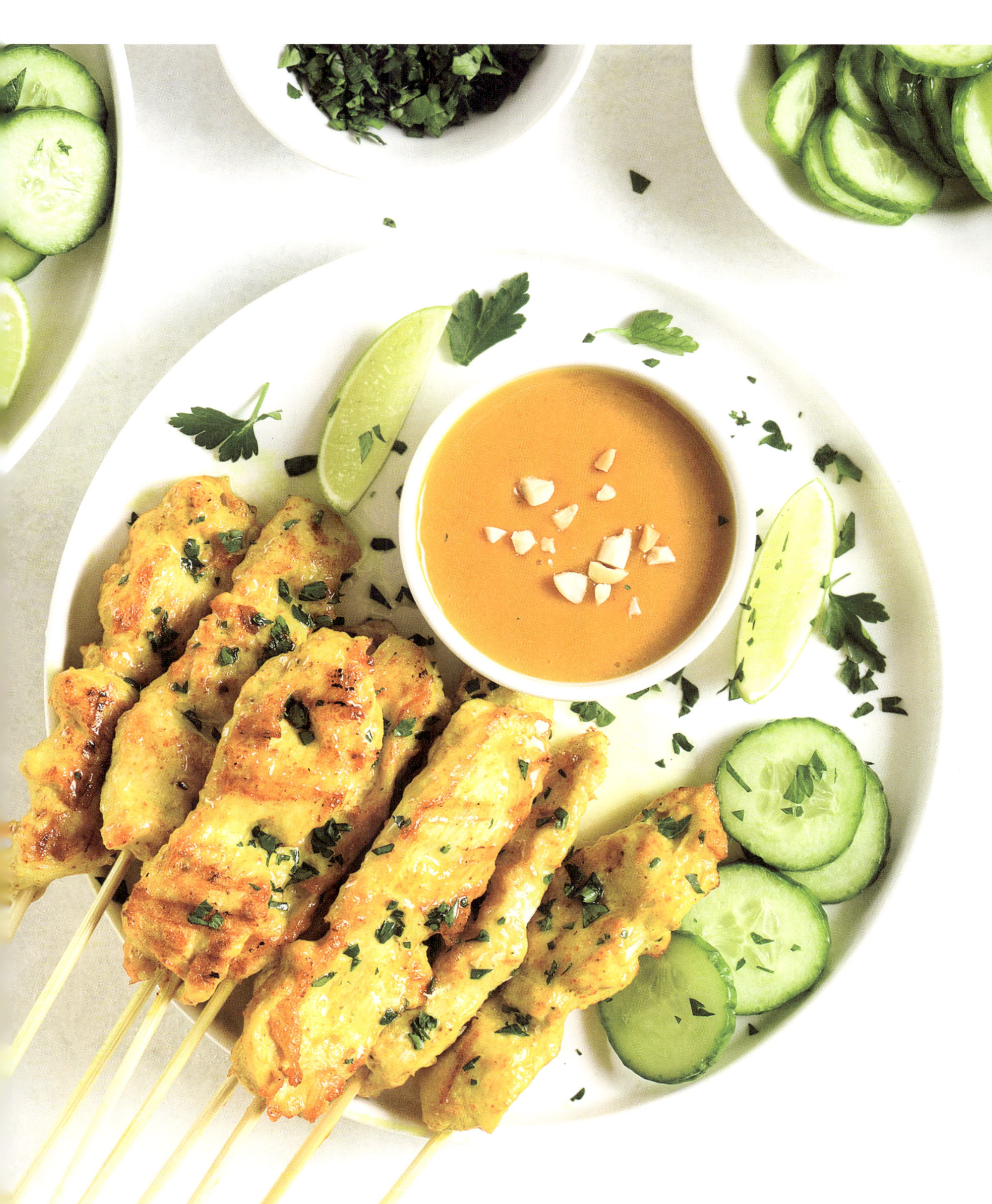

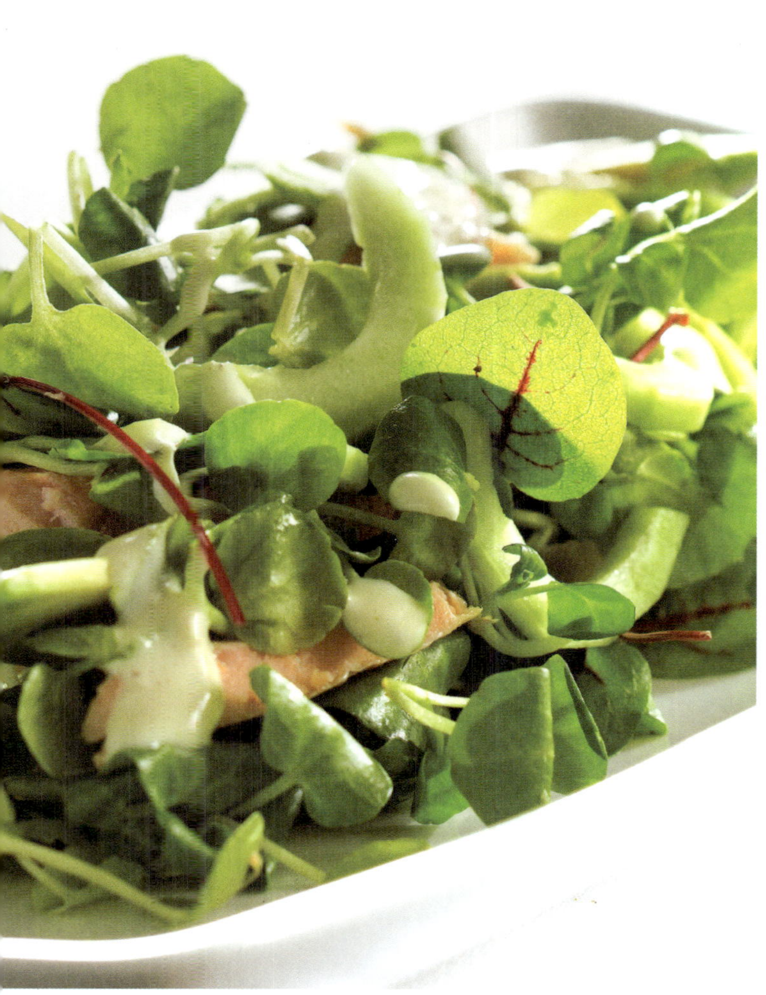

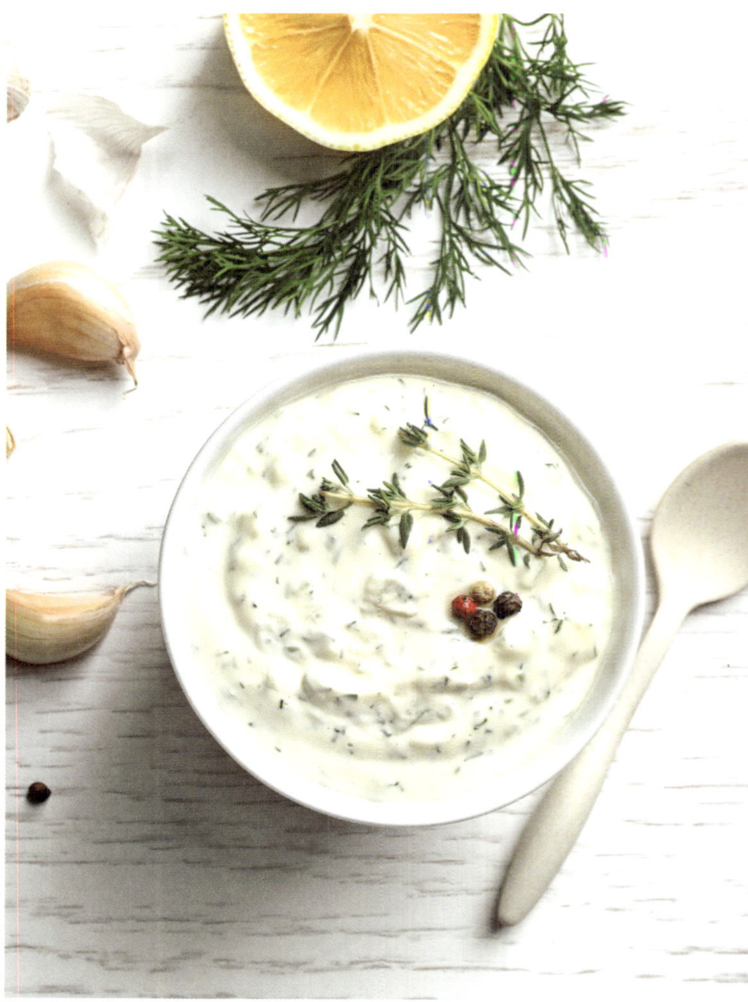

Smoked Trout Salad

SERVES 4

PREP + COOK TIME: 15 MINS

GLUTEN FREE • DAIRY FREE

Creme Fraiche Sauce

MAKES APPROXIMATELY 1 CUP

PREP + COOK TIME: 5 MINS + CHILLING

VEG • GLUTEN FREE

SMOKED TROUT SALAD

4 tbsps mayonnaise
1 tbsp warm water
Salt and pepper to taste
1 Continental cucumber
350g hot-smoked trout
2 ripe avocados, sliced
200g watercress, picked and washed
50g red-veined sorrel leaves or other strong-flavoured salad leaves

Place the mayonnaise and water together in a medium bowl. Season with salt and pepper, then whisk to make a light, runny dressing. Set aside.

Peel the cucumber, cut lengthways and scoop out the seeds. Slice into 1cm-thick slices.

Place the cucumber in a large bowl. Break the trout into bite-size pieces and add to the bowl with the avocado, watercress and sorrel.

Toss together gently, then divide between four bowls.

Drizzle with dressing and serve immediately.

CREME FRAICHE SAUCE

1 cup (240g) creme fraiche
1 tsp lemon zest
1 tbsp freshly squeezed lemon juice
2 tbsps chopped fresh dill
1 tbsp chopped fresh thyme
1 clove garlic, minced
Salt and pepper to taste

Combine all the ingredients in a bowl and mix well.

Refrigerate for 20 minutes before serving.

Broccoli Soup with Steamed Chicken

SERVES 4
PREP + COOK TIME: 45 MINS
GLUTEN FREE

1 tbsp butter
1 tbsp olive oil
1 onion, chopped
1 stalk celery, chopped
2 cloves garlic, chopped
1 tsp chopped fresh thyme
2 heads broccoli, chopped (stems and florets)
2 cups (500ml) water
4 cups (1L) chicken stock
2 chicken breasts
½ cup (125ml) cream
Salt and pepper to taste
Pinch of paprika
Handful of pea shoots to serve

Heat butter and oil in a large pan over medium heat until the butter melts. Add onion and celery; cook, stirring occasionally, for 5-7 minutes until soft and translucent. Add garlic and thyme; cook, stirring, for 30 seconds until fragrant.

Stir in broccoli, water and stock. Bring to a boil over high heat then reduce heat and simmer for 8 minutes until broccoli is very tender. Remove from the heat.

Meanwhile, cut the chicken breasts in half horizontally and place in a steamer basket over a pan of simmering water. Steam for 5-10 minutes or until just cooked through. Remove from the heat and set aside to rest.

Remove a few pieces of broccoli from the soup for garnish, if desired, using a slotted spoon. Set aside.

Puree the remaining soup with a stick blender until smooth. Stir in the cream and season with salt and pepper. Blend once more.

Spoon into bowls and top with the reserved broccoli pieces.

Season the chicken with salt and pepper and slice thinly. Lay the chicken pieces on top of the soup. Sprinkle with paprika and scatter with pea shoots if desired.

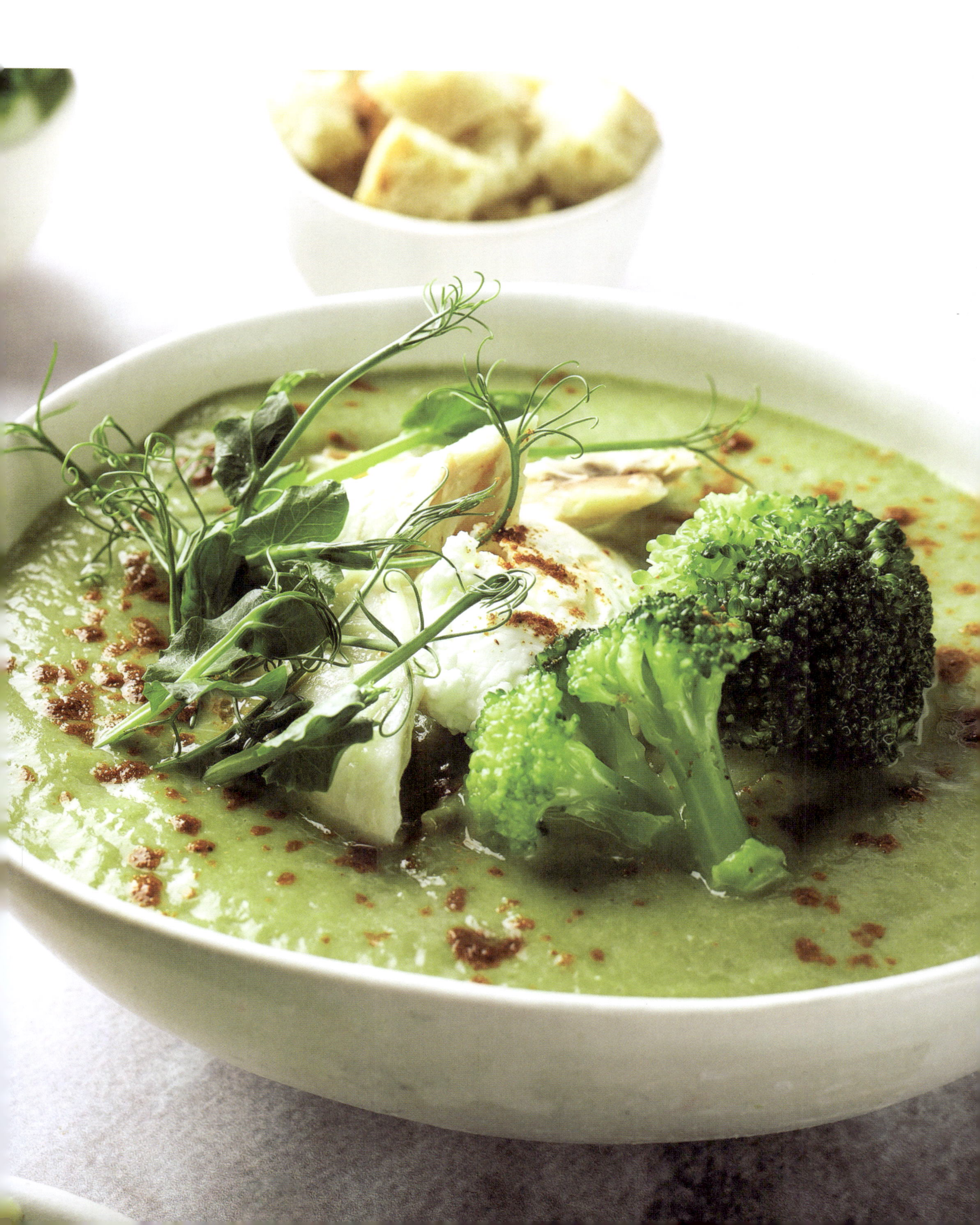

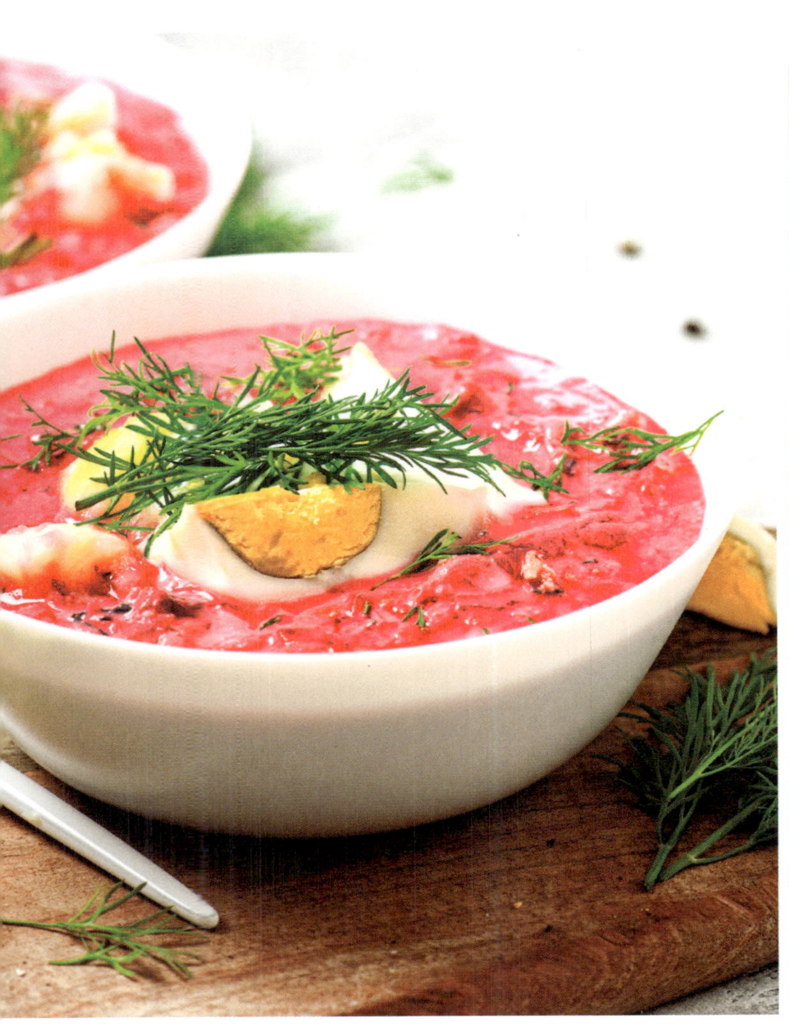

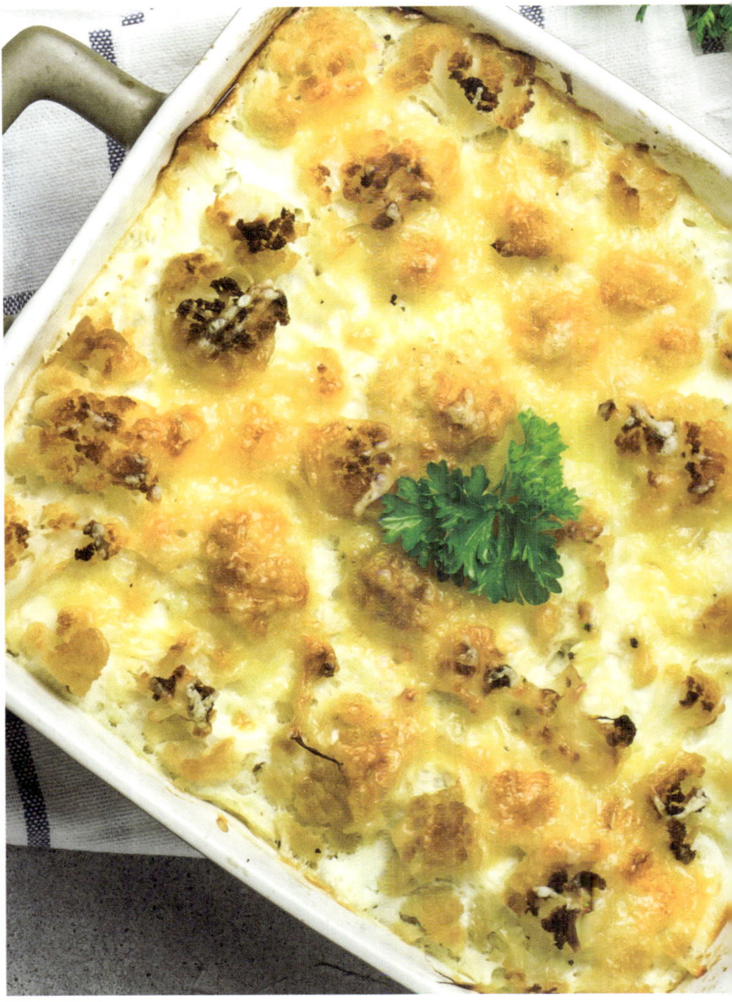

Cold Beetroot Soup

SERVES 6

PREP + COOK TIME: 15 MINS + COOLING AND CHILLING

VEG • GLUTEN FREE

Cauliflower Cheese

SERVES 8

PREP + COOK TIME: 1 HOUR 20 MINS

VEG • GLUTEN FREE

COLD BEETROOT SOUP

2 small beetroots
1⅔ cups (400ml) water or vegetable stock
3 tbsps lemon juice
3 cups (750ml) Greek yoghurt, buttermilk or kefir
3 tbsps dill, finely chopped + dill sprigs to serve
10 radishes, cut into thin batons
1 Lebanese cucumber, cut into thin batons
1 clove garlic, crushed
Salt and pepper to taste
3 eggs, to serve

Peel and coarsely grate the beetroots and place in a large pan with the water or vegetable stock and lemon juice. Cover the pan and bring to a boil. Simmer for 5 minutes, then remove from the heat and leave to cool completely.

When the beetroot mixture is cool add the yoghurt, buttermilk or kefir along with the dill, half the spring onions, the radishes, cucumber and garlic. Season to taste with salt and pepper and stir well to combine. Refrigerate for at least 30 minutes or up to 4 hours before serving.

Meanwhile bring a pan of water to the boil. Add the eggs and cook for 2½ minutes. Remove from the water with a slotted spoon. Run under cold water, peel and slice in quarters.

Serve the soup topped with eggs and dill sprigs.

CAULIFLOWER CHEESE

2 medium heads cauliflower, cut into florets
2 tbsps olive oil
Salt and pepper to taste
2 tbsps butter
3 leeks, white and light green parts only, sliced
1 cup (250ml) thickened cream
180g cream cheese, cut into cubes
4 cups (500g) grated Cheddar cheese
2 cups (250g) shredded mozzarella cheese
1 tsp Tabasco
¼ cup (25g) grated Parmesan cheese

Preheat oven to 190°C. Grease a large baking dish.

In a large bowl, toss cauliflower with 2 tablespoons oil and season with salt. Spread cauliflower onto two large baking trays and roast for 40 minutes until tender and lightly golden.

Meanwhile, melt butter in a large pan over medium heat. Add leeks and cook, stirring occasionally, for 10 minutes until soft. Add the cream and bring up to a simmer, then decrease heat to low and stir in cheeses until melted.

Remove from heat, add Tabasco and season with salt and pepper. Add the roasted cauliflower and stir to combine.

Transfer mixture to prepared baking dish. Sprinkle with Parmesan cheese.

Bake for 15 minutes until golden brown and bubbling.

Allow to cool for 5 minutes before serving.

FRESH GREENS SALAD

1 head broccoli, cut into florets
500g asparagus, trimmed and cut into 10cm lengths
250g snow peas
¼ cup (60ml) olive oil
2 tbsps red wine vinegar
1 tbsp fresh lemon juice
1 Asian shallot, minced
Salt and pepper to taste
1 tbsp capers
1 cup (30g) baby beetroot leaves or other salad leaves
¼ cup (5g) fresh herbs, such as chervil or parsley

Bring a large saucepan of salted water to a boil. Add the broccoli florets. Cook for 3 minutes then add the asparagus. Cook for 1 more minute then add the snow peas. Cook for 1 final minute. The vegetables should be bright green and tender. Drain and rinse under cold water. Dry on a clean tea towel.

In a medium bowl, whisk together the olive oil, vinegar, lemon juice and shallot. Season with salt and pepper, add the capers and whisk gently once more.

Combine the cooked vegetables with the salad leaves and herbs in a large bowl. Drizzle over the dressing and toss to combine. Serve immediately.

STUFFED ZUCCHINI ROLLS

2 medium zucchinis
Salt and pepper to taste
250g ricotta or cream cheese
1 tbsp sour cream
2 cloves garlic, minced
Small bunch of fresh basil, chopped + extra basil leaves to garnish
Small bunch of parsley, chopped
Olive oil for frying

Trim zucchinis and slice lengthwise into 3mm-thick strips using a sharp knife or a mandoline. Salt each slice of zucchini generously and arrange on a large plate. Set aside for 15-20 minutes.

In a large bowl mash ricotta or cream cheese with a fork, then add sour cream and stir well to combine. Add garlic, basil and parsley. Season with salt and pepper. Mix well.

Heat a grill pan over medium-high heat.

Rinse zucchini strips in cold water and pat dry with paper towels. Brush both sides with olive oil. Fry on the grill pan for 2-3 minutes per side until tender.

Spread the cream cheese mixture over each of the zucchini strips and roll up. Place seam-side down on a plate. Place a basil leaf in the end of each roll up, to serve, if desired.

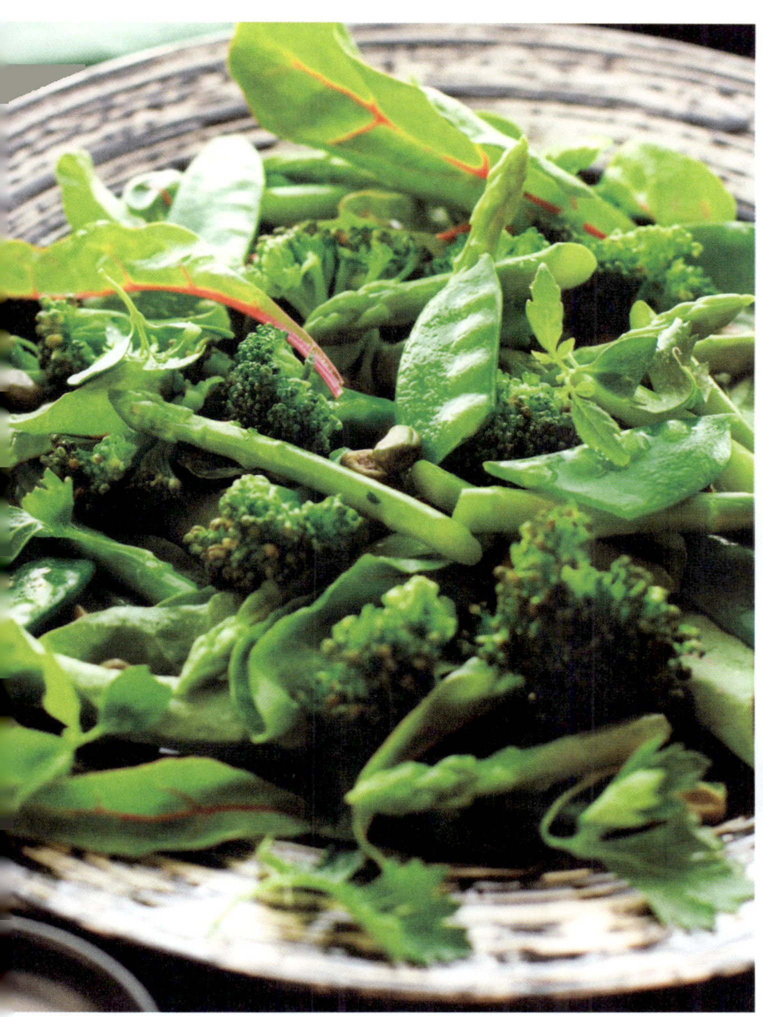

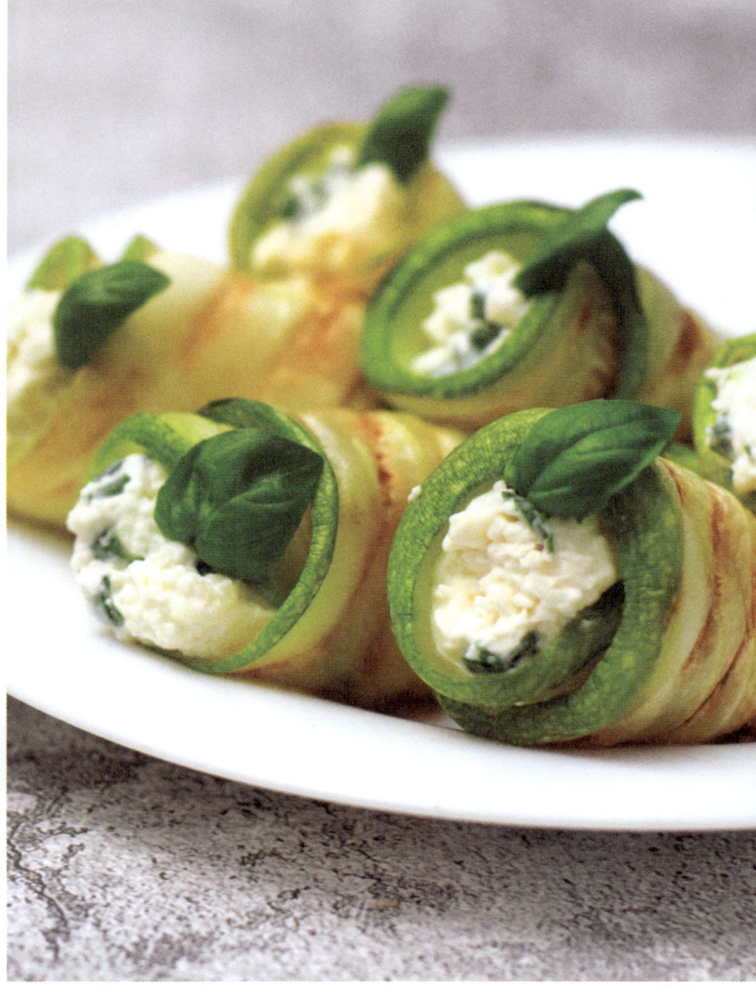

Fresh Greens Salad

SERVES 4

PREP + COOK TIME: 20 MINS

VEG • GLUTEN FREE • DAIRY FREE

Stuffed Zucchini Rolls

SERVES 4

PREP + COOK TIME: 40 MINS

VEG • GLUTEN FREE

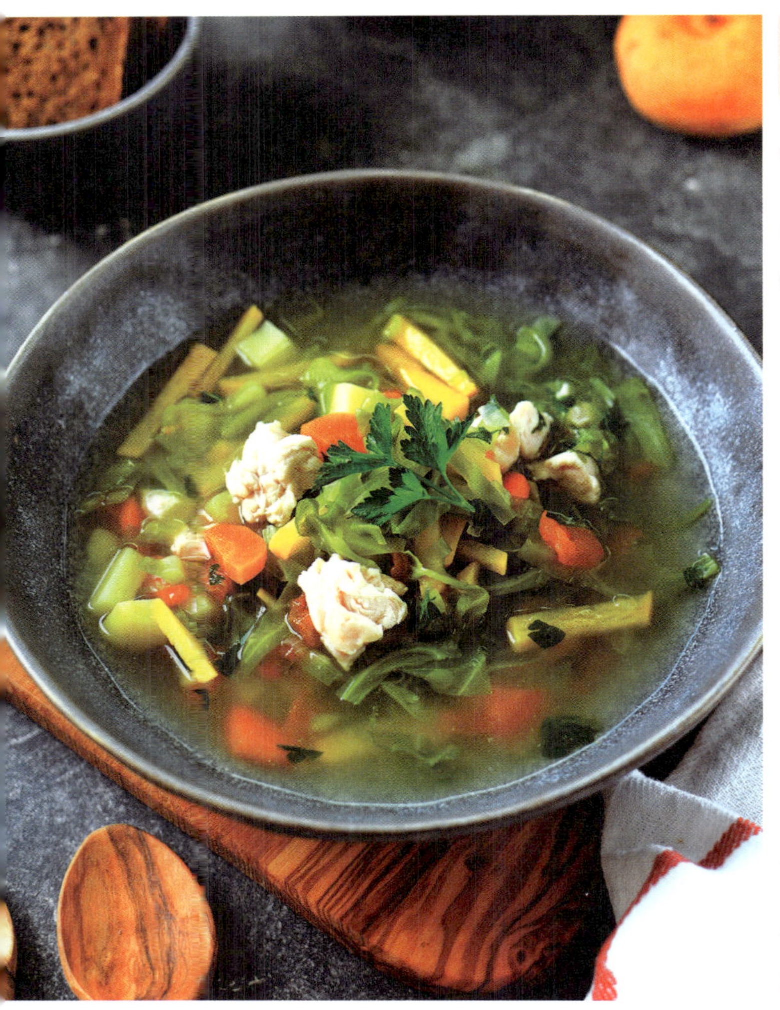

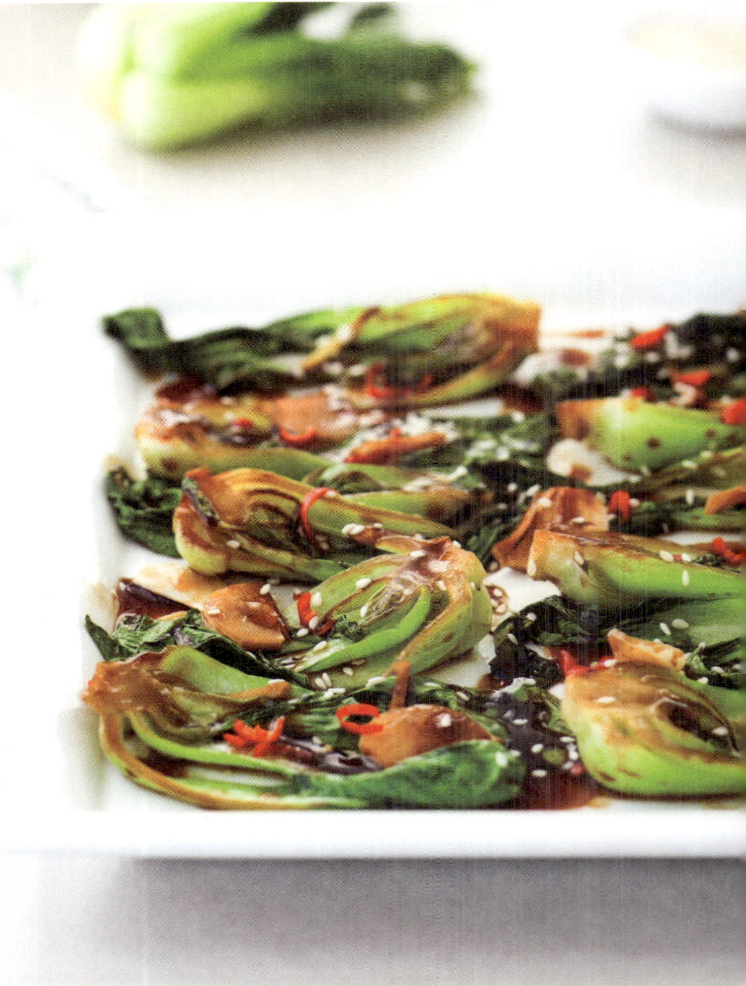

Chicken & Turnip Soup

SERVES 4

PREP + COOK TIME: 35 MINS

GLUTEN FREE • DAIRY FREE

Spicy Roasted Bok Choy

SERVES 6

PREP + COOK TIME: 15 MINS

VEG • GLUTEN FREE

CHICKEN & TURNIP SOUP

500g chicken thigh fillets, cut into bite-sized pieces
2 onions, quartered
4 turnips, chopped into 5 x 1 x 1cm lengths
3 medium carrots, chopped
2 stalks celery, chopped
6 cups (1.5L) chicken stock
Salt and pepper to taste
¼ small cabbage, chopped
1 bunch turnip leaves, chopped
Juice of 1 lemon
Parsley sprigs to garnish (optional)

Place the chicken, onion, turnips, carrots and celery into a large pan. Cover with chicken stock and season with salt and pepper.

Bring to boil over medium-high heat, then reduce to a simmer.

Simmer for about 20 minutes until the chicken is cooked and the turnips are tender.

Add the cabbage to the pan and cook for a further 3 minutes. Add the turnip leaves and cook for 2 minutes more.

Ladle soup into a bowls. Squeeze over the juice of the lemon and season once more with salt and pepper. Garnish with parsley to serve.

SPICY ROASTED BOK CHOY

6 heads bok choy
3 tbsps salted butter
1 tbsp avocado oil
2 cloves garlic, finely chopped
1 tsp dried chilli flakes
2 tbsps tamari
1 tsp sesame oil
1 tsp sesame seeds
¼ red chilli, finely sliced (optional)

Wash the bok choy and slice in half lengthways.

Place a large frying pan over high heat, add the butter and oil. As soon as the butter melts add garlic and chilli flakes. Cook for 1 minute until fragrant.

Add the bok choy flat-side down in the pan. Cook for 4 minutes until bok choy starts to colour. Flip the bok choy and cook for another 1-2 minutes. Add tamari and sesame oil to the pan and toss to coat.

Serve onto plates, drizzle with the sauce from the pan and scatter with sesame seeds and sliced chilli, if desired.

Keto Bagels with Smoked Salmon & Cream Cheese

MAKES 8
PREP + COOK TIME: 45 MINS
GLUTEN FREE

1¾ cups (210g) almond meal, finely ground
1 tbsp baking powder
3 cups (375g) mozzarella cheese, shredded
60g cream cheese, softened
3 large eggs
1 tbsp sesame seeds

TO SERVE

250g cream cheese
300g smoked salmon
2 tbsps capers

Preheat oven to 200°C. Line a large baking tray with greaseproof paper.

Place the almond meal and baking powder in a food processor and pulse once or twice to combine.

In a microwave-safe bowl, add the mozzarella and cream cheese. Microwave the cheeses in 30-second bursts, stirring between each burst, until mostly melted. Whisk together until smooth. Transfer the melted cheese mixture to the food processor with the almond meal mixture and add two eggs. Pulse until a smooth dough forms. Dust a clean work surface with almond meal. Transfer the dough to the prepared work surface and divide into eight equal portions. Roll out each piece of dough into a thick sausage shape. Connect the ends of the sausage shapes to form bagels. Place the bagels onto the prepared baking tray.

Whisk the remaining egg in a small bowl. Brush the top of each bagel with beaten egg then sprinkle with sesame seeds. Bake the bagels for 12-15 minutes until firm and golden on top.

Remove the bagels from the oven and let them cool completely before slicing and serving. Fill each bagel with cream cheese, smoked salmon and capers.

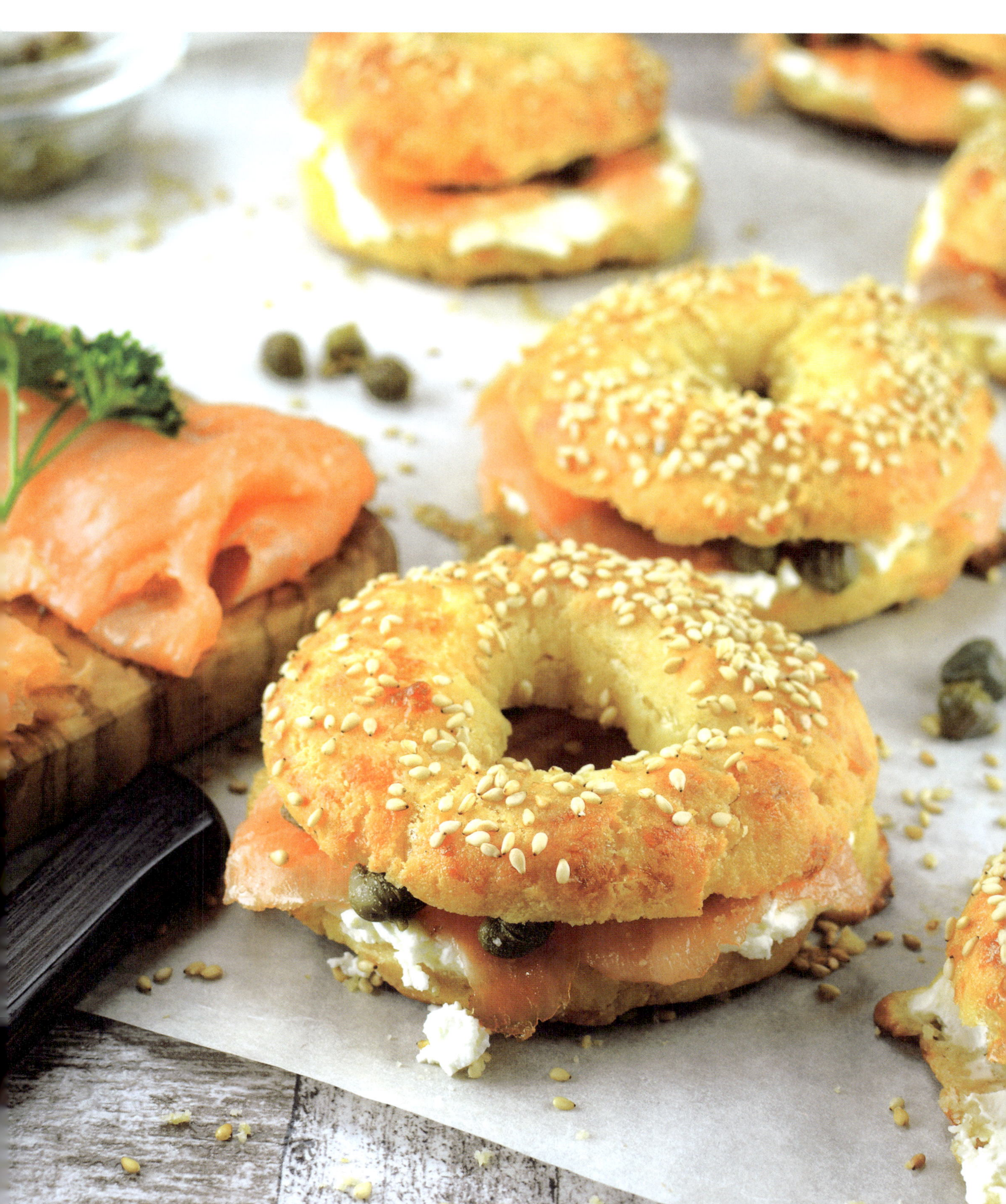

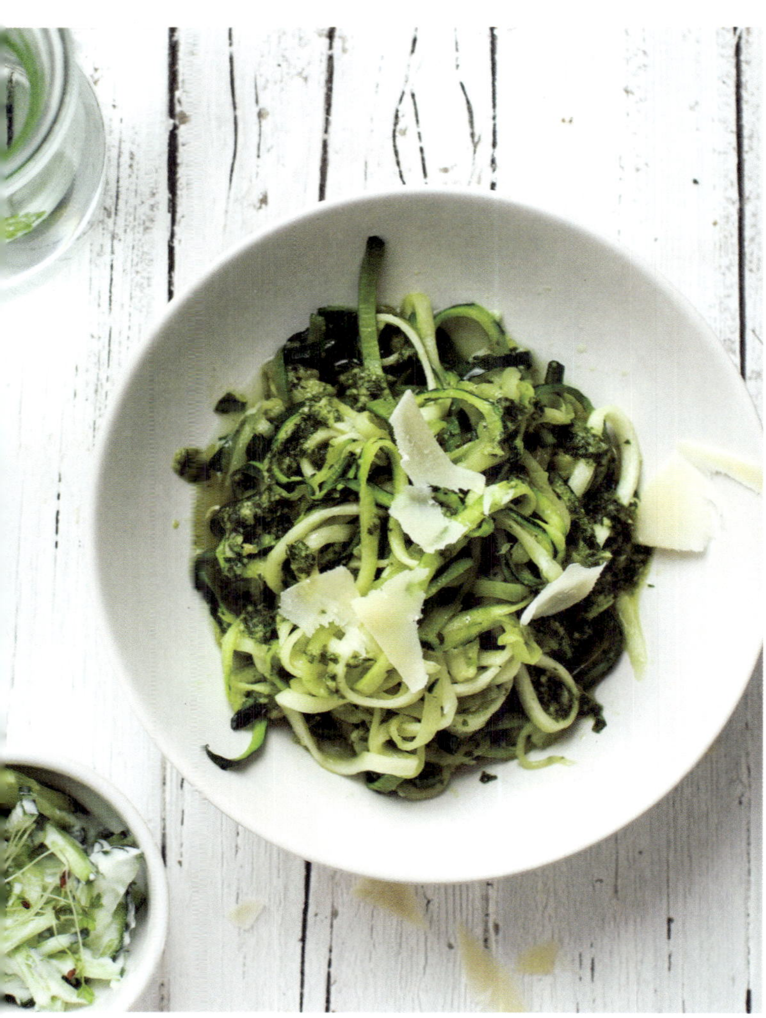

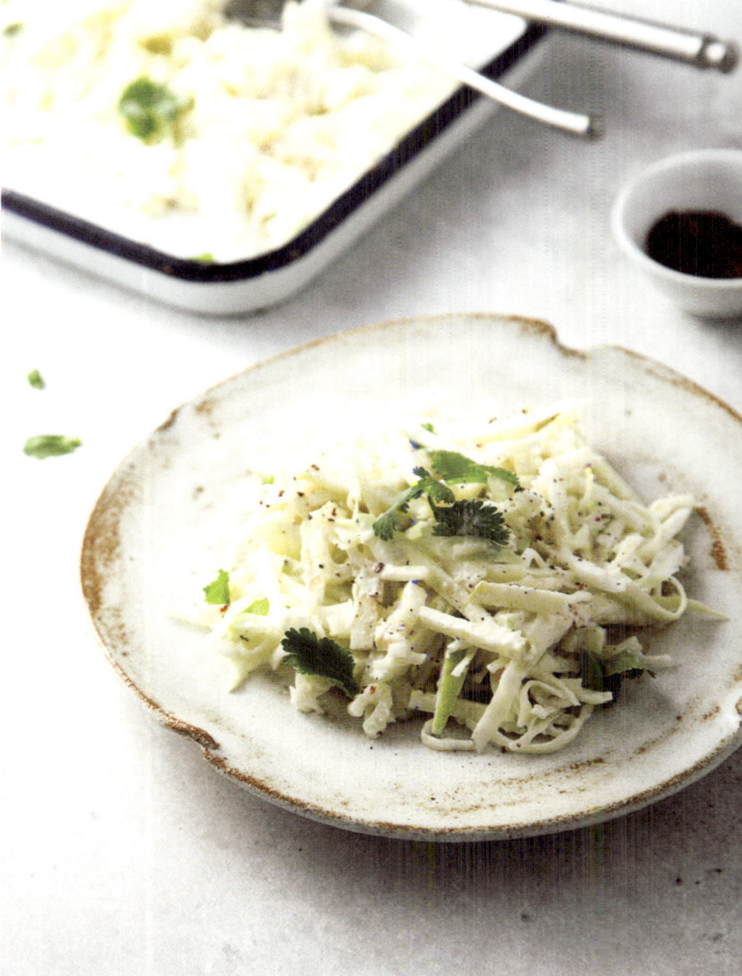

Zoodles with Pesto

SERVES 4

PREP + COOK TIME: 15 MINS

VEG • GLUTEN FREE

Cabbage Salad

SERVES 4

PREP + COOK TIME: 15 MINUTES

VEG • GLUTEN FREE • DAIRY FREE

ZOODLES WITH PESTO

4 small zucchinis, ends trimmed

1 tbsp olive oil

1 jar (190g) store-bought pesto

¼ cup (25g) shaved Parmesan cheese

Use a julienne peeler or mandoline to slice the zucchinis into noodles. Set aside.

Heat the olive oil in a large pan over medium heat. Add the zucchini noodles and cook, tossing regularly with tongs, for 3-4 minutes until warmed through. Add the pesto and toss to coat.

Serve into bowls and top with Parmesan shavings.

CABBAGE SALAD

1 cup (245g) mayonnaise (see recipe page 22)

Zest and juice of 1 lemon

2 tbsps apple cider vinegar

2 tbsps Dijon mustard

Salt and pepper to taste

½ white cabbage, finely chopped

2 stalks celery, thinly sliced

½ green apple, chopped into matchsticks (optional)

Fresh coriander leaves to serve (optional)

Place mayonnaise, lemon zest and juice, vinegar and mustard in a small bowl. Season well with salt and pepper and whisk to combine.

Place the cabbage, celery and apple into a large bowl.

Pour the dressing over the salad and toss to combine.

Adjust seasoning as necessary.

Refrigerate until ready to serve. Scatter with coriander leaves, if desired, before serving.

Tip:

While apple is not recommended on a keto diet the small amount in this salad should not kick you out of ketosis. Feel free to leave the apple out completely if you wish.

Baked Mussels with Cheese

SERVES 2-3
PREP + COOK TIME: 40 MINS
GLUTEN FREE

1kg mussels, well scrubbed with beards removed

2 cups (500ml) water

115g unsalted butter

7 cloves garlic, minced

250g cream cheese

½ tbsp tamari

¼ cup (10g) chopped coriander leaves + more to garnish

1 cup (125g) grated Cheddar cheese

Preheat oven to 180°C. Line two baking trays with scrunched up foil. (The foil helps to keep the mussels level.)

Place the mussels in a large pan with the water over medium-high heat. Cover with a lid and allow the liquid to come to a boil. Cook for a further minute until the mussels open. Drain and set aside to cool slightly.

In a small pot, melt the butter over medium-low heat. Add the garlic and cook for 1- 2 minutes, stirring regularly, until fragrant. Transfer garlic butter to a medium bowl. Add cream cheese and mash with a fork to combine. Add tamari and chopped coriander and mix well. Remove the empty halves of the mussels shells. Place the half shells containing the mussels onto the foil-lined baking trays. Ensure the mussels are level. Spread approximately 1 heaped teaspoon of garlic cream cheese on each mussel, then sprinkle with Cheddar cheese.

Transfer to the oven and bake for 10-15 minutes until the cheese melts. You can place under the grill for a final minute to brown the cheese if you wish.

Scatter with coriander leaves to serve.

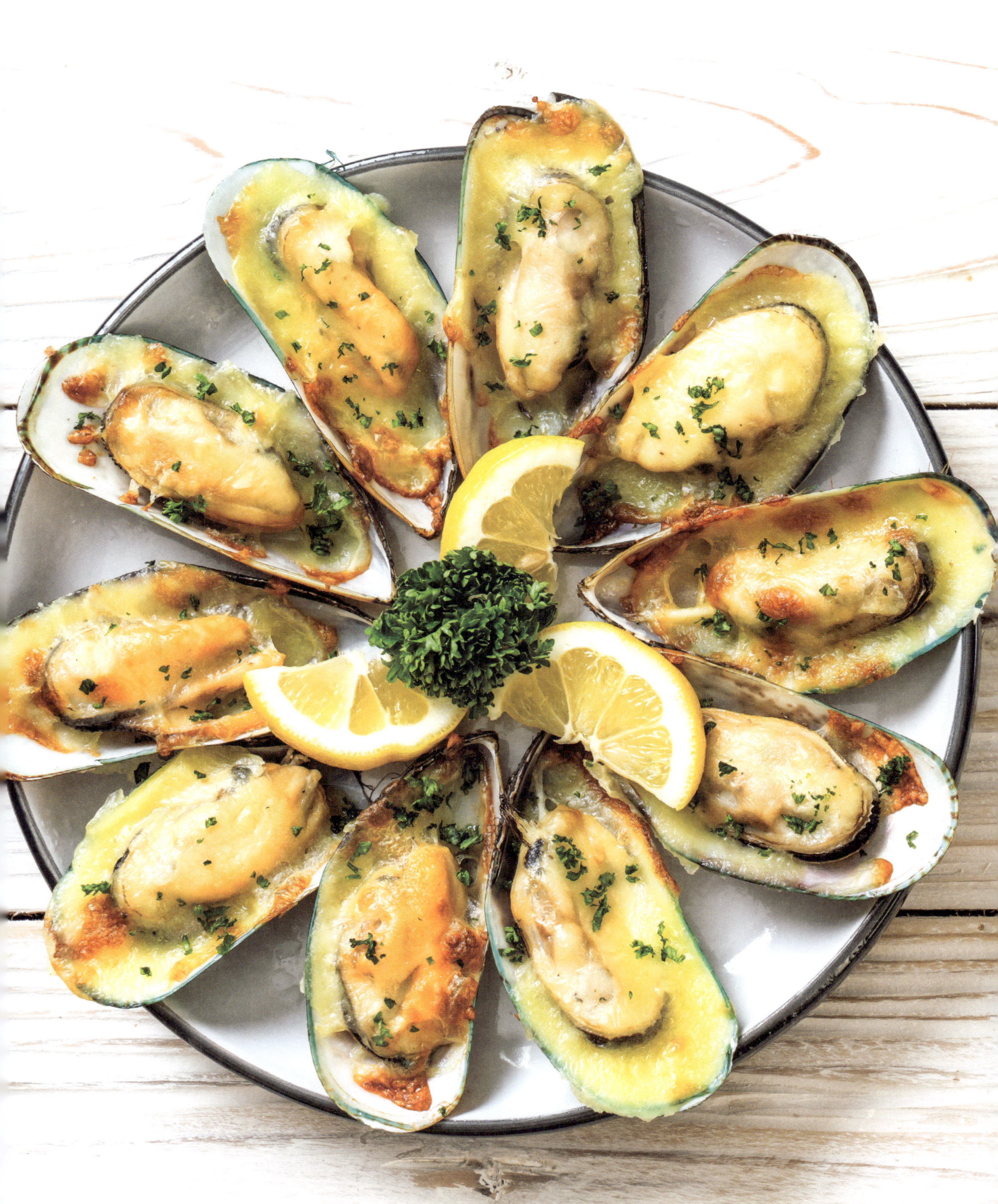

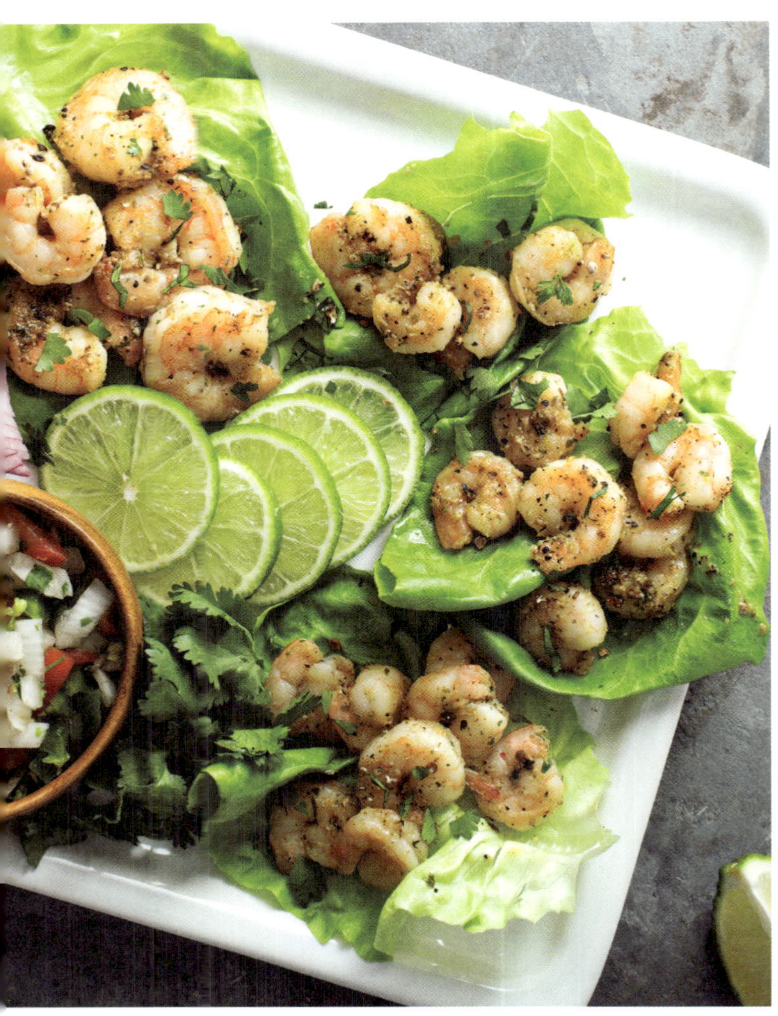

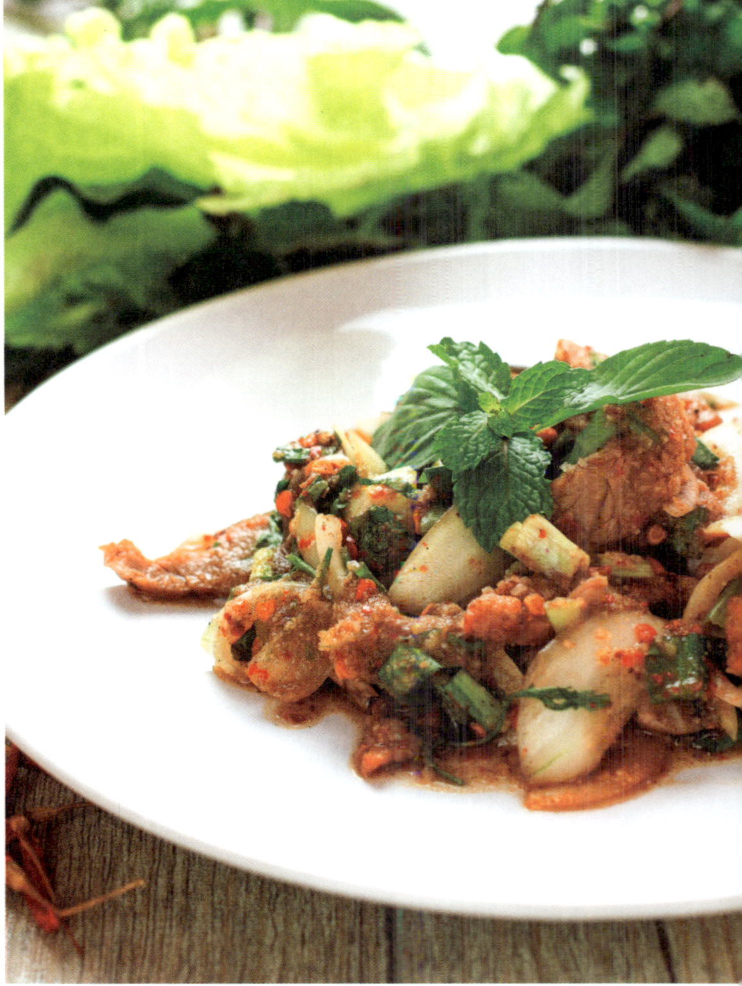

Spicy Prawn Lettuce Wraps

SERVES 4

PREP + COOK TIME: 15 MINS

GLUTEN FREE • DAIRY FREE

Chilli Pork Salad

SERVES 2

PREP + COOK TIME: 20 MINS

GLUTEN FREE • DAIRY FREE

SPICY PRAWN LETTUCE WRAPS

Zest of 1 lime + ¼ cup (60ml) lime juice + lime wedges to serve

1-3 tsps chilli powder (according to taste)

½ cup (10g) fresh coriander leaves + 2 tbsps finely chopped

2 cloves garlic, minced

¼ cup (60ml) + 1 tbsp olive oil

½ tsp each salt and pepper

500g raw prawns, peeled and deveined

12 large lettuce leaves

Pico de gallo to serve (see recipe page 116)

In a large bowl mix together the lime zest and juice, chilli powder, chopped coriander, garlic, ¼ cup olive oil, salt and pepper. Add the prawns and toss to coat. Set aside for between 5 and 20 minutes.

Heat 1 tablespoon oil in a large frying pan over high heat. Add the prawns and fry for 2 minutes until just turning pink.

Divide the prawns between lettuce leaves. Serve with coriander, lime wedges and pico de gallo.

CHILLI PORK SALAD

2 tbsps fish sauce

2 tsps dried chilli flakes

½ red chilli, chopped

1½ tbsps lime juice

2 spring onions, chopped

2 Asian shallots, sliced

1 tbsp coconut oil

450g pork fillet, sliced

¼ cup (10g) mint leaves, chopped + mint sprigs, to garnish

In a small bowl place the fish sauce, chilli flakes, chopped chilli and lime juice. Stir to combine.

Add the spring onions and shallots and allow to sit for 5 minutes.

Heat the oil in a large frying pan over medium-high heat. Add the pork to the pan and stir-fry for 5 minutes or until just cooked through.

Remove the pan from the heat.

Pour the spring onions and shallots into the pan along with the marinade.

Add the mint leaves and toss to coat.

Serve on two plates and garnish with mint sprigs.

SPINACH GRATIN

2 tbsps butter

1 small onion, diced

2 cloves garlic, minced

500g frozen spinach, defrosted and water squeezed out

½ tsp salt

¼ tsp ground nutmeg

1 cup (250ml) thickened cream

¼ cup (25g) grated Parmesan cheese

½ cup (60g) grated Gruyere cheese

Preheat oven to 200°C.

Heat butter in a large, deep frying pan over medium-high heat. Add the onion and saute for 3-5 minutes until soft and translucent. Add the garlic and cook for 1 minute until fragrant. Add the spinach and season with salt and nutmeg. Cook, stirring, for 2-3 minutes, then add the cream and bring to a simmer. As soon as the mixture is simmering add half the Parmesan and half the Gruyere cheeses.

Remove from the heat and spoon the mixture into one casserole dish or six individual ramekins. Top with the remaining cheese.

Bake for 15-20 minutes until browned and bubbly.

Serve immediately.

BURRATA PROSCIUTTO SALAD

500g cherry tomatoes or baby Roma tomatoes (varied colours)

Salt and pepper to taste

1 shallot, minced

½ clove garlic, minced

½ red chilli, minced

1 tsp chopped fresh oregano

1 tbsp red wine vinegar

3 tbsps olive oil

½ cup (10g) basil leaves

100g prosciutto

350g burrata

Halve the tomatoes and place in a colander. Sprinkle with salt and set aside for 15 minutes to drain.

Meanwhile prepare the vinaigrette. Mix shallot, garlic, chilli, oregano, red wine vinegar and olive oil in a small bowl. Season with salt and pepper and whisk to combine.

Add tomatoes to a large bowl. Pour over the vinaigrette and toss to coat. Add the basil leaves and toss once more.

Divide the salad between four bowls. Top each bowl with pieces of prosciutto and with a quarter of the burrata. Season once more with salt and pepper.

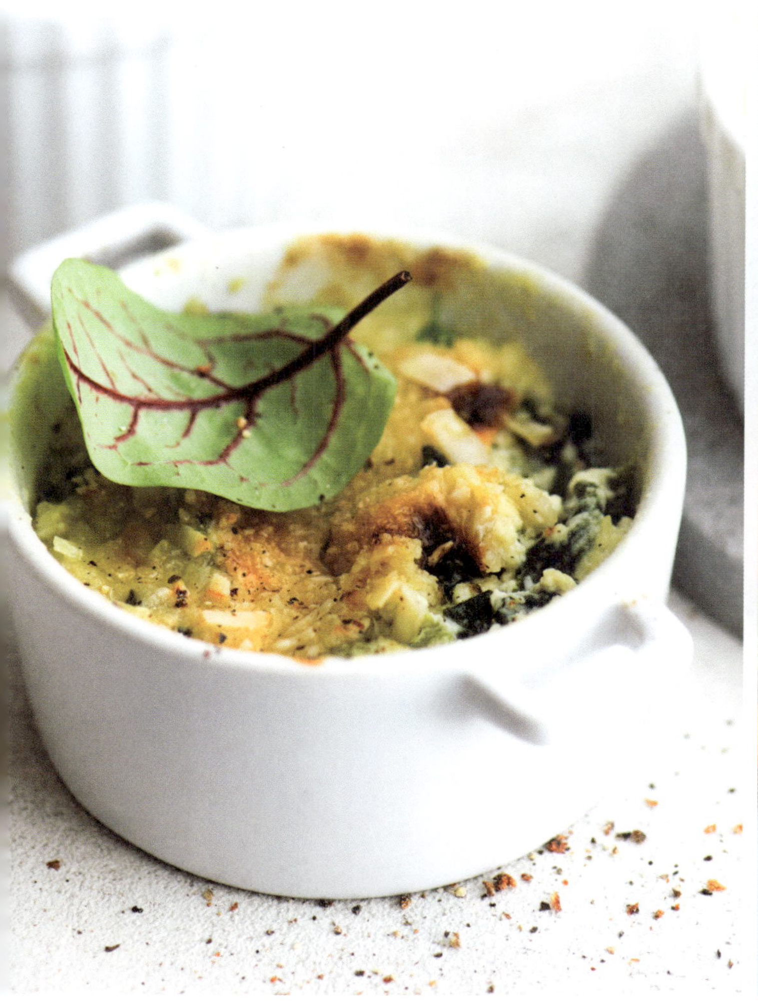

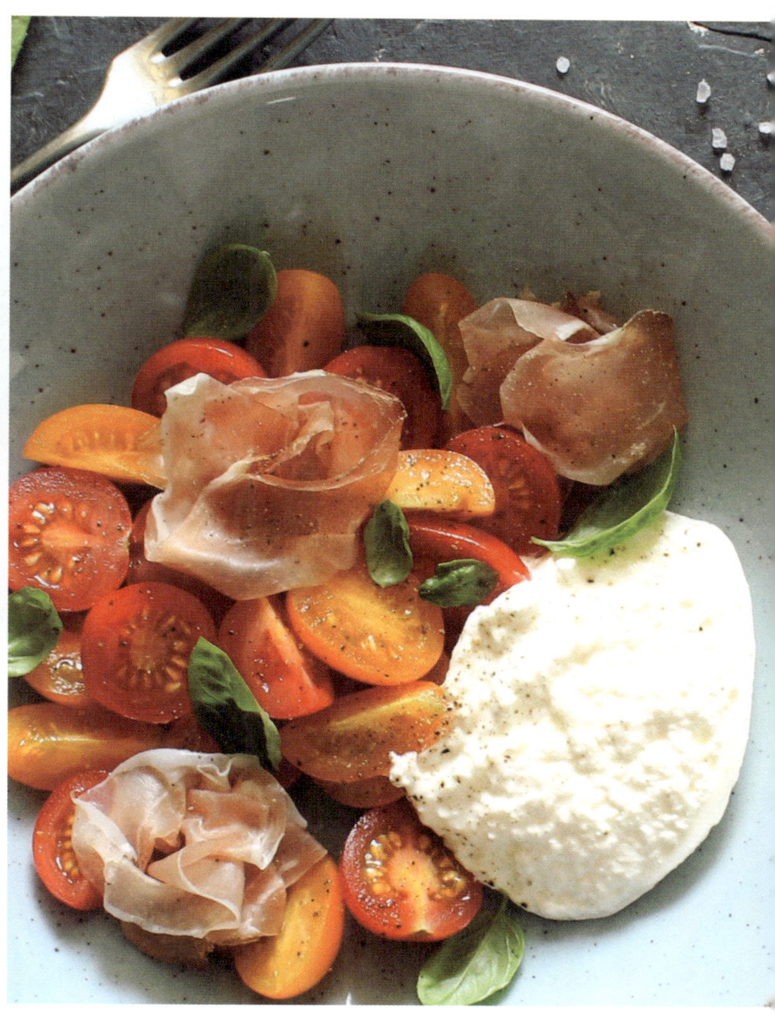

Spinach Gratin

SERVES 6

PREP + COOK TIME: 40 MINS

VEG • GLUTEN FREE

Burrata Prosciutto Salad

SERVES 4

PREP + COOK TIME: 25 MINS

GLUTEN FREE

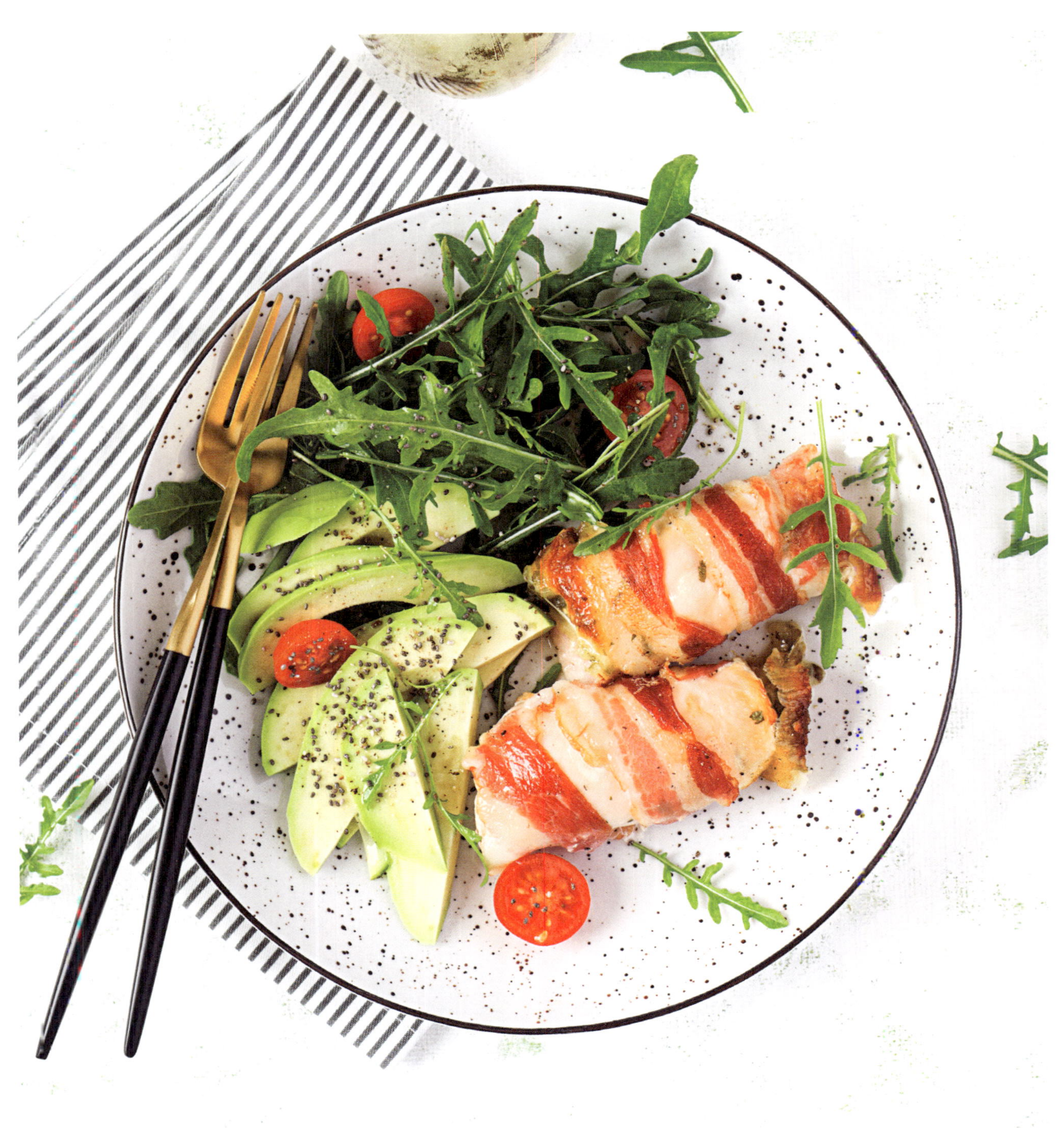

Chicken Wrapped in Bacon

SERVES 4

PREP + COOK TIME: 30 MINS

GLUTEN FREE • DAIRY FREE

CHICKEN WRAPPED IN BACON

1kg chicken tenderloins
1 tsp paprika
1 tsp chilli powder
1 tsp cumin
1 tsp onion powder
1 tsp garlic powder
Salt and pepper to taste
12 rashers streaky bacon
150g rocket
½ cup (110g) cherry tomatoes, halved
2 avocados, sliced
2 tbsps olive oil
1 tbsp lemon juice
1 tsp chia seeds

Preheat oven to 200°C.

Place the chicken tenders in a large mixing bowl.

Add the paprika, chilli powder, cumin, onion powder and garlic powder to the bowl. Season lightly with salt and pepper. Toss to combine.

Wrap each seasoned chicken tender in a strip of bacon, and place them on a wire rack in a roasting tin. Bake for 20-22 minutes until the chicken is cooked through and the bacon begins to crisp. Remove from the oven.

Divide the rocket and tomatoes evenly between four plates. Place half a sliced avocado on each plate. Drizzle the salad with olive oil and lemon juice and season with salt and pepper. Scatter over chia seeds.

Add the bacon-wrapped chicken to each plate and serve.

Kelp Noodle Salad with Sesame Seeds

SERVES 4

PREP + COOK TIME: 20 MINS

VEG • GLUTEN FREE • DAIRY FREE

- 4 servings kelp noodles
- 2½ tbsps coconut oil, divided
- 3 small cloves garlic, crushed
- 2 small bunches bok choy, cut into 1cm-thick slices
- 2 cups (220g) carrot, grated
- ¼ cup (60ml) tamari
- ¼ tsp liquid stevia
- Salt and pepper to taste
- 2 tbsps white and black sesame seeds

Cook the noodles according to packet directions, toss with ½ tablespoon of the oil and set aside.

Heat the rest of the oil in a large wok over high heat. Fry the garlic for 30 seconds, then add the bok choy and stir-fry for 2 minutes.

Stir through the carrot and cook for 1 minute. Add the noodles, tamari and stevia. Heat through for 2 minutes.

Season to taste and serve garnished with sesame seeds.

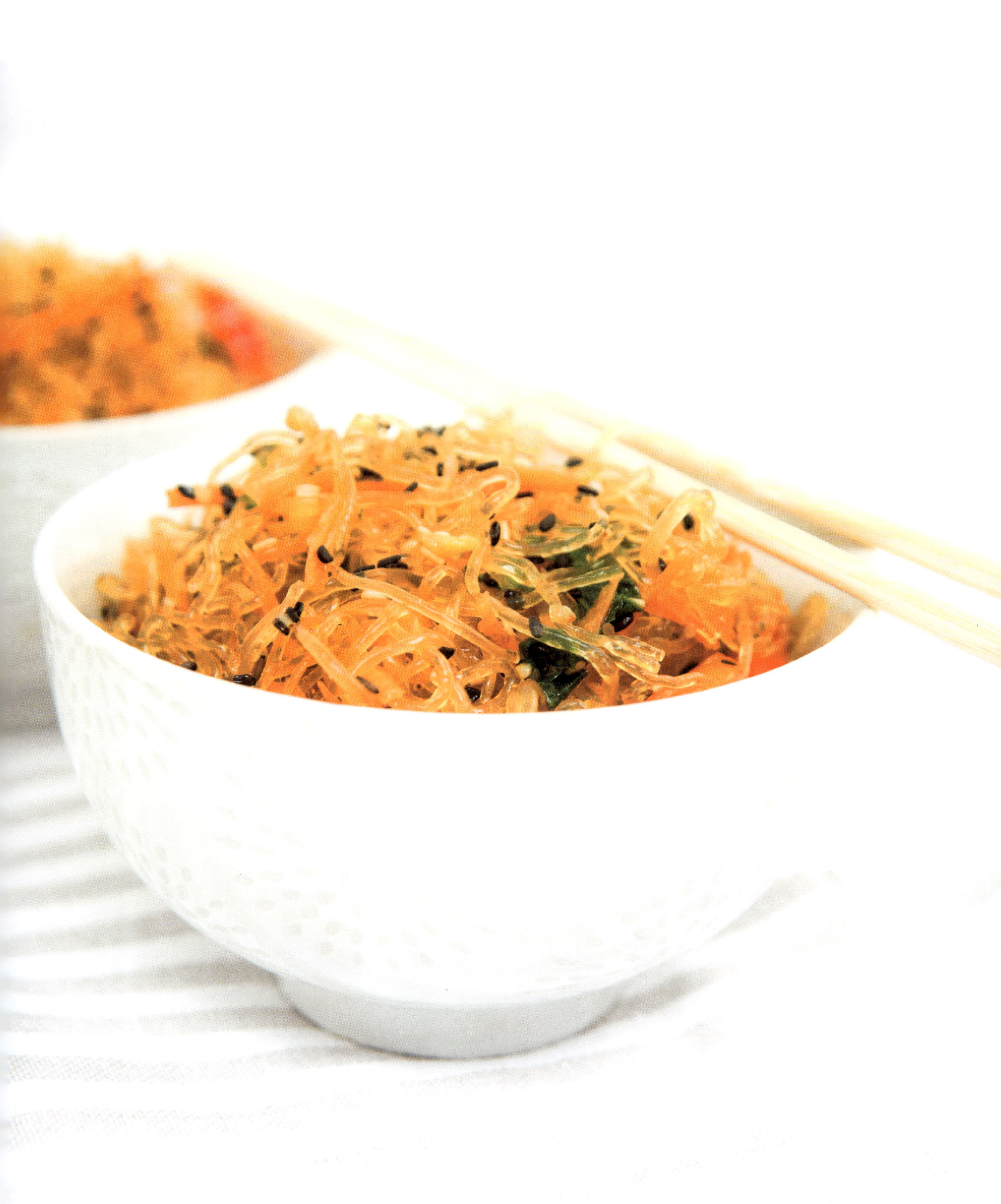

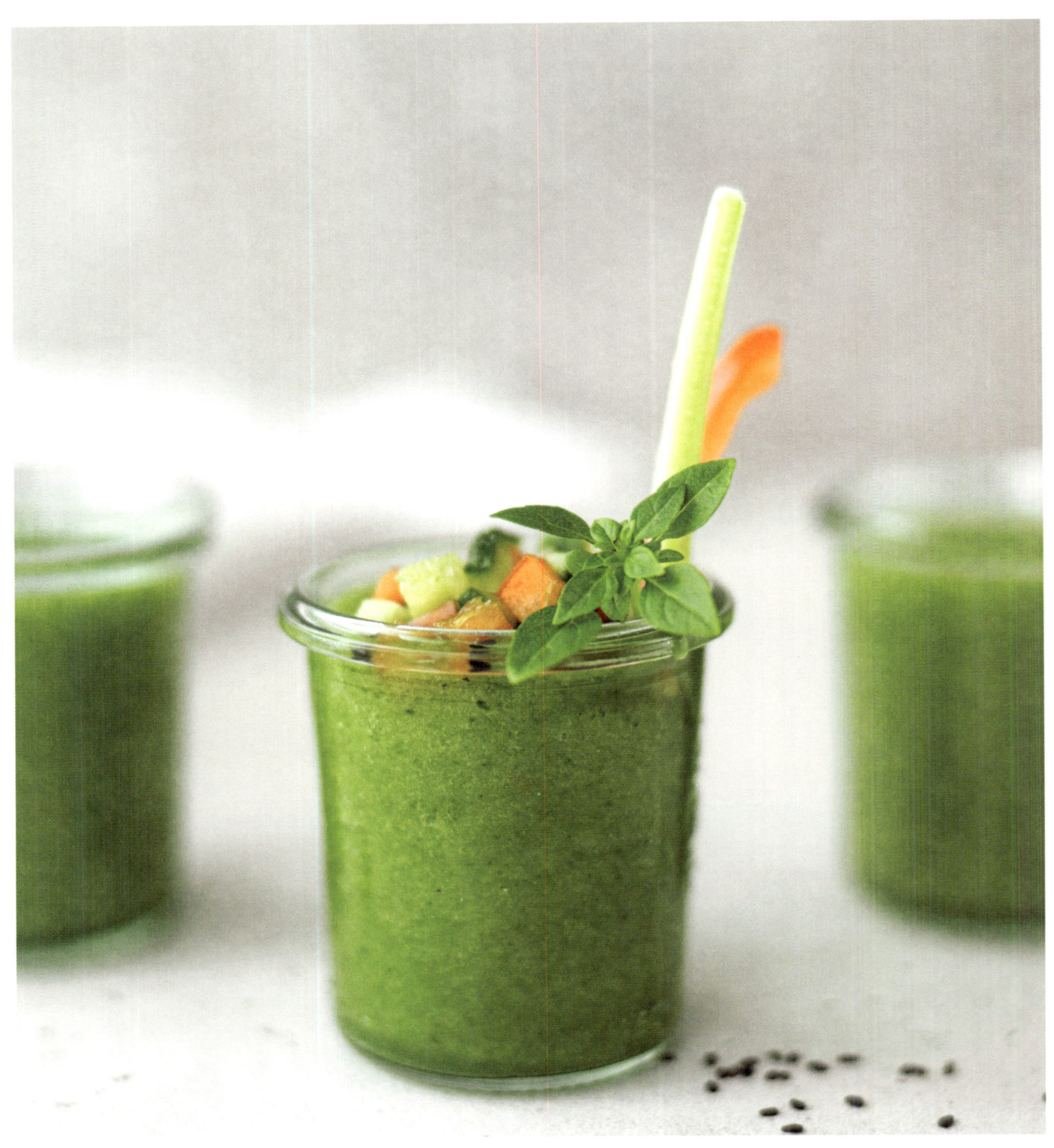

Avocado Chilled Summer Soup

SERVES 4

PREP + COOK TIME: 15 MINS

VEG • GLUTEN FREE

AVOCADO CHILLED SUMMER SOUP

2 Lebanese cucumbers
2 small stalks celery
2 medium, ripe avocados
2 cups (300g) ice cubes
1 cup (250ml) Greek yoghurt
1 cup (250ml) vegetable stock
2½ tbsps lime juice
Handful of basil + more to serve
¼ tsp garlic powder
½ tsp salt
1 tbsp diced orange capsicum, to garnish

Peel and chop the cucumbers and celery and place in a food processor or blender, reserving a few pieces for garnish.

Scoop the avocado flesh into the food processor and add the ice cubes, yoghurt, vegetable stock, lime juice, basil, garlic powder and salt. Pulse a few times, then process until smooth.

Serve in glasses topped with diced celery, cucumber and capsicum.

Coconut Fish Curry

SERVES 4

PREP + COOK TIME: 35 MINS

GLUTEN FREE • DAIRY FREE

4 small red chillies, chopped
Small piece ginger, grated
Small piece fresh turmeric, grated
2 tbsps coconut oil
1 onion, finely chopped
2 tsps ground coriander
2 tsps ground turmeric
1 tsp ground cumin
¼ tsp ground cloves
6 green cardamon pods, cracked
12 curry leaves
1 x 400ml can coconut milk
1 cup (250ml) fish or vegetable stock
600g firm white fish fillets, cut into 5cm pieces
Juice of 1 lime
Salt to taste

Using a mortar and pestle or food processor pound or blend the garlic, chilli, ginger and turmeric to a paste.

Heat oil in a large, deep frying pan over medium heat. Cook onion, stirring, for 5-7 minutes until soft and translucent.

Add garlic-chilli paste and cook, stirring, for 3-4 minutes until fragrant.

Add ground spices, cardamon pods and curry leaves and cook, stirring, for a further 2 minutes.

Add coconut milk and stock, then bring to a simmer.

Cook, stirring occasionally, for 10 minutes or until slightly reduced

Add fish and cook for 4 minutes or until just cooked. Remove from heat. Season with lime juice and salt to taste.

Tip:

Spanish mackerel, snapper, barramundi or cod are good firm white fish to use in this recipe.

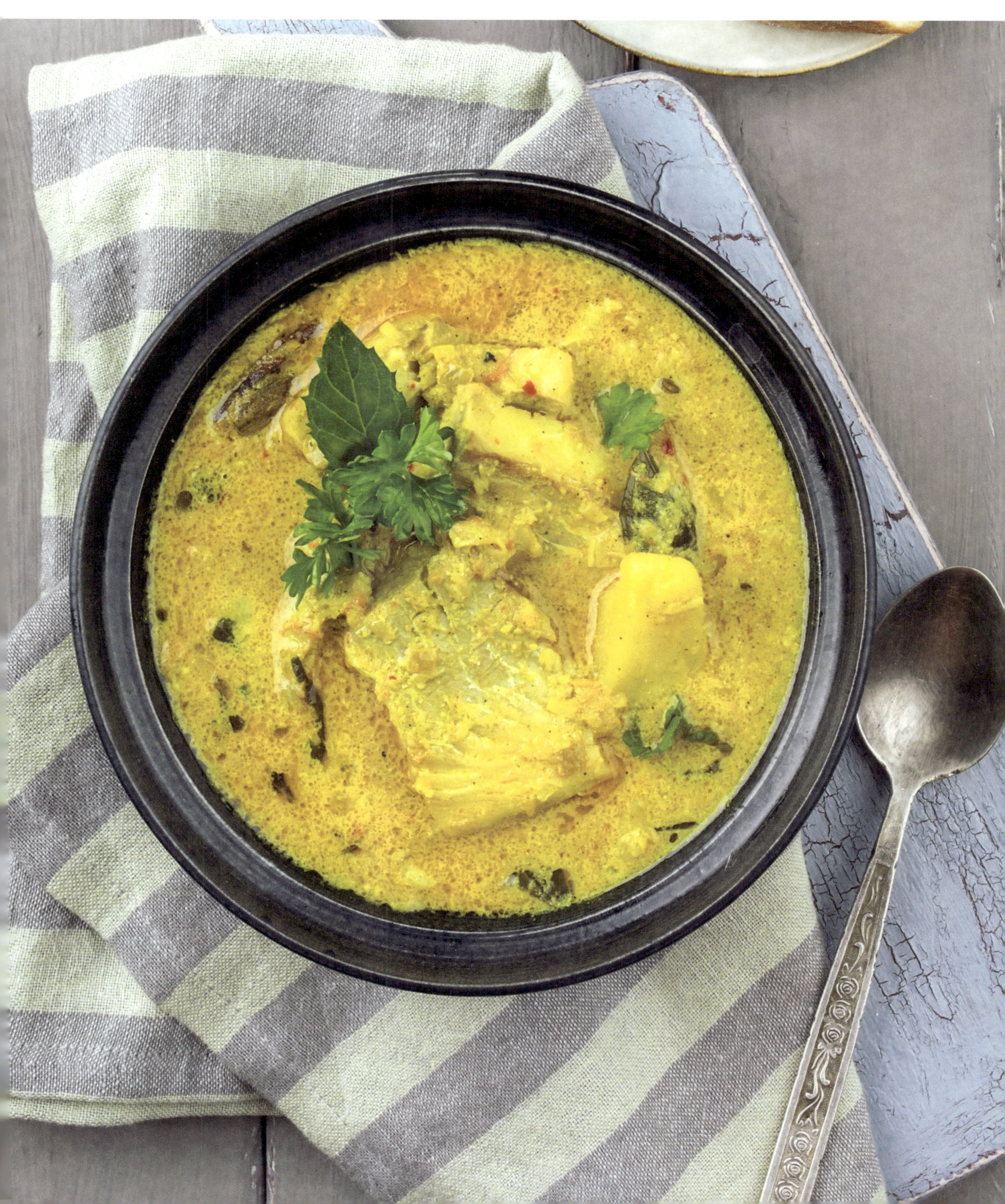

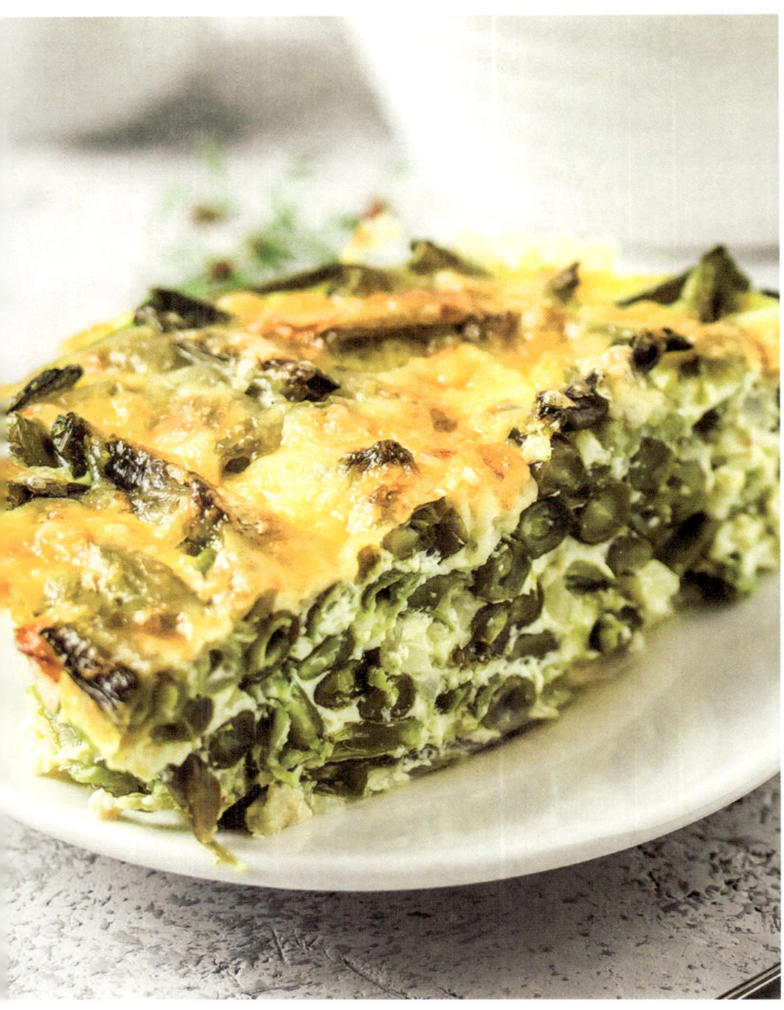

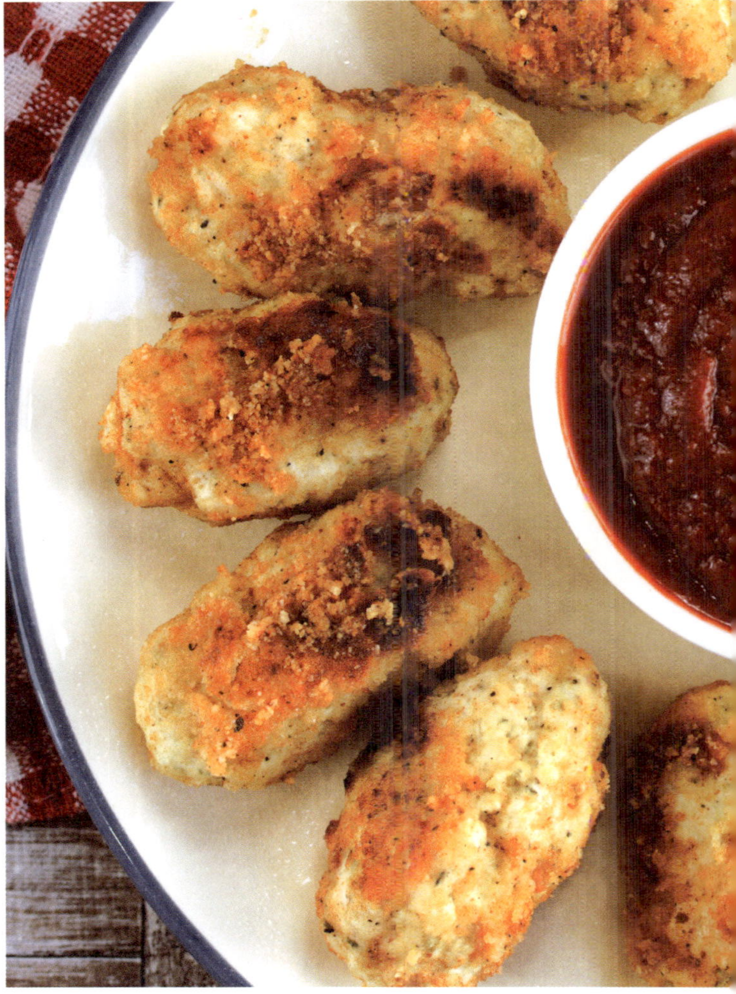

Cheesy Green Bean Casserole

SERVES 4

PREP + COOK TIME: 35 MINS

VEG • GLUTEN FREE

Chicken Nuggets

SERVES 6

PREP + COOK TIME: 25 MINS

GLUTEN FREE • DAIRY FREE

CHEESY GREEN BEAN CASSEROLE

1kg green beans, trimmed
1 cup (250ml) thickened cream
2 cloves garlic, thinly sliced
2 tsps lemon zest
Salt to taste
Pinch of dried chilli flakes
1 cup (125g) grated mozzarella cheese
1 cup (100g) grated Parmesan cheese

Preheat oven to 200°C.

Place green beans into a baking dish.

Pour cream over beans and scatter with garlic and lemon zest. Season with salt and chilli flakes.

Sprinkle with mozzarella and ⅔ cup Parmesan and toss to combine. Sprinkle with remaining Parmesan.

Transfer baking dish to the oven and bake for 25-30 minutes until beans are tender and cheese is melted.

CHICKEN NUGGETS

1 egg, whisked
6 tbsps avocado oil
1 cup (120g) almond meal
½ tsp salt
½ tsp garlic powder
1 tsp onion flakes
¼ tsp paprika
850g chicken breast or chicken thigh fillets

Mix the egg and 4 tablespoons oil together with a fork in a shallow dish.

In another shallow dish combine the almond meal, salt, garlic powder, onion flakes and paprika.

Cut the chicken breast or thigh fillets into nugget-sized pieces. Dip each piece first in the egg mixture then in the almond meal mixture and turn to coat fully.

Heat remaining avocado oil in a large frying pan over medium heat. Fry each chicken nugget for 4-6 minutes on both sides, until golden and cooked thoroughly in the centre.

Serve with sugar-free tomato sauce (see recipe on page 105) or garlic mayonnaise.

Prawn, Avocado & Cucumber Salad

SERVES 4

PREP + COOK TIME: 15 MINS

GLUTEN FREE • DAIRY FREE

2½ tbsps olive oil

600g prawn tails, peeled, deveined and patted dry

2 large avocados, diced

2 small Lebanese cucumbers, diced

1 large lime, juiced

1 medium red onion, finely chopped

⅓ cup (15g) fresh parsley leaves, roughly chopped

2 tbsps apple cider vinegar

Salt and pepper, to taste

Heat the oil in a large frying pan over medium heat. Fry the prawns in batches for 3 minutes until pink and cooked through. Remove to a large salad bowl.

Add the rest of the ingredients and gently toss to combine.

Season to taste and serve.

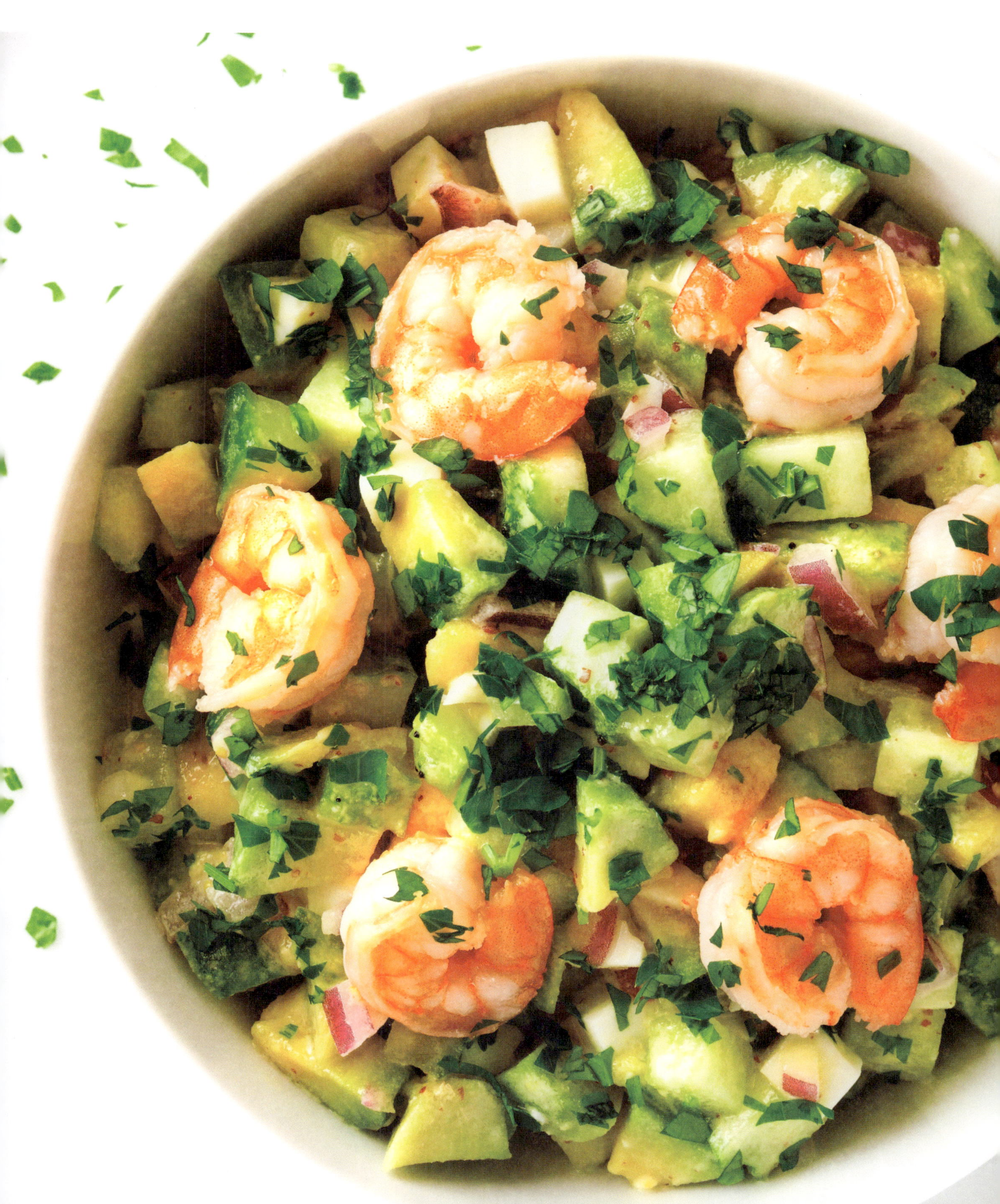

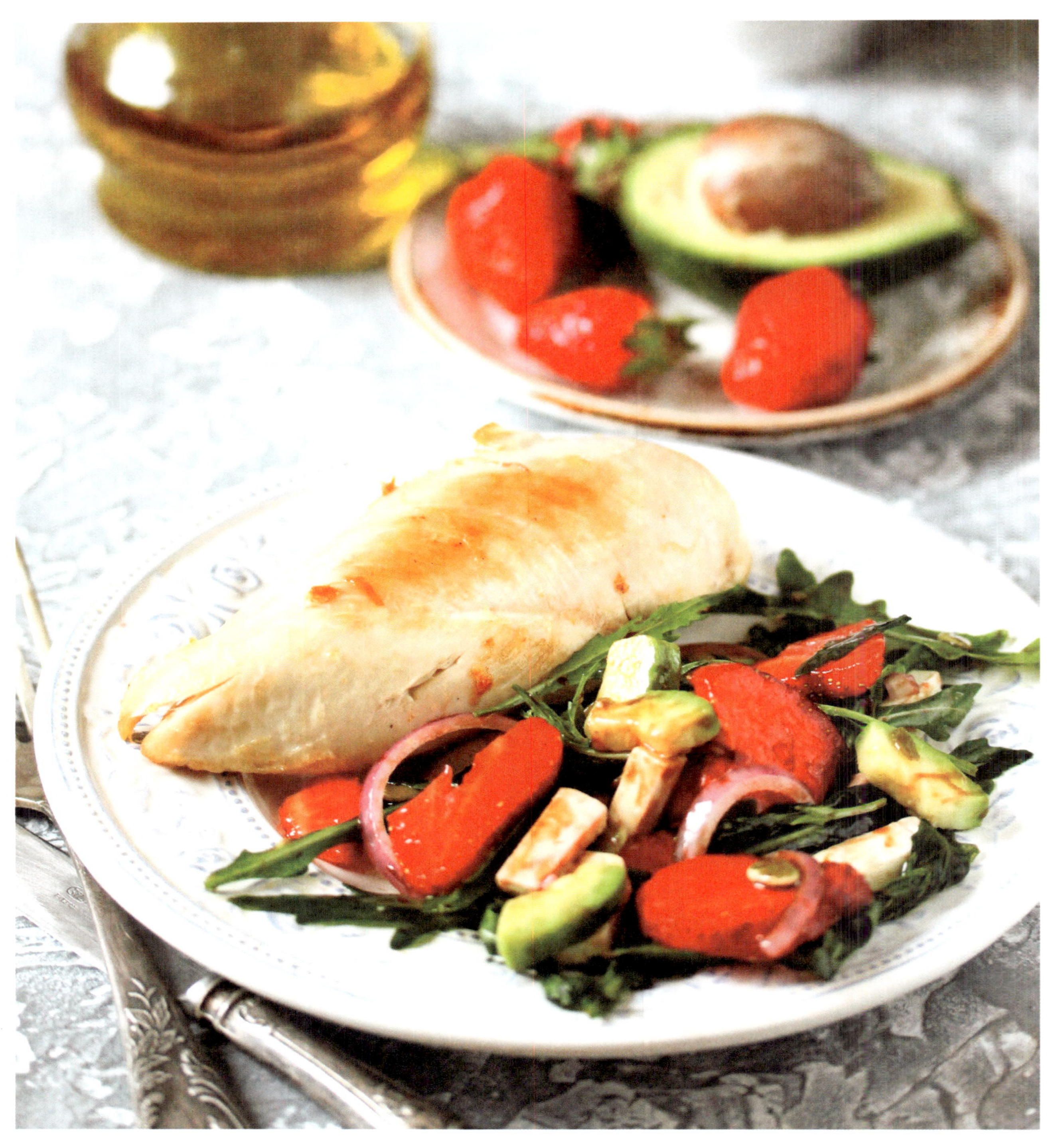

Chicken Strawberry Salad

SERVES 4
PREP + COOK TIME: 35 MINS
GLUTEN FREE

CHICKEN STRAWBERRY SALAD

4 chicken breasts
Salt and pepper to taste
1 tbsp olive oil
50g butter

SALAD

150g rocket leaves
1¼ cups (250g) strawberries, sliced
1 avocado, chopped
¼ red onion, sliced
100g feta cheese, cubed

DRESSING

2 tbsps olive oil
2 tsps balsamic vinegar

Preheat the oven to 180°C.

Season chicken breasts with salt and pepper.

Heat oil in a large ovenproof pan over a high heat, add chicken breasts and cook for 5 minutes or until golden. Flip over and add butter. Once melted, baste the chicken with the butter.

Place in the oven and cook for 15-20 minutes, until firm and white and the juices run clear. Set aside to rest.

Place the salad ingredients in a bowl. Combine oil and vinegar and drizzle over salad. Season with salt and pepper and toss to combine.

Serve each chicken breast with a portion of salad.

Lettuce Wedge Salad

SERVES 4
PREP + COOK TIME: 30 MINS
GLUTEN FREE

- 8 rashers bacon
- ¼ cup (50ml) buttermilk
- ¼ cup (50ml) sour cream
- ¼ cup (50g) mayonnaise
- 1 tsp lemon juice
- 75g blue cheese, crumbled
- Salt and pepper to taste
- 1 iceberg lettuce, washed and quartered
- ⅔ cup (150g) baby Roma tomatoes, halved
- ¼ red onion, thinly sliced
- 1 spring onion, chopped

Preheat oven to 200°C.

Place a wire rack on a baking tray and lay the bacon on top of the wire rack. Cook the bacon in the oven for 15-20 minutes until crispy.

Make the blue cheese dressing in a medium-sized bowl by combining the buttermilk, sour cream, mayonnaise, lemon juice and 50g of the blue cheese. Season with salt and pepper and whisk well. Refrigerate until ready to serve.

Place the lettuce quarters on four serving plates. Pour half the dressing over the lettuce wedges. Scatter over the tomatoes, red onion and spring onion. Crumble over the remaining blue cheese and the crispy bacon. Serve the rest of the dressing on the side.

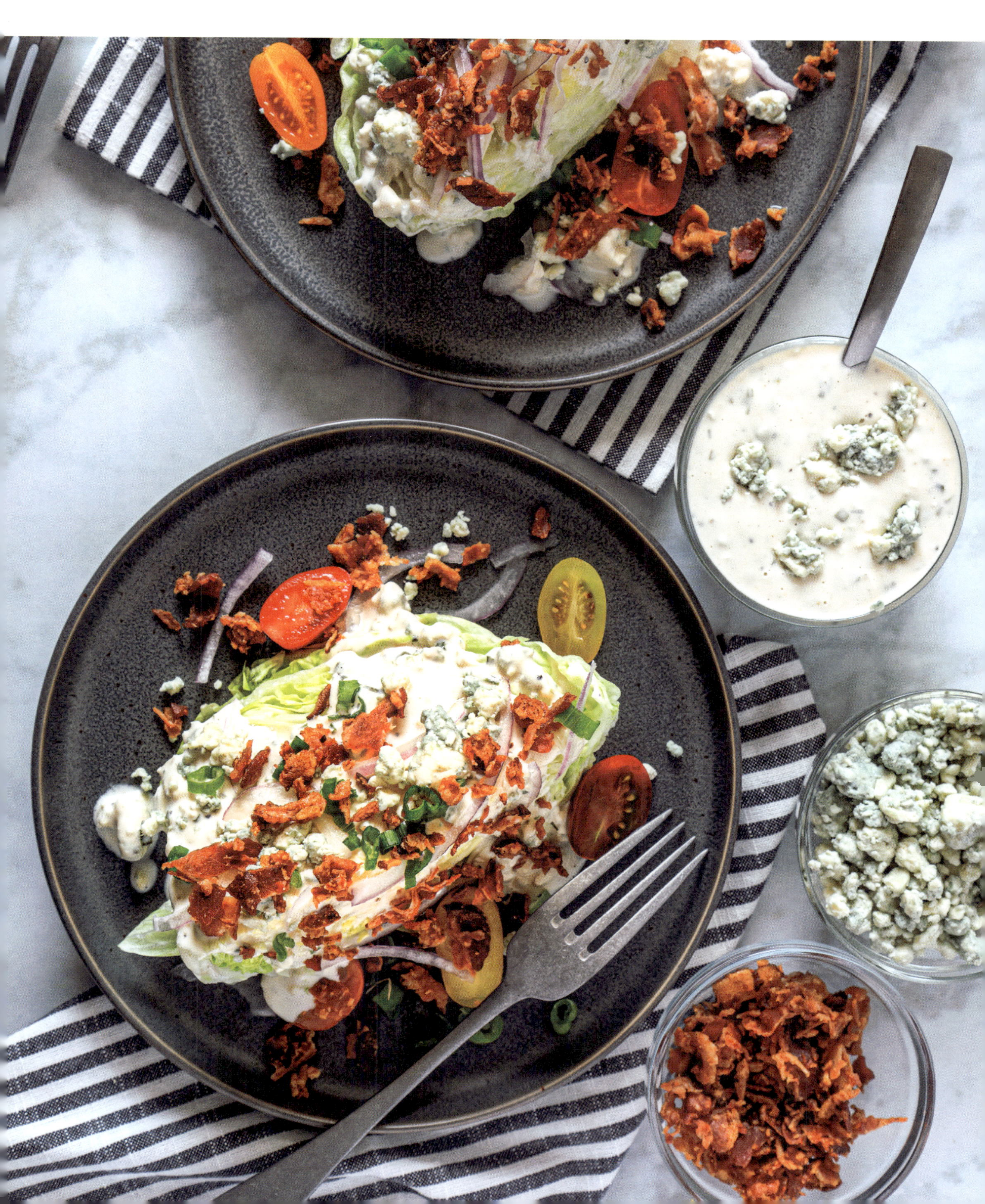

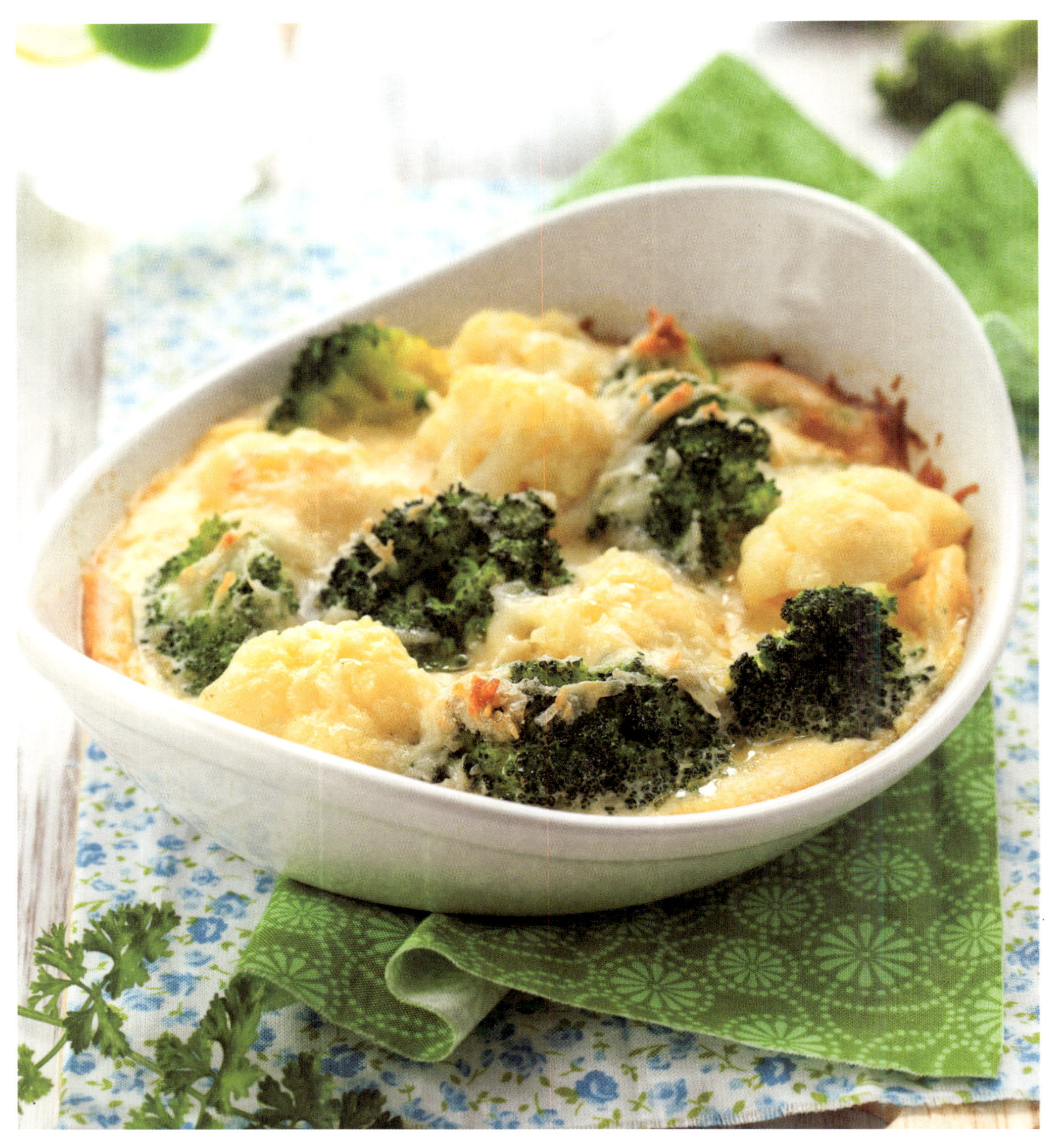

Broccoli & Cauliflower Bake

SERVES 6

PREP + COOK TIME: 45 MINS

VEG • GLUTEN FREE

BROCCOLI & CAULIFLOWER BAKE

1 medium head cauliflower, cut into florets
1 medium head broccoli, cut into florets
½ cup (125ml) sour cream
¼ cup (60ml) thickened cream
1⅔ cups (200g) grated sharp Cheddar cheese
½ cup (50g) grated Parmesan cheese
1 tsp Dijon mustard
1 tsp garlic powder
1 tsp paprika
Salt and pepper to taste

Preheat oven to 190°C.

Steam cauliflower for 5-6 minutes and broccoli for 3-4 minutes over a pan of simmering water until tender-crisp.

In a large bowl, combine sour cream, thickened cream, cheeses, mustard, garlic powder and paprika. Season with salt and pepper and stir to combine.

Add cauliflower and broccoli and mix well.

Pour mixture into a baking dish and spread into an even layer.

Cover the pan with foil and bake for 25-30 minutes. Remove the foil and bake for 5 minutes more.

Tip:

Try adding a little cooked bacon for some extra crispy saltiness.

Grilled Pork Kebabs

SERVES 4
PREP + COOK TIME: 30 MINS
GLUTEN FREE • DAIRY FREE

- 500g pork loin
- Salt and pepper to taste
- 1 tsp dried oregano
- 1 tsp smoked paprika
- Finely grated zest and juice of 2 lemons
- ¼ cup (60ml) olive oil
- 1 red capsicum
- 1 yellow capsicum
- Chopped parsley to serve

Cut pork into 3cm cubes and place in a large bowl.

Season with salt and pepper then sprinkle with oregano, paprika and lemon zest. Drizzle with olive oil. Toss to coat. Set aside for 10 minutes to marinate.

Cut capsicums into 3cm dice.

Thread pork and capsicum onto metal skewers.

Preheat a grill pan or barbecue over medium-low heat.

Cook for kebabs for 3-4 minutes each side until cooked through, drizzling occasionally with lemon juice as they cook.

Scatter with chopped parsley to serve.

Tip:

Add other vegetables such as mushrooms or zucchini to the kebabs if you wish.

Creamy Greek yoghurt flavoured with garlic is a great accompaniment.

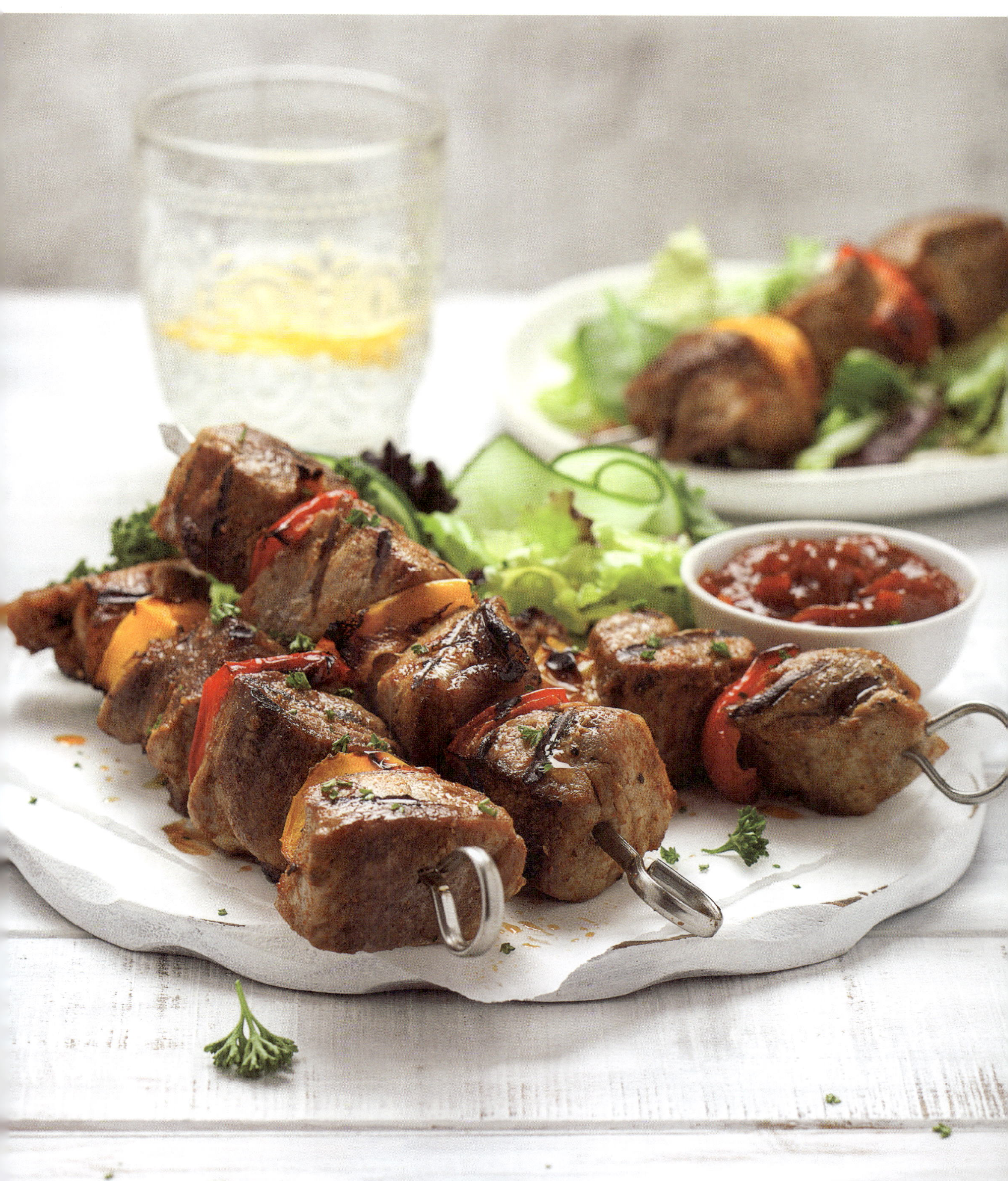

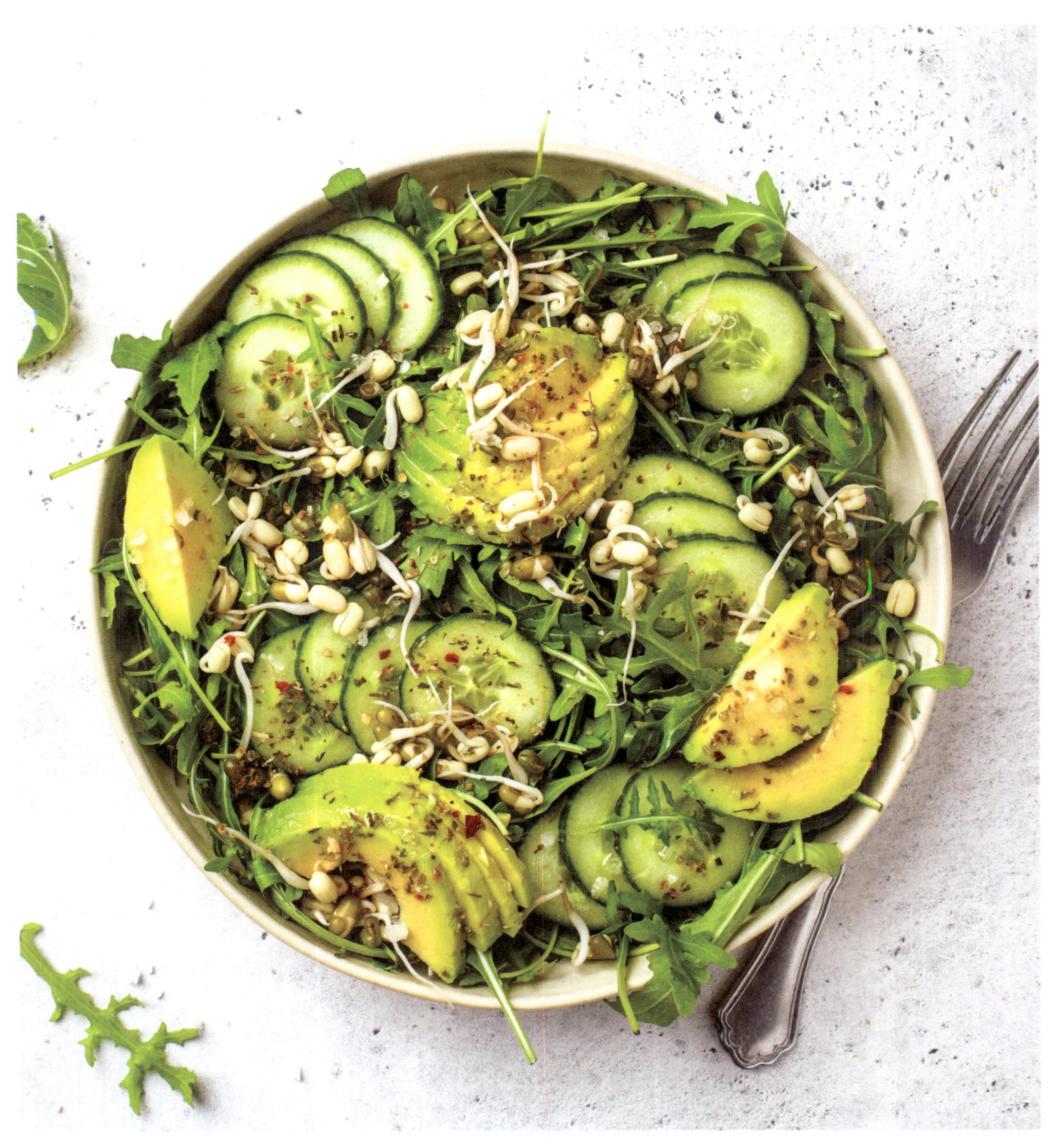

Avocado Sprout Salad

SERVES 4

PREP + COOK TIME: 10 MINS

VEG • GLUTEN FREE • DAIRY FREE

AVOCADO SPROUT SALAD

200g rocket leaves
2 Lebanese cucumbers, sliced
2 avocados, sliced
1 cup (110g) mung bean sprouts
¼ cup (60ml) olive oil
3 tbsps lemon juice
1 tsp dried mixed herbs
¼ tsp dried chilli flakes
Salt and pepper to taste

Divide the rocket leaves, cucumber, avocados and bean sprouts between four bowls.

Combine the remaining ingredients in a small bowl or sealable jar with a lid. Stir or shake to combine.

Drizzle dressing over the salad and serve immediately

CREAMY COCONUT PRAWNS

500g prawns, peeled and deveined
Salt and pepper to taste
1 tbsp olive oil
2 tbsps butter
6 cloves garlic, minced
½ cup (125ml) chicken stock
1½ cups (375ml) cream
½ cup (50g) freshly grated Parmesan cheese

Season the prawns with salt and pepper.

Heat the oil in a large frying pan over medium-high heat. Cook the prawns for 1-2 minutes each side until just turned pink. Remove from the heat, and set aside in a covered bowl.

Melt the butter in the same pan. Fry the garlic, stirring for about 1 minute. Pour in the chicken stock and allow the sauce to reduce by about half. Stir occasionally, scraping off any bits from the base of the pan.

Reduce heat to medium-low. Pour in the cream and bring to a gentle simmer, stirring occasionally. Season with salt and pepper to taste.

Add the cheese and gently simmer for a further 2 minutes until cheese melts and the sauce has thickened.

Return the prawns to the pan. Season with salt and pepper, stir and serve.

HERBED CAULIFLOWER RICE

1 medium zucchini, finely grated
1 medium head of cauliflower, broken into small florets
2½ tbsps coconut oil
1 small onion, finely chopped
1 small carrot, finely grated
2½ tbsps mixed dried herbs
⅓ cup (15g) fresh parsley leaves, finely chopped
Salt and pepper to taste

Place the grated zucchini in a clean tea towel and squeeze to remove excess liquid. Set aside.

Place the cauliflower florets in a food processor and pulse until the cauliflower resembles grains of rice. You may need to do this in batches.

Heat the oil in a large wok over medium heat. Add the onion and fry for 2 minutes. Add the carrot, zucchini and herbs and fry for 2 more minutes.

Add the cauliflower and parsley and stir-fry for 3 minutes until the cauliflower is cooked through.

Season to taste and serve warm.

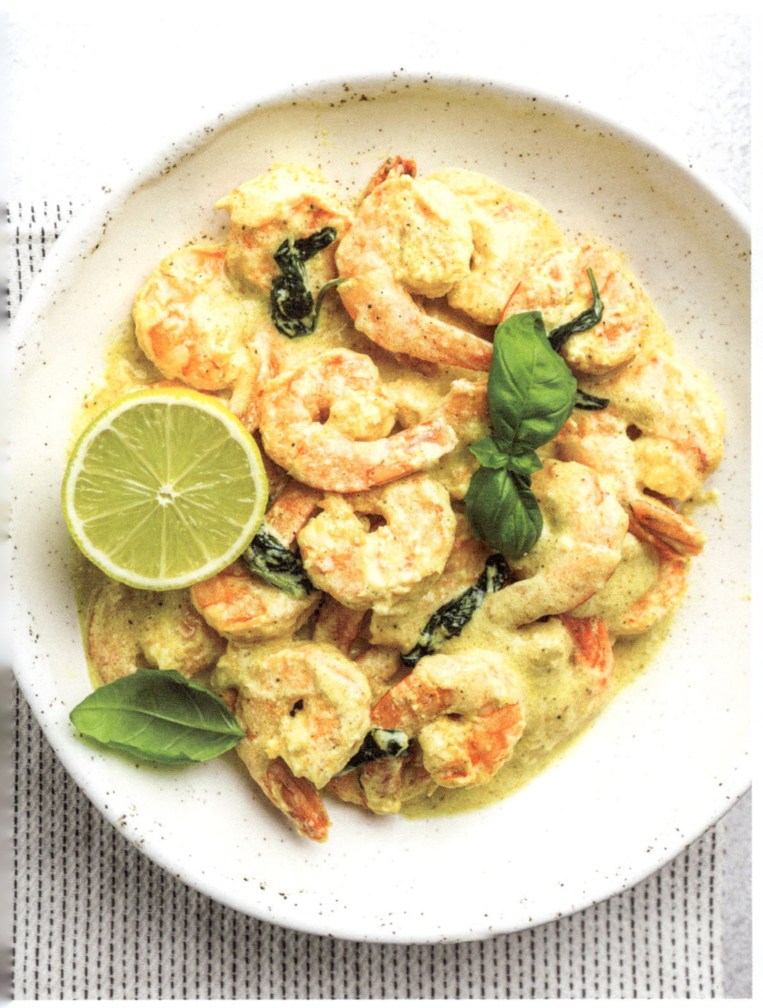

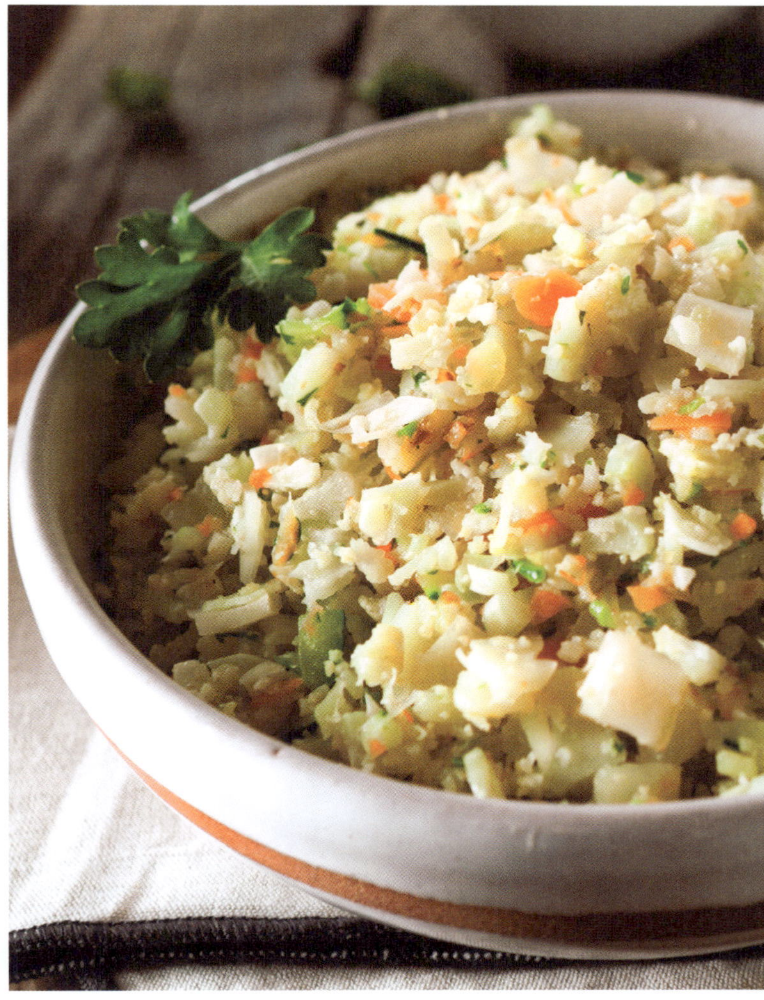

Creamy Coconut Prawns

SERVES 4

PREP + COOK TIME: 20 MINS

GLUTEN FREE

Herbed Cauliflower Rice

SERVES 4

PREP + COOK TIME: 20 MINS

VEG • GLUTEN FREE • DAIRY FREE

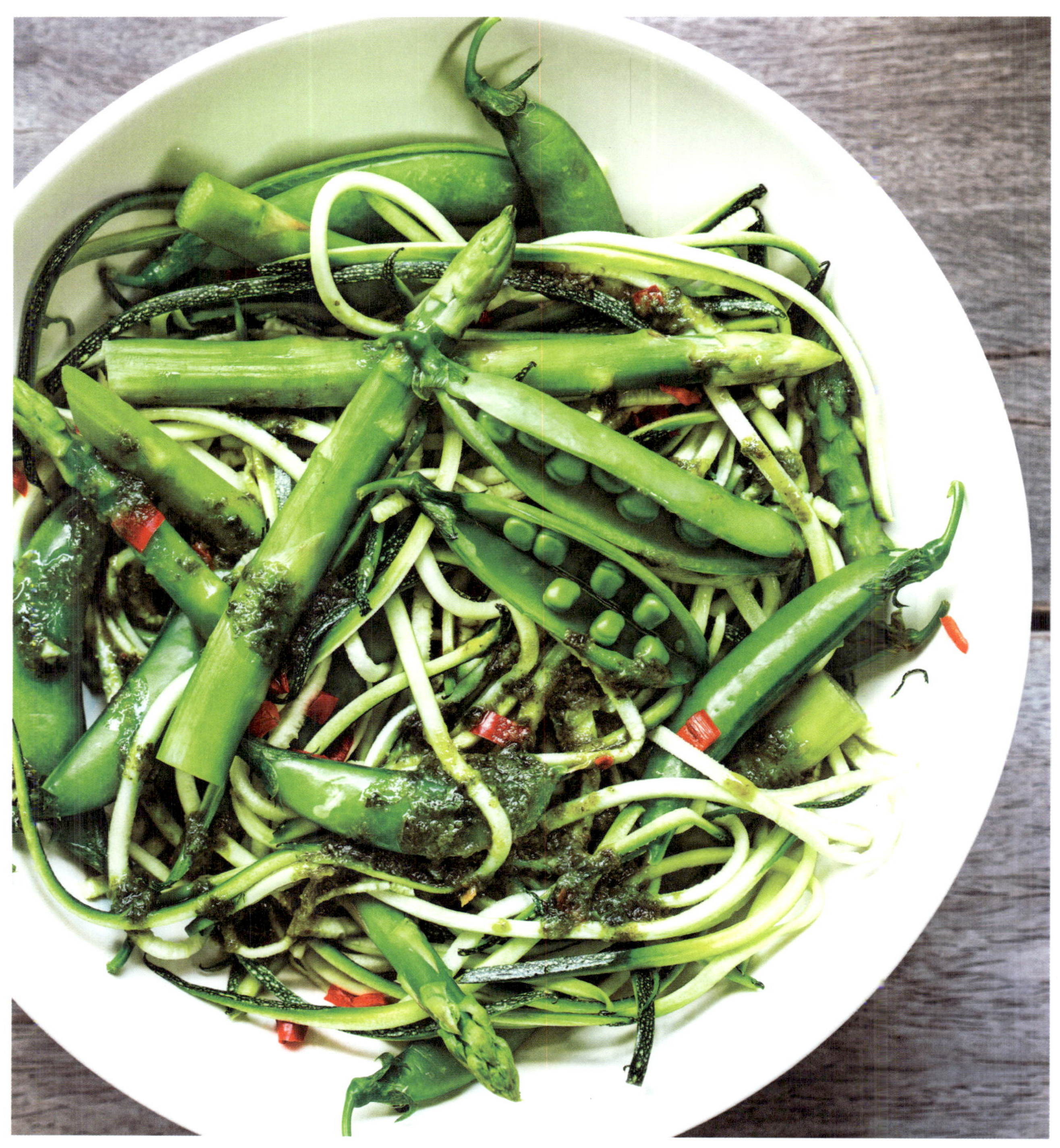

Green Zoodle Pasta with Chilli & Basil Dressing

SERVES 4

PREP + COOK TIME: 30 MINS

VEG • GLUTEN FREE • DAIRY FREE

GREEN ZOODLE PASTA WITH CHILLI & BASIL DRESSING

6 large zucchinis, ends trimmed, cut into thin noodle strands
Salt and pepper to taste
4 cups (60g) fresh basil leaves, roughly torn
3 small cloves garlic, crushed
⅓ cup (100ml) + 2½ tbsps olive oil
16 large asparagus spears, ends trimmed, cut into 3cm lengths
500g sugar snap peas
2 large red chillies, seeds removed, finely chopped

Place the zucchini noodles in a large colander and gently toss with 1 teaspoon salt. Let drain for 30 minutes, then gently squeeze to remove excess liquid.

Place the basil and garlic in a food processor and pulse a few times, then drizzle in the ⅓ cup oil and blend until you have a thin basil sauce. Season to taste and set aside.

Heat the remaining oil in a large, deep-sided frying pan over medium heat. Fry the zucchini noodles for 2 minutes then remove to a large bowl.

Steam the asparagus and sugar snap peas for 2 minutes until tender. Add to the noodles.

Gently toss the noodles and vegetables with the basil sauce and chillies.

Serve warm.

Tip:

Due to the sugar snap pea content, this recipe may not be suitable for those on a very low-carb diet.

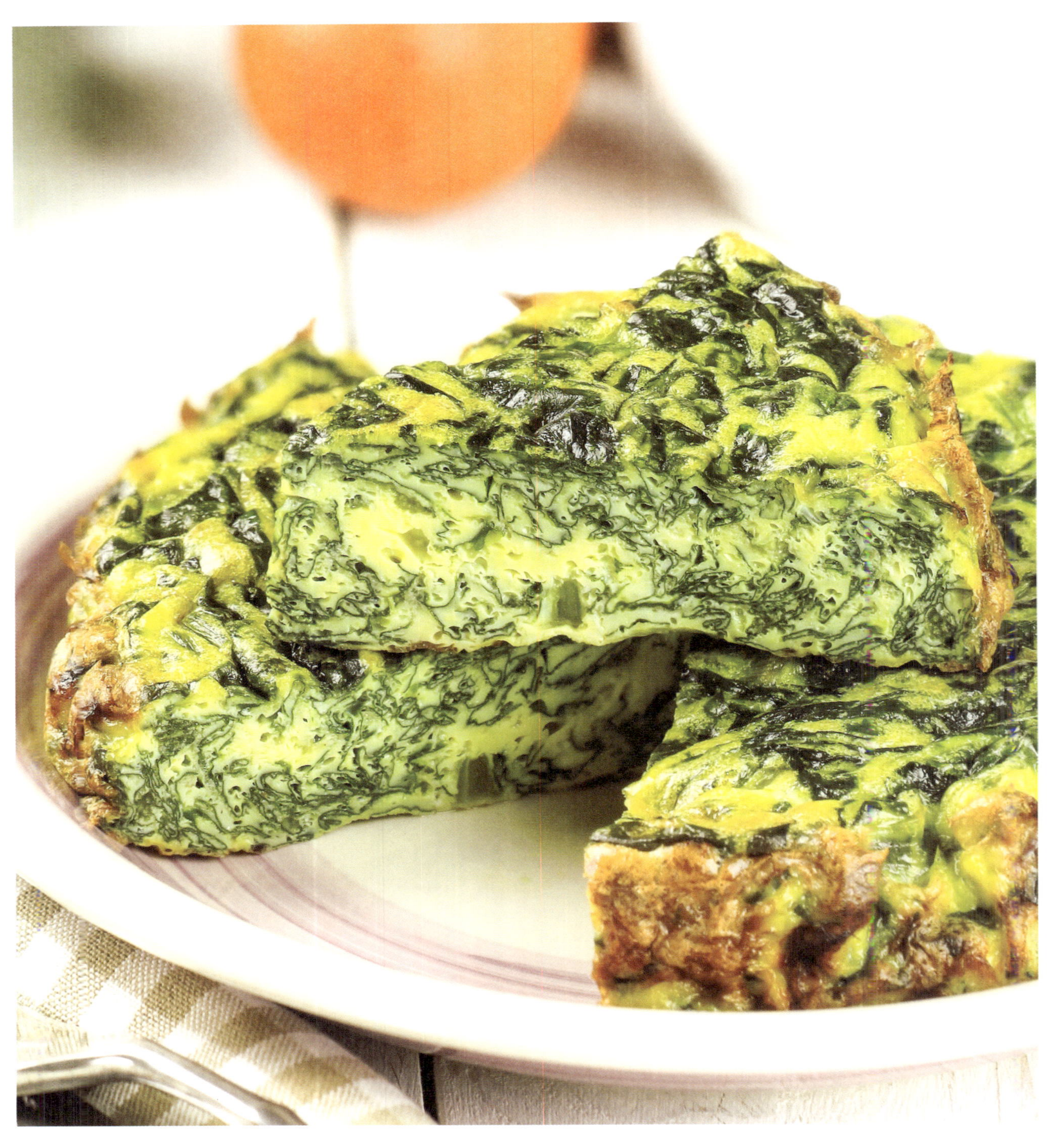

Spinach Frittata

SERVES 4

PREP + COOK TIME: 35 MINS

VEG • GLUTEN FREE

SPINACH FRITTATA

2 tbsps olive oil
1 onion, thinly sliced
150g baby spinach
Salt and pepper to taste
8 large eggs
⅓ cup (80ml) thickened cream
¾ cup (90g) grated Cheddar cheese
½ cup (50g) grated Parmesan cheese
¼ cup (10g) chopped fresh basil

Preheat the oven to 160°C.

Heat the oil in a large ovenproof frying pan over medium heat. Add the onion and cook, stirring frequently, for 3-5 minutes until soft and translucent. Add half of the spinach and cook for 1 minute until wilted, then add the remaining spinach and continue cooking for a further minute until all of the spinach is wilted. Season with salt and pepper.

In a large bowl, whisk together the eggs, cream, cheeses and basil. Season with salt and pepper. Add the egg mixture to the cooked spinach mixture, and stir to combine. Transfer the pan to the centre of the oven and bake for 20 minutes until set.

Use a rubber spatula to loosen the edges and slide the frittata onto a serving platter. Slice into wedges and serve.

Chapter Four

Dinner

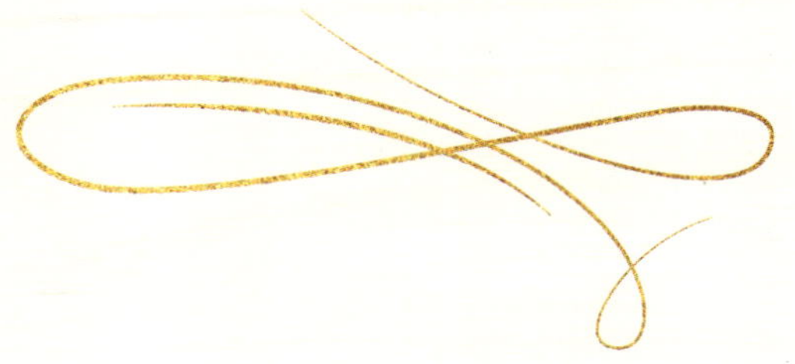

Broccoli, Mozzarella & Mushroom Pizza on Spinach Crust

SERVES 4

PREP + COOK TIME: 1 HOUR

VEG • GLUTEN FREE

1 tbsp coconut oil
150g spinach leaves, roughly chopped
½ cup (50g) grated Parmesan cheese
½ cup (60g) almond meal
¾ cup (75g) coconut flour
2 tsps baking powder
Salt and pepper to taste
1 large egg, beaten
1 cup (75g) broccoli florets
100g button mushrooms, halved and sliced
1¼ cups (150g) grated mozzarella cheese

Preheat oven to 180°C.

Heat 1 teaspoon of the oil in a large frying pan and cook the spinach for 3 minutes until wilted. Place in a colander and press to remove excess liquid. Place in a blender and puree until smooth.

Transfer to a large bowl and mix thoroughly with the Parmesan, almond meal, flour, baking powder, a pinch each of salt and pepper, egg and remaining coconut oil.

Line a large, flat baking tray with baking paper and smooth out the mixture into a pizza base around 1cm thick. Bake for 25 minutes, then remove and let cool for 10 minutes.

Steam the broccoli for 5 minutes until just tender. Chop and scatter over the pizza base, then add the mushrooms and the mozzarella.

Bake for 20 minutes until the cheese is golden and bubbling.

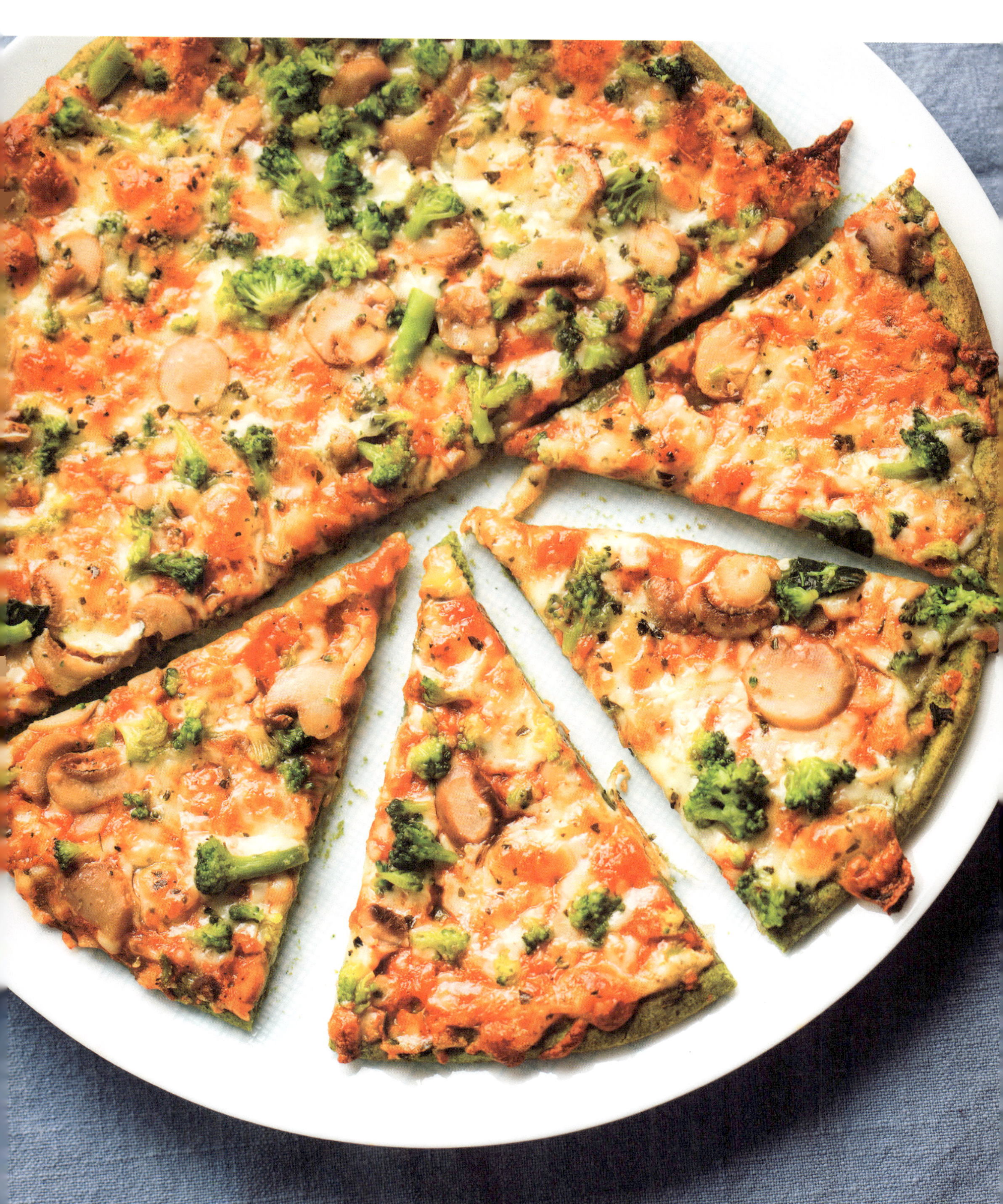

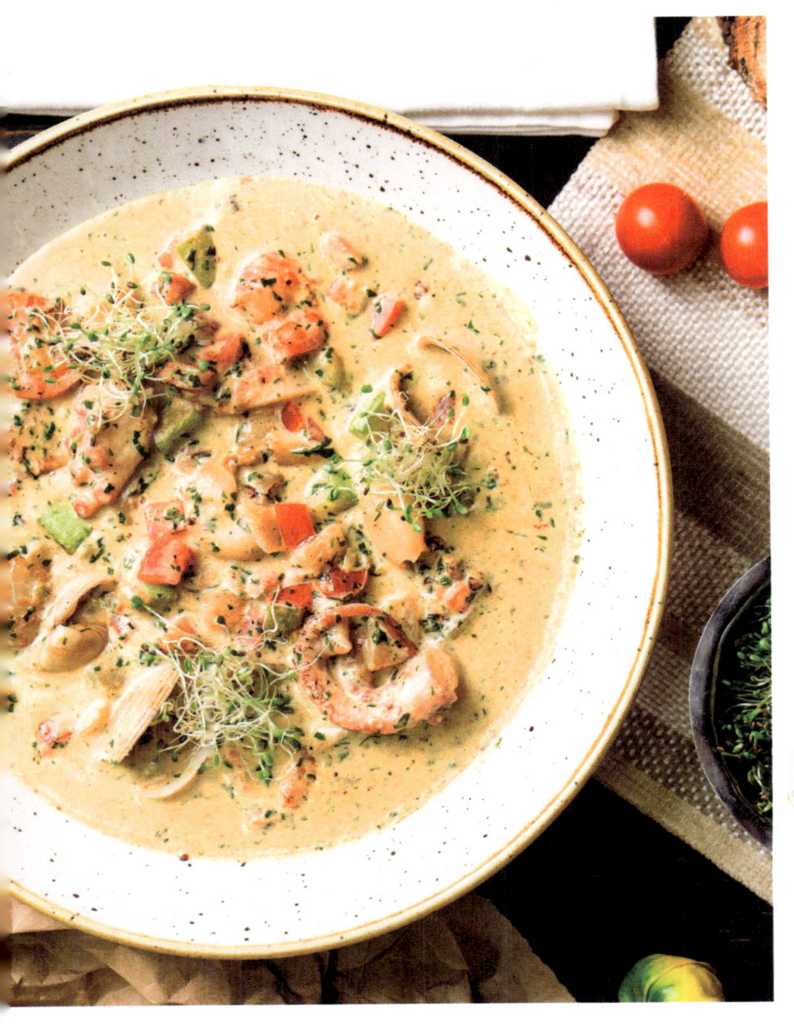

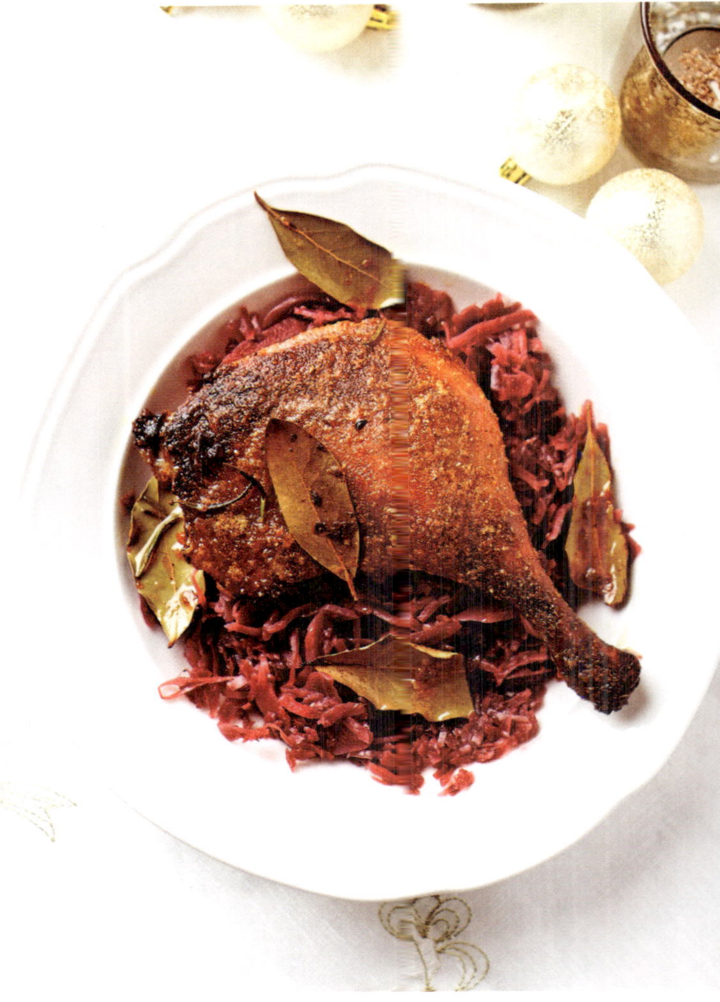

Creamy Seafood Chowder

SERVES 4
PREP + COOK TIME: 50 MINS
GLUTEN FREE

Roasted Duck with Red Cabbage

SERVES 4
PREP + COOK TIME: 3 HOURS 5 MINS + MARINATING
GLUTEN FREE

CREAMY SEAFOOD CHOWDER

100g butter
1 large onion, finely chopped
¾ cup (75g) celery, chopped
4 cups (1L) chicken stock (or fish stock)
800g mixed seafood, prawns, scallops, octopus, clams
1 cup (200g) tomato, chopped
1 cup (250ml) cream
Salt and pepper to taste
1 cup (100g) alfalfa sprouts, to garnish

Heat the butter in a large pot over medium heat. Fry the onion and celery for 5 minutes until the onion is softened.

Add the stock and bring to a boil. Reduce to a simmer and add the seafood.

Simmer for 20 minutes, then add the tomatoes and simmer for a further 10 minutes.

Stir through the cream and heat without boiling.

Season to taste and serve garnished with alfalfa sprouts, if desired.

ROASTED DUCK WITH RED CABBAGE

4 duck Marylands (or legs)
1 tbsp orange zest
1 tbsp rosemary leaves
2 small cloves garlic, crushed
Salt and pepper to taste
1 tbsp butter
½ red cabbage, shredded
4-6 bay leaves
Pinch of stevia powder
¼ cup (60ml) balsamic vinegar

Place the duck legs on a roasting tray. Mix together the zest, rosemary, half the garlic and ½ teaspoon each of salt and pepper and rub into the duck legs. Let sit in the refrigerator for at least 2 hours.

To make the cabbage, heat the butter in a large, deep-sided frying pan over medium heat. Add the cabbage in batches and saute for 10 minutes. Add the bay leaves, the remaining garlic, stevia and vinegar and stir through.

Reduce the heat to low and cook for 40 minutes. Season to taste and set aside.

Preheat oven to 140°C. Roast the duck for 2 hours, basting with the duck fat as needed. After 2 hours, turn the temperature up to 220°C for 15 minutes to crisp the skin.

Serve the duck on top of the cabbage.

Lemon Garlic Chicken

SERVES 2
PREP + COOK TIME: 50 MINS
GLUTEN FREE

500g chicken breast or thighs
Salt and pepper to taste
2 tbsps olive oil
1 tbsp butter
6 cloves garlic, whole
2 cups (500ml) chicken stock
2 lemons; 1 sliced, 1 juiced
½ cup (125ml) cream
1 sprig rosemary, broken into pieces.
1 tsp whole black peppercorns

Preheat oven to 170°C.

Season the chicken with salt and pepper.

Heat olive oil in an ovenproof pan over medium heat. Add the chicken and sear both sides until golden brown, about 2-3 minutes per side. Remove and set aside.

While the chicken is resting, melt the butter in the same pan, over medium-low heat. Add garlic and cook, stirring, for about 2 minutes until fragrant.

Stir in chicken stock, lemon juice and cream.

Bring to a boil then reduce heat to a gentle simmer. Cook, stirring occasionally, for 5-7 minutes until the sauce has thickened slightly.

Return the chicken to the pan. Decorate with lemon slices, rosemary sprigs and peppercorns.

Cover and transfer to oven. Cook for 25-30 minutes until the chicken is cooked through.

Allow to rest for 5 minutes before serving

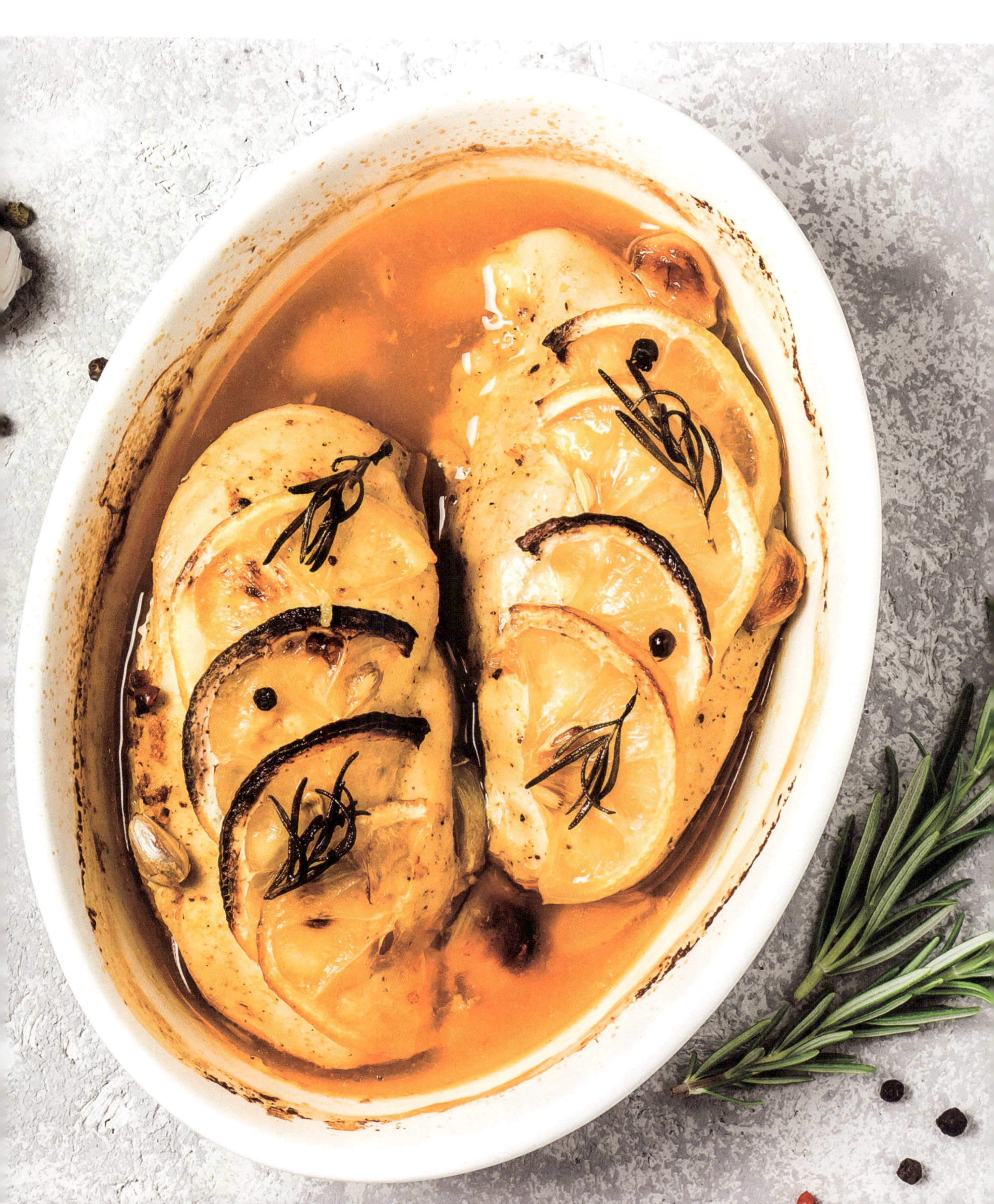

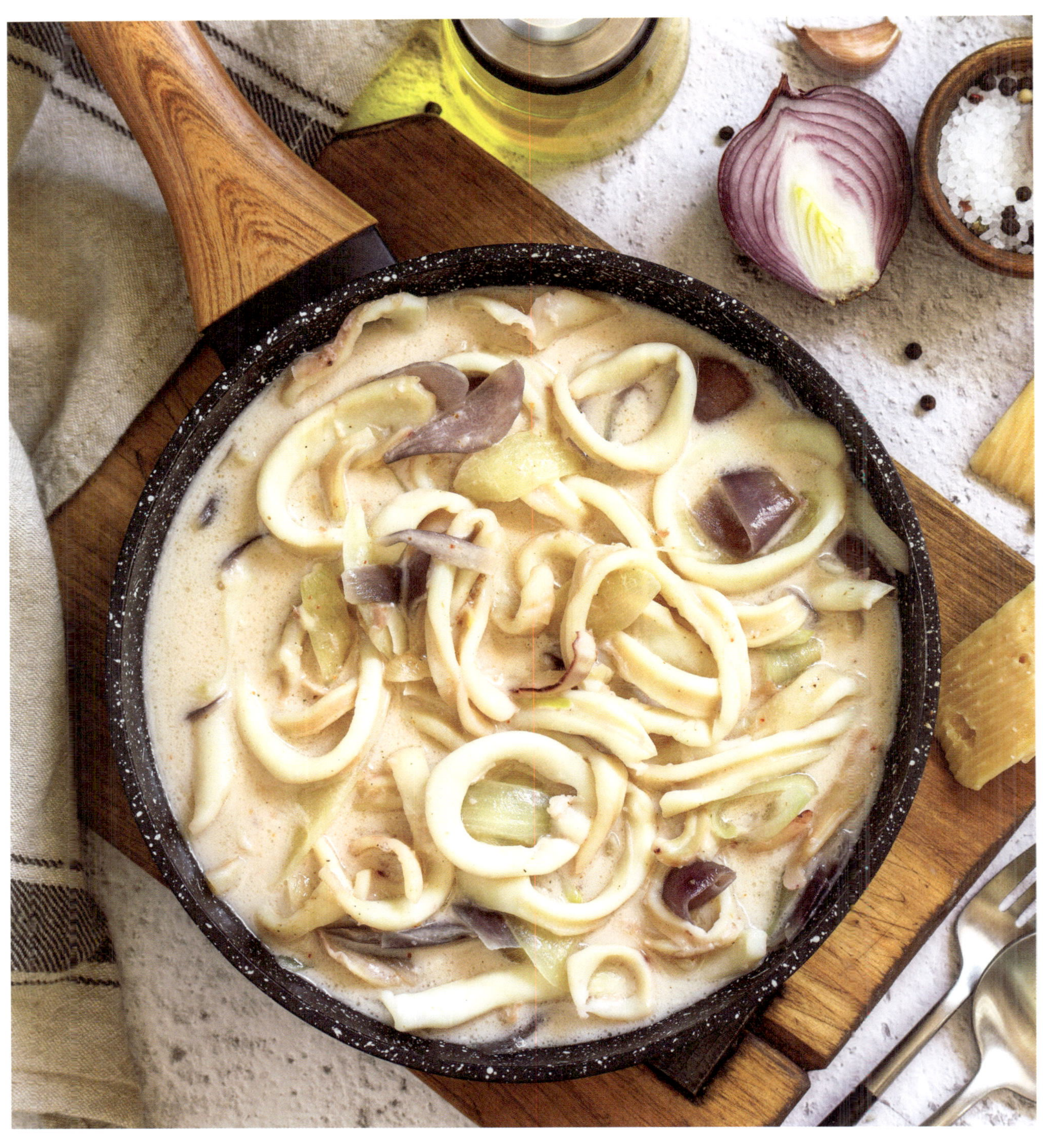

Sour Cream Squid

SERVES 4

PREP + COOK TIME: 30 MINS

GLUTEN FREE

SOUR CREAM SQUID

3 tbsps butter
1 small red onion, sliced
2 cloves garlic, minced
400g fresh squid rings
1 tsp ground cumin
Salt and pepper to taste
⅔ cup (150ml) sour cream
½ cup (60g) grated mature Cheddar cheese

Heat 2 tablespoons butter in a large frying pan over medium heat.

Add onion and cook for 5-7 minutes until soft and translucent. Add garlic and cook for 1 minute until fragrant. Reduce the heat to low. Add the remaining tablespoon butter and the squid rings.

Cook for 3-4 minutes, stirring occasionally, until the squid is opaque. Add cumin and a pinch of salt and stir to combine. Add sour cream and cheese and simmer for 3 minutes until the cheese is melted.

Do not overcook or the squid will become tough. Season with salt and pepper to serve.

VEAL IN TUNA CAPER SAUCE

20g butter

8-12 (600g) veal schnitzels (uncrumbed and thinly sliced)

SAUCE

1 x 100g can tuna in olive oil, drained

60g capers + more to garnish

4 anchovy fillets

4 egg yolks

1 lemon, juiced

Pepper to taste

⅔ cup (150ml) olive oil

SALAD

Handful of rocket leaves

½ cup (100g) cherry tomatoes, chopped

1 tbsp olive oil

Place tuna, capers, anchovies, egg yolks, lemon juice and pepper in a food processor and blitz for 30 seconds. Turn food processor to lowest speed and add olive oil, slowly, in a single stream. Set aside.

Heat the butter in a large frying pan over medium-high heat. Cook the veal for 2-3 minutes each side. Cook in batches as needed and keep warm.

Pour the sauce over the veal. Top with rocket and tomatoes, decorate with capers and drizzle with olive oil to serve.

SEARED TUNA STEAKS

1½ tsps salt

1 tsp ground coriander

½ tsp paprika

¼ tsp cayenne pepper

4 x 150g sushi-grade tuna steaks

4 tbsps fresh coarsely ground pepper

2 tbsps olive oil

In a small bowl, combine the salt, coriander, paprika and cayenne pepper.

Lay the tuna steaks out on a plate and sprinkle the spice mixture evenly on both sides.

Then coat the tuna on both sides with the pepper and gently press it in so that it sticks to the surface.

Place a heavy-bottomed frying pan over medium-high heat, until very hot.

Add the oil and sear the tuna steaks for about 2 minutes per side, or until desired doneness is reached.

Serve with a green salad.

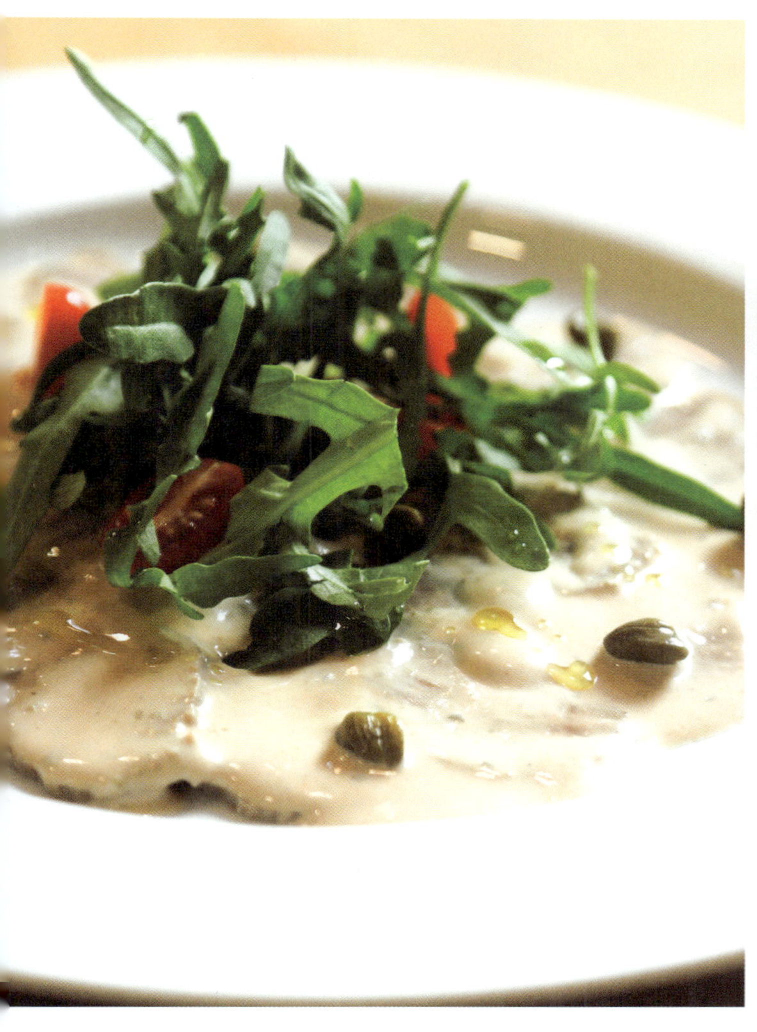

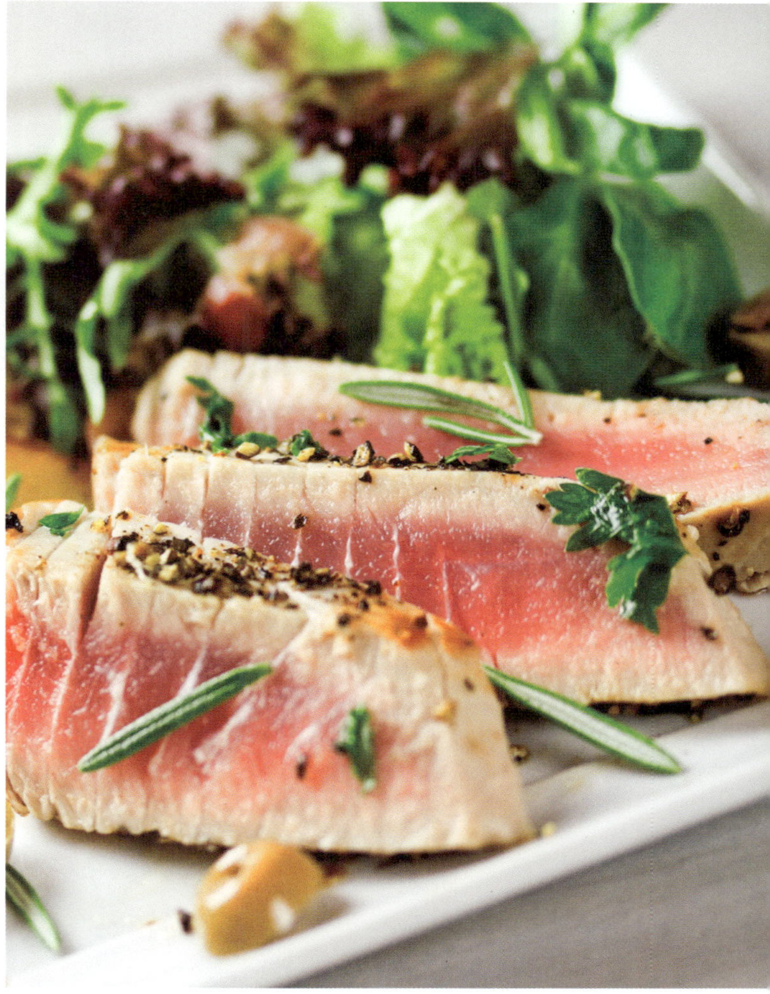

Veal in Tuna Caper Sauce

SERVES 4

PREP + COOK TIME: 30 MINS

GLUTEN FREE • DAIRY FREE

Seared Tuna Steaks

SERVES 4

PREP + COOK TIME: 10 MINS

GLUTEN FREE • DAIRY FREE

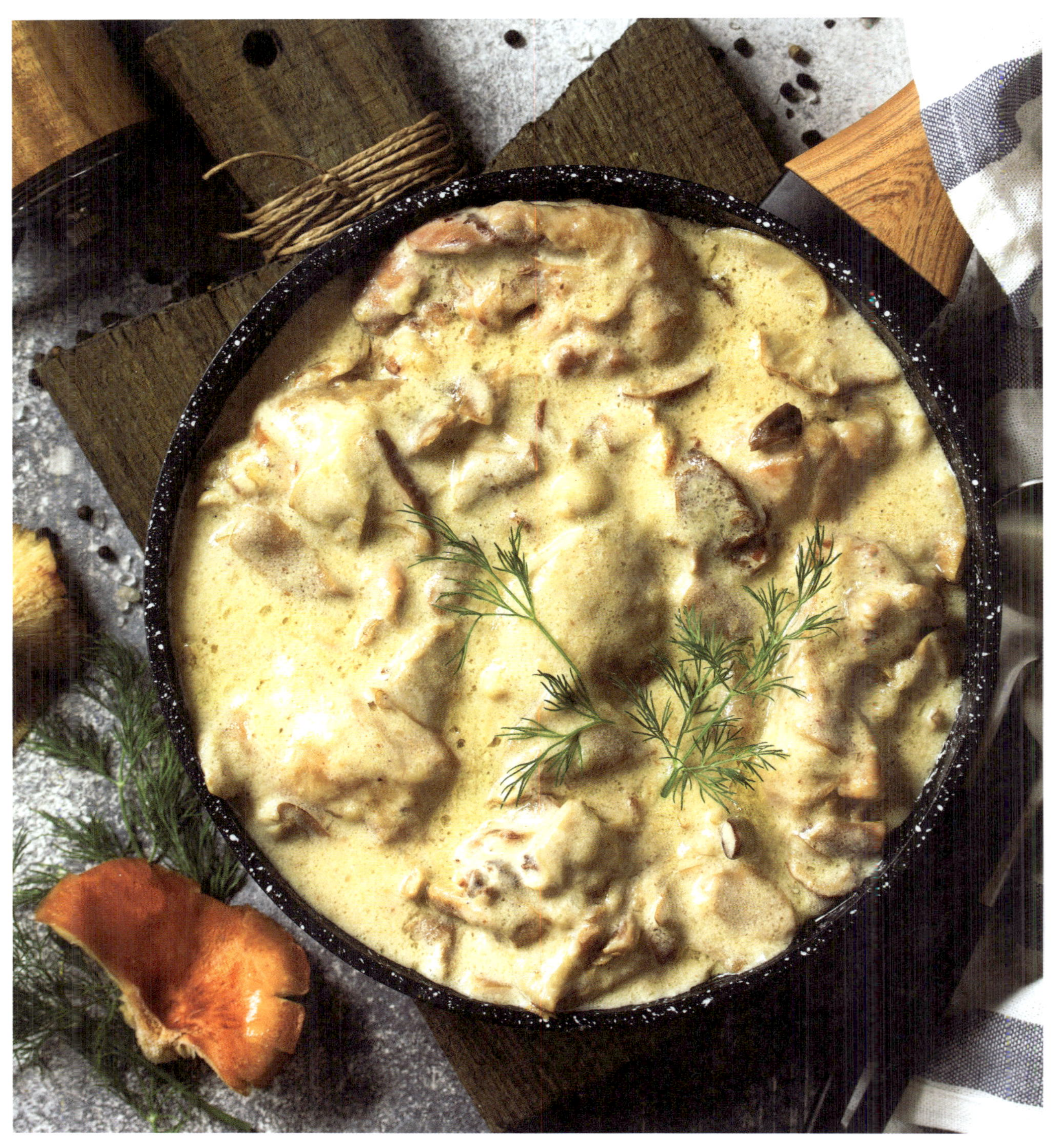

Chicken Fricassee

SERVES 6

PREP + COOK TIME: 45 MINS

GLUTEN FREE

CHICKEN FRICASSEE

1 tbsp olive oil
1kg chicken thighs or legs
1 small onion, chopped
1 carrot, finely diced
1 stalk celery, finely chopped
2 cloves garlic, minced
150g mushrooms, sliced
1 tsp dried thyme
½ cup (125ml) dry white wine
1 cup (250ml) chicken stock
½ cup (125ml) thickened cream
¼ cup (25g) grated Parmesan cheese
Salt and pepper to taste

Heat the oil in a large pan over medium heat. Season the chicken all over with salt and pepper. Brown the chicken pieces for about 4 minutes per side until golden. Transfer to a plate and set aside.

In the same pan, saute the onion, carrot, celery and garlic for 5-7 minutes until the onion is soft and translucent.

Add the sliced mushrooms and thyme, then cook for another 2-3 minutes until the mushrooms begin to soften.

Add the white wine, scraping up the brown bits from the bottom of the pan with a spatula. Allow the wine to bubble for 3 minutes then pour in the chicken stock and cream. Stir through the Parmesan and season with salt and pepper to taste.

Return the chicken to the pan and simmer for about 15 minutes until the chicken is completely cooked through and the sauce is thickened.

Chicken Broccoli Casserole

SERVES 8
PREP + COOK TIME: 45 MINS
GLUTEN FREE

500g broccoli, cut into florets
1 x 700g roast chicken, meat shredded
250g cream cheese
¾ cup (185ml) thickened cream
½ cup (125ml) milk
1 tbsp Dijon mustard
1 tsp garlic powder
½ tsp salt
¼ tsp pepper
¼ cup (10g) chopped fresh parsley
1 cup (125g) grated Cheddar cheese

Preheat oven to 200°C.

Place a saucepan of water over high heat and bring to a boil. Add the broccoli florets and cook for 2 minutes until al dente. Drain well and add to a large mixing bowl along with the shredded chicken.

In a small saucepan, add the cream cheese, cream, milk, mustard, garlic powder, salt and pepper and place over low heat. Whisk until the sauce is smooth. Pour the warm sauce into the broccoli and chicken mixture, add the parsley, and mix well. Pour the mixture into a casserole dish and top with grated cheese.

Bake in the oven for 20-30 minutes, until bubbling and golden brown.

Allow to cool for 5 minutes before serving.

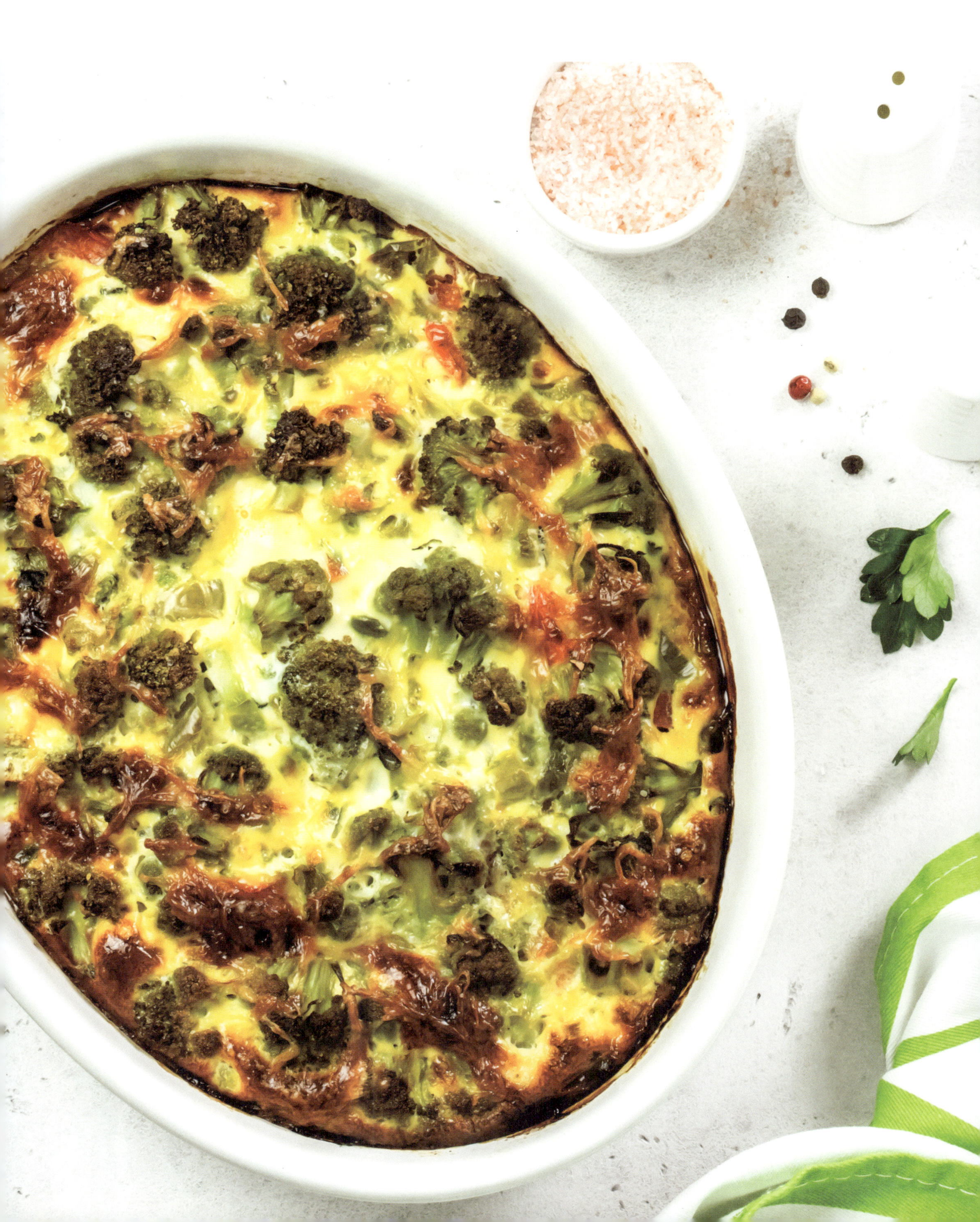

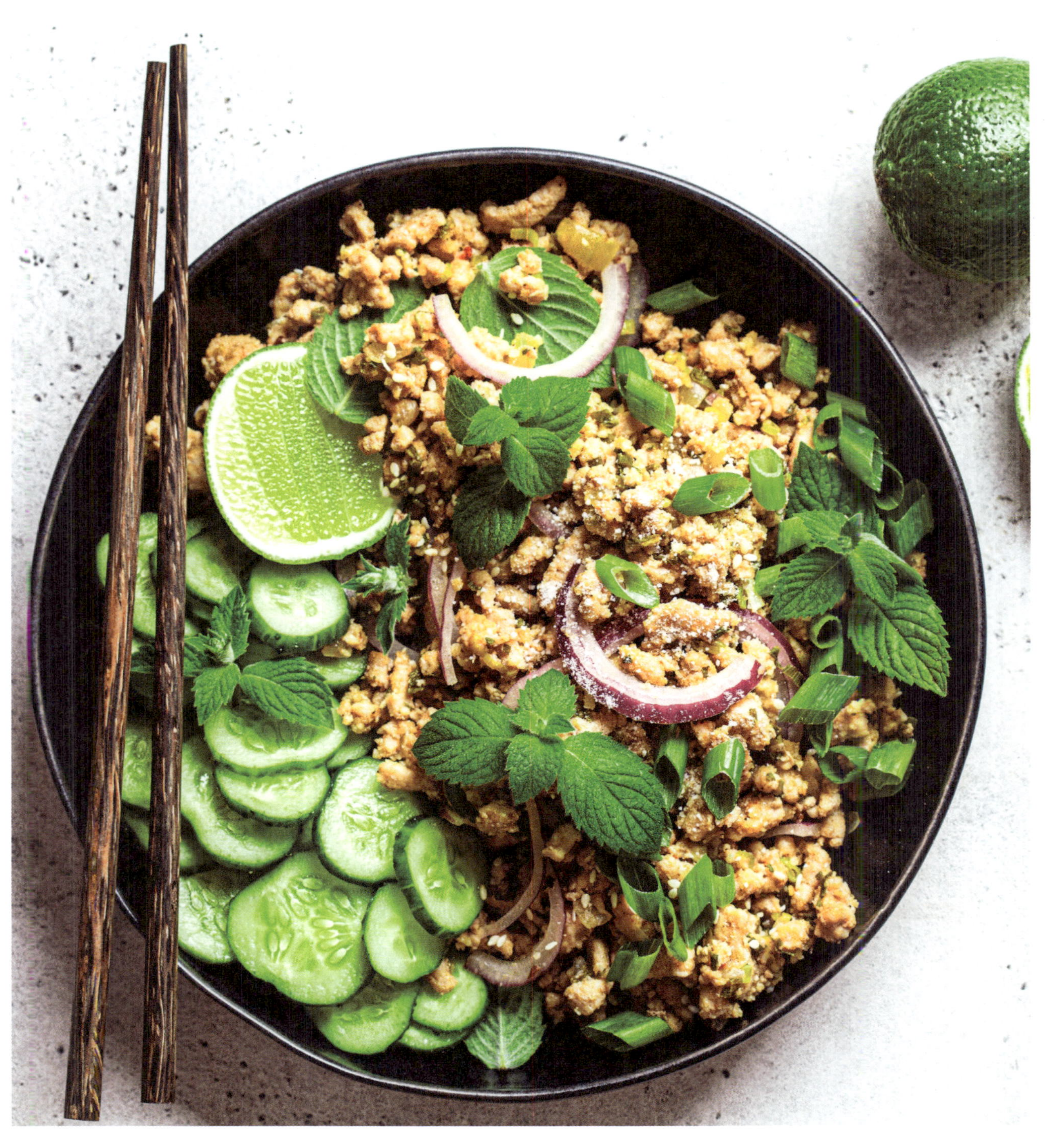

Chicken Larb Bowls

SERVES 4

PREP + COOK TIME: 20 MINS

GLUTEN FREE • DAIRY FREE

CHICKEN LARB BOWLS

2 tbsps sesame seeds

1 tbsp cooking oil

¼ red onion, sliced (reserve some for garnish)

2 spring onions, thinly sliced (reserve some for garnish)

2 tbsps fish sauce

1 tbsp water

500g chicken mince

2 tbsps sesame oil

1 tbsp ground lemongrass

3 small cloves garlic, crushed

1 tsp ground galangal (substitute with ground ginger if needed)

1 lime, juiced

½ cup (10g) fresh mint leaves + extra sprigs to garnish

Cucumber slices to serve

Lime wedges to serve

Place a large saucepan over medium heat. Add the sesame seeds and toast until evenly golden. Using a spice grinder (or mortar and pestle) grind the seeds to a fine breadcrumb consistency. Set aside.

Heat the pan again, this time over high heat, and add the cooking oil. When hot add the red onion and spring onion and saute for 2 minutes. Add the fish sauce, water and chicken mince. Break up the chicken with a wooden spoon, and saute for 3-5 minutes until cooked through but not brown.

Add the sesame oil, lemongrass and garlic to the pan and stir to combine well. Cook for a further minute before removing the pan from the heat.

Stir through the galangal and lime juice. Allow the mixture to cool for about 5 minutes before adding the mint and ground sesame seeds. Mix well.

Spoon the mixture evenly into bowls and serve with cucumber slices, reserved red and spring onions, fresh lime and mint sprigs.

SHREDDED CHILLI BEEF

1.2kg beef chuck steak, cut into 10cm pieces
Salt and pepper to taste
2 tbsps olive oil
2 onions, finely chopped
2 cloves garlic, finely chopped
2 tsps ground cumin
1½ tsps smoked paprika
1 tsp ground allspice
2 cups (450g) passata
1½ cups (375ml) water
1 red chilli, deseeded and chopped
1 tbsp dried red chillies
3 dried bay leaves
Parsley, chopped, to serve

Season beef with salt and pepper. Heat oil in a large pan or casserole over high heat. Cook beef for 3 minutes each side or until golden. Transfer to a plate.

Reduce heat to medium-low. Add onion and cook, stirring, for 10 minutes. Add garlic, cumin, paprika and allspice and cook, stirring, for 30 seconds or until fragrant. Add passata, water, fresh and dried chillies and bay leaves. Return beef to the pan and bring to a boil. Reduce heat to low. Cover and cook, stirring occasionally, for 2 hours.

Uncover and cook, stirring occasionally, for 1½ hours or until beef is very tender. Transfer beef to a chopping board. Use a fork to shred. Return to pan and mix through.

Top with parsley and serve.

MUSSELS SOUP WITH SAFFRON CREAM

3 tbsps unsalted butter
4 Asian shallots, finely chopped
2 cloves garlic, minced
½ tsp saffron threads
2kg mussels, well scrubbed with beards removed
Tabasco sauce to taste
¼ cup (10g) finely chopped fresh parsley leaves
2 sprigs thyme
1½ cups (375ml) dry white wine
3 cups (750ml) thickened cream
Salt and pepper to taste
1 tbsp chopped chives to serve

Melt the butter in a large pan over medium-high heat. Add the shallots, garlic and saffron. Cook, stirring, for 3-5 minutes until soft and translucent.

Add the mussels, Tabasco, parsley, thyme and wine. Cover and cook for 3-5 minutes until the mussels open.

Add the cream and bring to a boil. Season with salt and pepper.

Scatter with chopped chives to serve.

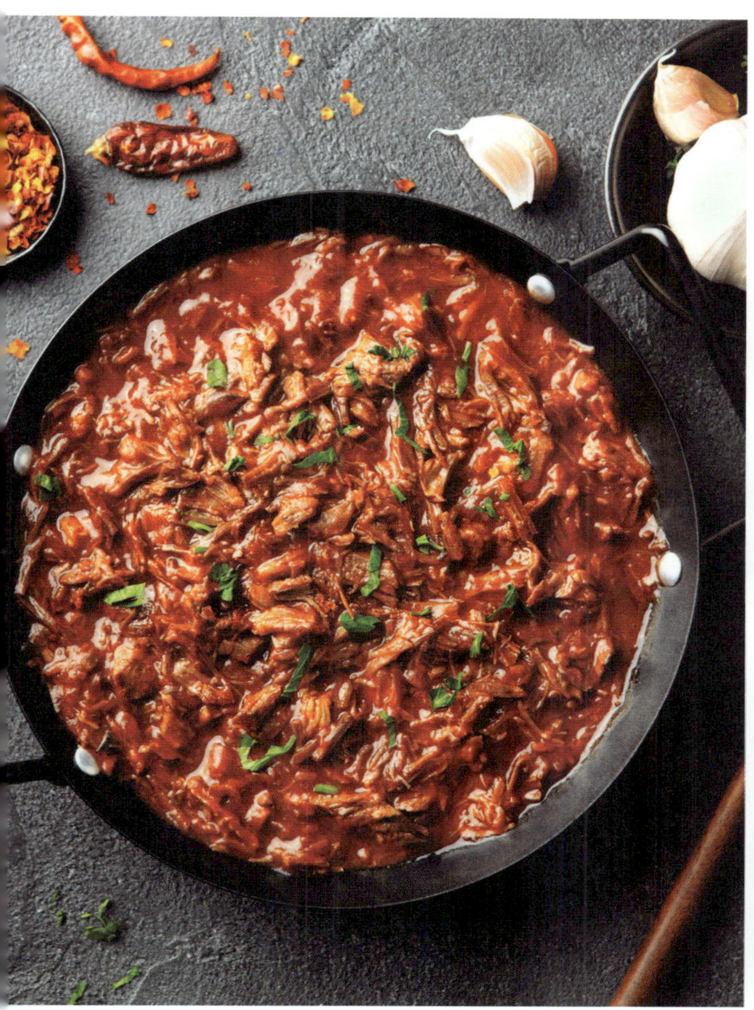

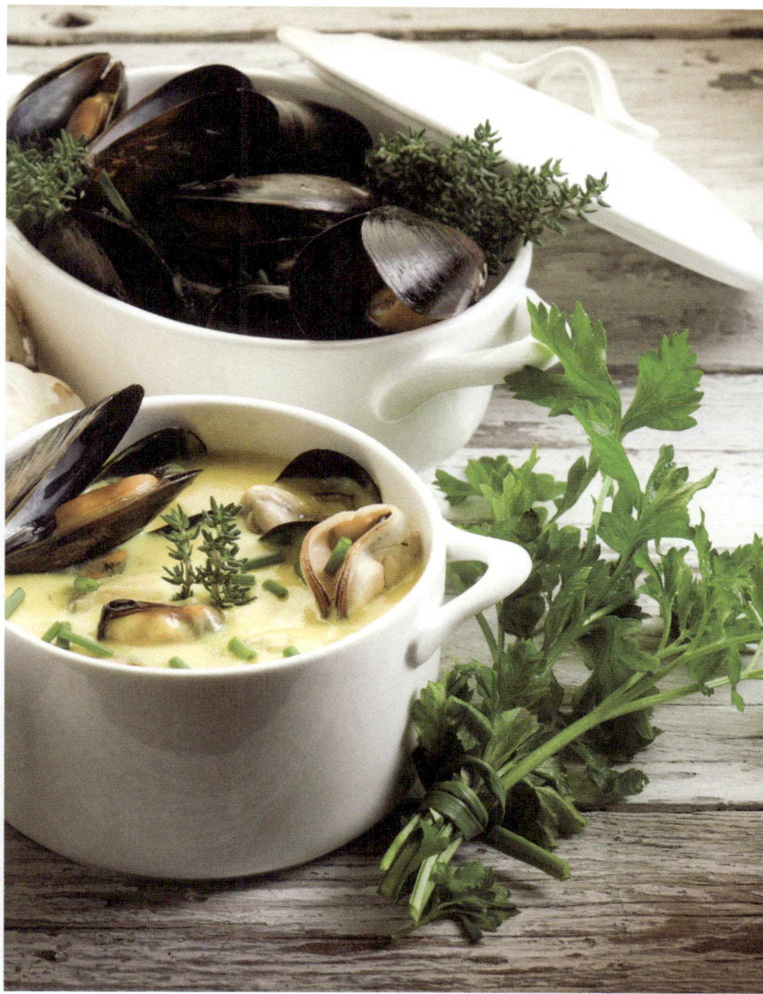

Shredded Chilli Beef

SERVES 4

PREP + COOK TIME: 4 HOURS

GLUTEN FREE • DAIRY FREE

Mussels Soup with Saffron Cream

SERVES 4

PREP + COOK TIME: 15 MINS

GLUTEN FREE

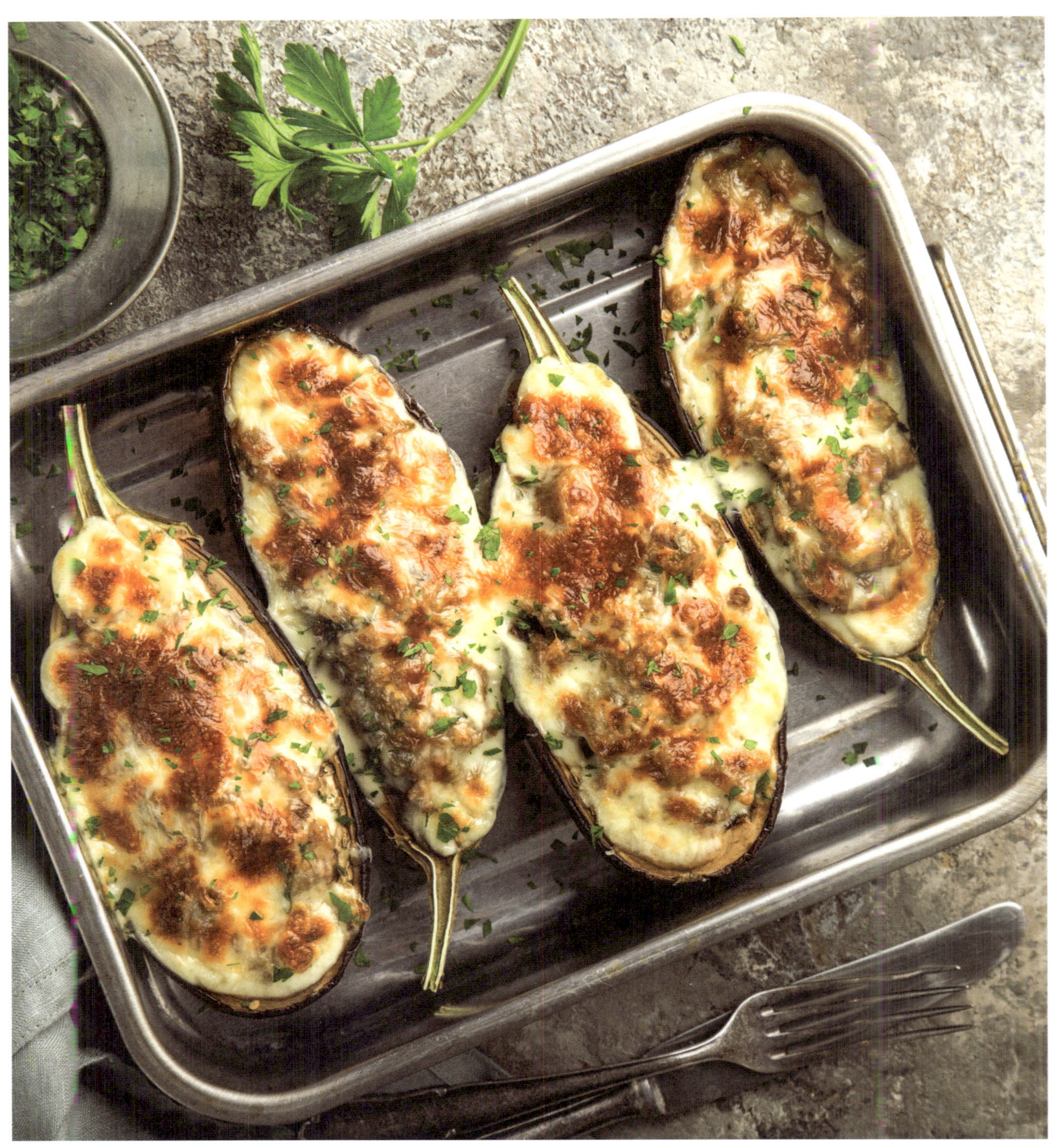

Stuffed Eggplant

SERVES 4

PREP + COOK TIME: 1 HOUR

GLUTEN FREE

STUFFED EGGPLANT

2 medium eggplants
2 tbsps olive oil
350g mushrooms, sliced
Juice of 1 lemon
500g beef mince
1 egg
½ medium onion, finely chopped
3 cloves garlic, minced
¼ cup (10g) chopped parsley + more to garnish
3 tbsps grated Parmesan cheese
1 tsp Sriracha
1 tsp dried chilli flakes
Salt and pepper to taste
1 cup (125g) shredded mozzarella cheese
½ cup (125ml) water

Preheat oven to 180°C.

Cut eggplants in half lengthwise. Scoop out the pulp with a spoon leaving about 1cm thickness of eggplant flesh in the skin. Chop eggplant pulp.

Heat oil in a large frying pan over medium heat. Add chopped eggplant and mushrooms and cook for 10 minutes, stirring regularly, until eggplant and mushrooms are soft. Transfer to a large bowl. Pour in lemon juice and set aside to cool.

In a large bowl, mix beef, egg, onion, garlic, parsley, Parmesan, Sriracha and chilli flakes. Season with salt and pepper to taste. Add in mushroom and eggplant mixture and mix well to combine.

Generously stuff eggplant shells with stuffing. Top with mozzarella. Place eggplants in a large baking dish and pour water in the bottom.

Bake uncovered for 30 minutes, until meat is cooked through. Place under the grill for an additional 2-3 minutes until cheese is golden brown. Scatter with parsley to serve.

Keto Carbonara with Zoodles

SERVES 4
PREP + COOK TIME: 30 MINS
GLUTEN FREE

1kg zucchinis
25g butter
300g bacon, cut into small strips
1¼ cups (310ml) thickened cream
Salt and pepper to taste
4 egg yolks + 4 eggs
1 cup (90g) grated Parmesan cheese

Use a spiraliser or vegetable peeler to create zucchini noodles (zoodles).

In a large frying pan, melt butter over a medium heat. Add bacon and fry for 4-5 minutes until crispy. Remove from the heat and set aside.

Pour cream into a saucepan over medium-high heat and bring to a boil. Add a pinch of salt. Reduce the heat and continue to gently boil until the cream has reduced down by approximately one quarter.

Remove the saucepan from the heat and allow the cream to reduce in temperature, stirring occasionally to prevent a skin from forming.

While the cream is reducing, in a separate bowl combine the egg yolks, cooked bacon including the fat, and Parmesan cheese. Add to the cream, stirring continuously to ensure the egg does not scramble. Add salt and pepper to taste.

Return the saucepan to medium-low heat to gently warm the sauce. Add the zoodles to the saucepan and warm through for 1-2 minutes.

Meanwhile bring a pan of water to the boil. Stir the water to create a gentle whirlpool then break the eggs into the centre. Cook for 3-4 minutes until the white is set but the yolk is still runny.

Serve the zoodles into four bowls. Top each with a poached egg and season with salt and pepper.

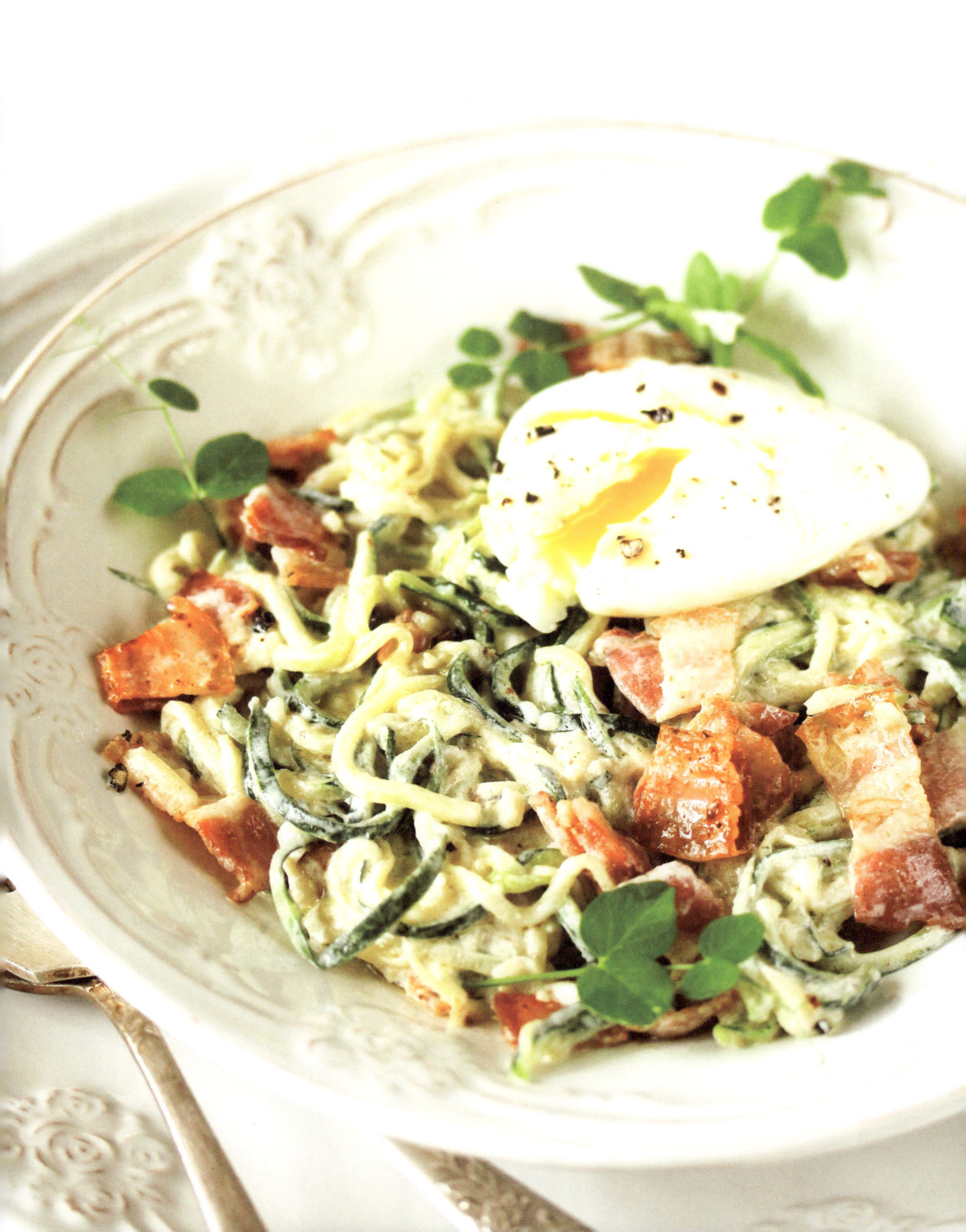

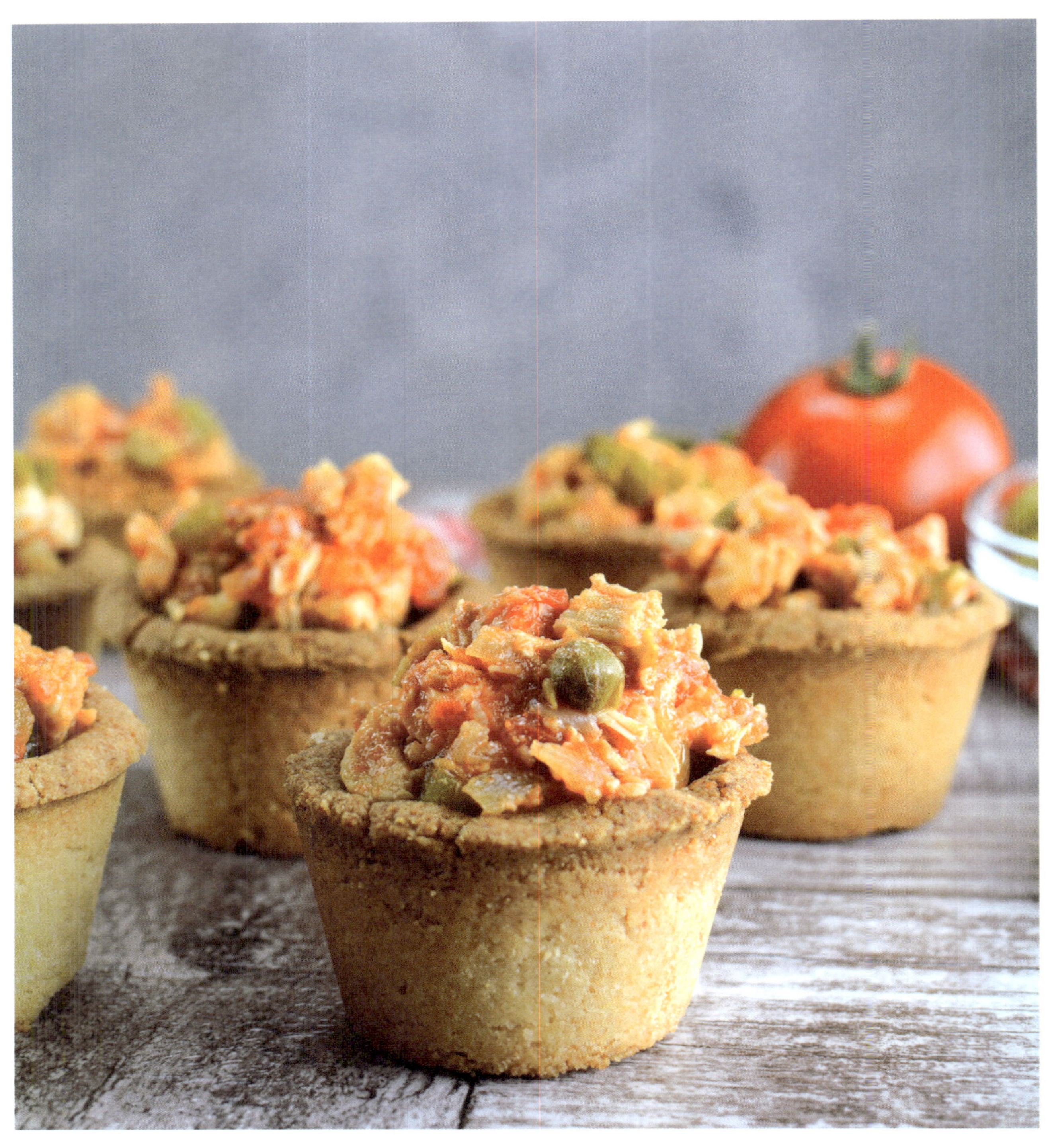

Mediterranean Chicken & Veg Almond Cups

MAKES 12

PREP + COOK TIME: 50 MINS

GLUTEN FREE

MEDITERRANEAN CHICKEN & VEG ALMOND CUPS

PASTRY

3¾ cups (450g) almond meal

½ tsp salt

115g butter, melted

1 large egg

FILLING

3 tbsps olive oil

2 chicken breasts

1 onion, chopped

3 cloves garlic, chopped

1 green capsicum, finely chopped

2 large tomatoes, diced

½ cup (70g) green olives, sliced

2 tbsps capers, rinsed

Pinch of dried chilli flakes

Salt and pepper to taste

Preheat the oven to 180°C. Grease a 12-hole muffin tin.

In a large bowl, mix together the almond meal and salt. Stir in the melted butter and egg until the mixture is well combined.

Press the dough into the holes of the prepared muffin tin. Carefully poke holes in the base of each with a fork to prevent bubbling.

Bake for 10-12 minutes, until golden brown.

Meanwhile heat 2 tablespoons oil in a large frying pan over medium-high heat. Add the chicken breasts and cook for 4-5 minutes on each side until cooked through. Set aside to rest for 5 minutes, then cut into 2cm pieces.

Meanwhile heat the remaining oil in the same frying pan over medium-high heat. Add the onion and cook for 3-5 minutes, stirring regularly, until soft and translucent. Add the garlic and cook for 1 minute until fragrant. Add capsicum and cook, stirring, for 4 minutes until soft. Add the tomatoes and cook for a further 4 minutes until starting to break down. Add chicken, olives, capers, tomatoes and dried chilli flakes. Season with salt and pepper. Allow to cook for 4-5 minutes to allow the flavours to meld.

Spoon the mixture into the prepared cups and serve immediately. Or, if serving cold, allow the mixture to cool, then transfer to the fridge to chill before serving in the prepared cups.

Turkey Meatballs Zoodle Soup

SERVES 4

PREP + COOK TIME: 30 MINS + CHILLING

GLUTEN FREE

500g turkey mince

2 large cloves garlic, crushed

1 tbsp coconut flour

Salt and pepper to taste

1 tbsp butter

4 cups (1L) hot chicken stock

1 cup (250ml) water

1 medium carrot, cut into thin rounds

1 tbsp sesame oil

4 large zucchinis, ends trimmed, cut into thin noodle strands

Place the turkey, garlic, coconut flour and a teaspoon each of salt and pepper in a large bowl and mix together thoroughly. Form dessertspoons of the mix into balls and place in the refrigerator to chill and firm up for at least 30 minutes.

Heat the butter in a large frying pan over medium-high heat. Fry the meatballs for at least 8 minutes, turning every 2 minutes to cook them evenly.

Bring the stock and water to a boil in a medium saucepan. Reduce to a simmer. Add the meatballs, carrot and sesame oil. Simmer for 5 minutes.

Add the zucchini and simmer for 2 more minutes. Season to taste and serve.

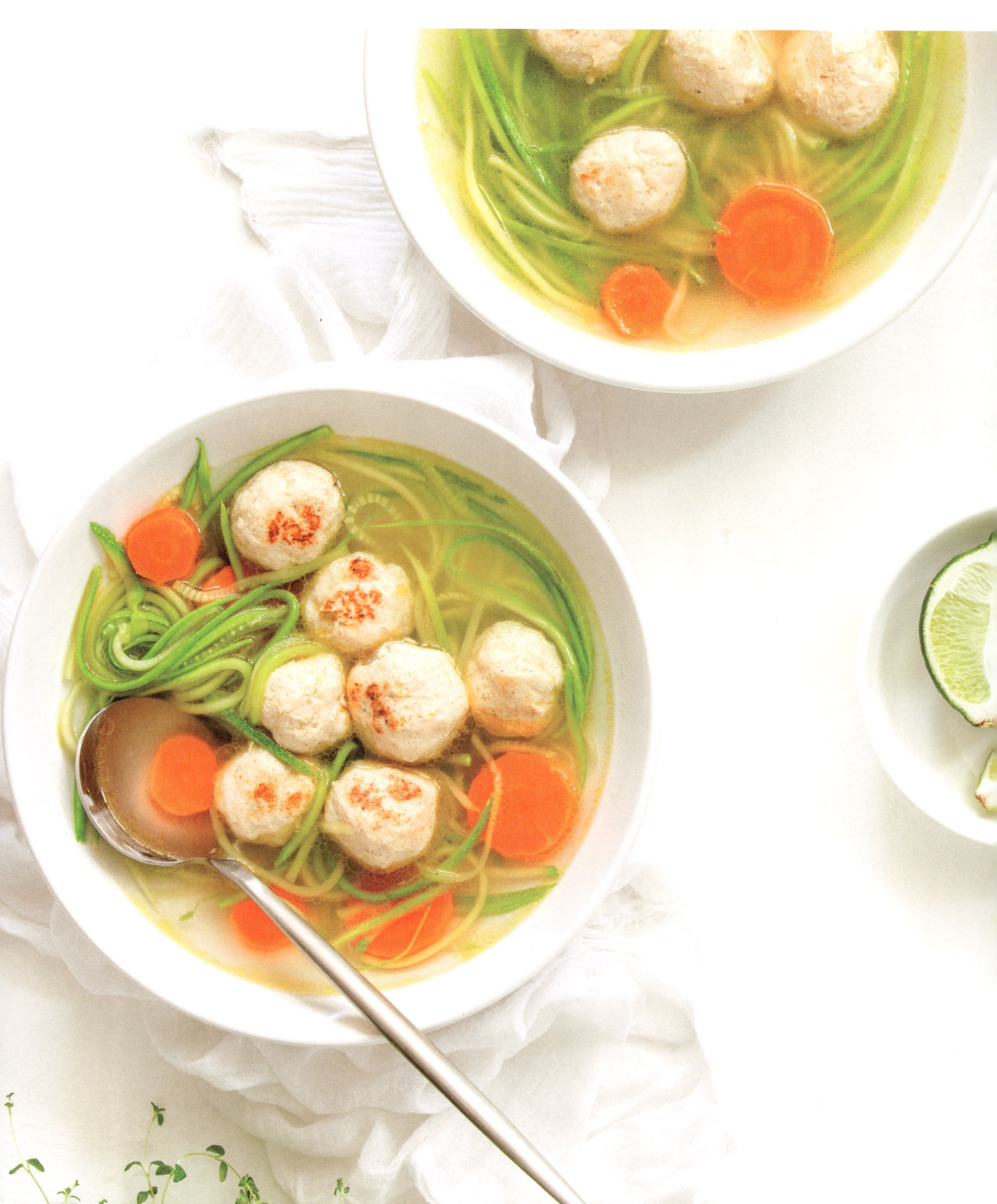

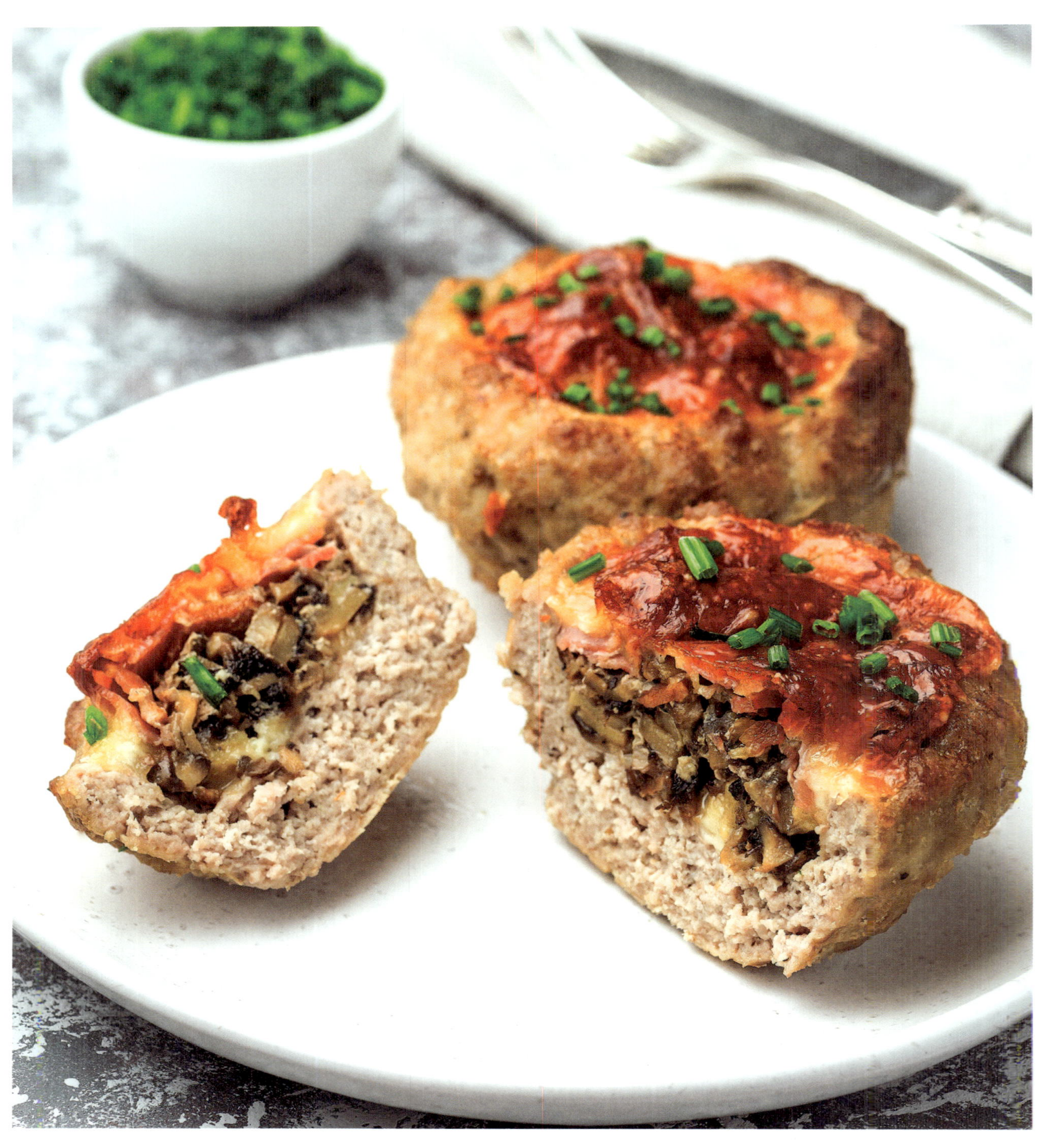

Burger Cups

SERVES 6

PREP + COOK TIME: 45 MINS

GLUTEN FREE

BURGER CUPS

1 tbsp + 1 tsp olive oil
250g mushrooms, quartered
Salt and pepper to taste
6 rashers bacon, chopped
1kg beef mince
1 tsp garlic powder
1 tsp smoked paprika
2 tsps Dijon mustard
2 tbsps sugar-free tomato sauce (see recipe on page 93)
2 cups (250g) grated Cheddar cheese
¼ onion, finely diced
Chopped chives to serve (optional)

Preheat oven to 200°C.

Heat 1 tablespoon olive oil in a large frying pan over medium-high heat. Add the mushrooms and season with salt and pepper. Cook, stirring regularly, for 7-8 minutes until tender. Transfer to a bowl and set aside to cool.

Heat 1 teaspoon oil in a frying pan over medium heat. Add bacon and cook, stirring, for 3-4 minutes until soft and cooked through. Transfer to a plate to cool.

In a large bowl, combine the beef mince, garlic powder, paprika, mustard and tomato sauce. Season with 1½ teaspoons salt and ½ teaspoon pepper. Mix well. Divide the mixture into 12 balls and press into 12 holes of a muffin pan. Press the mixture evenly along the bottom and up the sides to form a cup shape. Place a small amount of cheese in the base of each cup then layer in the mushrooms and bacon. Sprinkle with chopped onion, then top with the remaining cheese.

Bake for 15-20 minutes until the cups shrink away from the sides and the cheese is bubbling and golden brown.

Use a fork to carefully remove from the muffin tin. Scatter with chopped chives to serve, if desired.

SPICY STEAMED EGGPLANT

6 Japanese eggplants, ends trimmed and cut into thick 4cm-long matchsticks

3 large cloves garlic, crushed

3 large spring onions, roughly chopped

2 small red chillies, seeds removed, roughly chopped

2½ tbsps sesame oil

Pinch of stevia powder

¼ cup (60ml) tamari

Salt and pepper to taste

Steam the eggplant for 15 minutes until softened.

Remove to a large bowl and toss with the rest of the ingredients.

Return to the steamer and cook for a further 5 minutes to absorb the sauce.

Season to taste with salt and pepper.

SWEDISH MEATBALLS

500g beef mince

½ cup (75g) grated onion

¼ cup (30g) almond meal

1 egg

½ tsp garlic powder

¼ tsp allspice

Salt and pepper to taste

2 tbsps olive oil

1 tbsp fresh chopped parsley

CREAM SAUCE

1 cup (250ml) chicken or beef stock

½ cup (125ml) cream

1 tsp Dijon mustard

2 tsps Worcestershire sauce

In a mixing bowl, combine beef mince, grated onion, almond meal, egg, garlic powder and allspice. Season with ½ teaspoon each of salt and pepper. Mix well to combine. Roll into 20 walnut-sized meatballs.

Heat olive oil in a large frying pan over medium-high heat. Add the meatballs in batches and cook, turning every few minutes, until browned all over. Transfer to a plate with a slotted spoon and set aside while you prepare the sauce.

Add stock and cream to the pan and whisk over medium-low heat. Add Dijon mustard and Worcestershire sauce and bring to a simmer. Cook for 5-6 minutes until the sauce is thickened. Season with salt and pepper to taste. Return the meatballs to the pan and simmer for another 1-2 minutes.

Scatter with chopped parsley to serve.

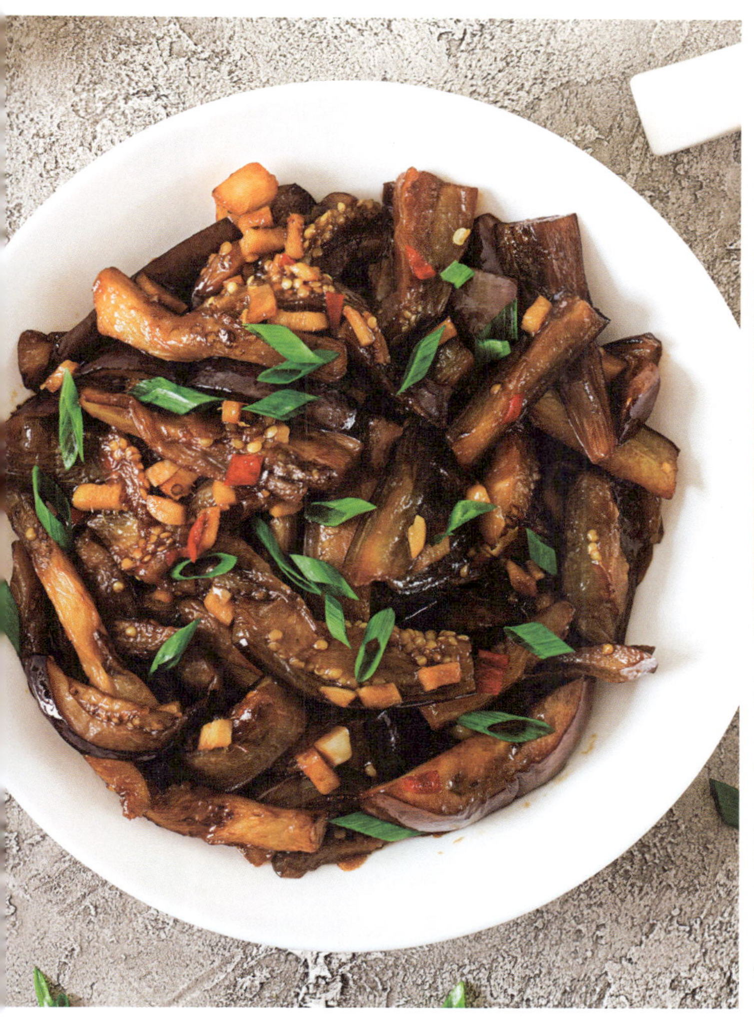

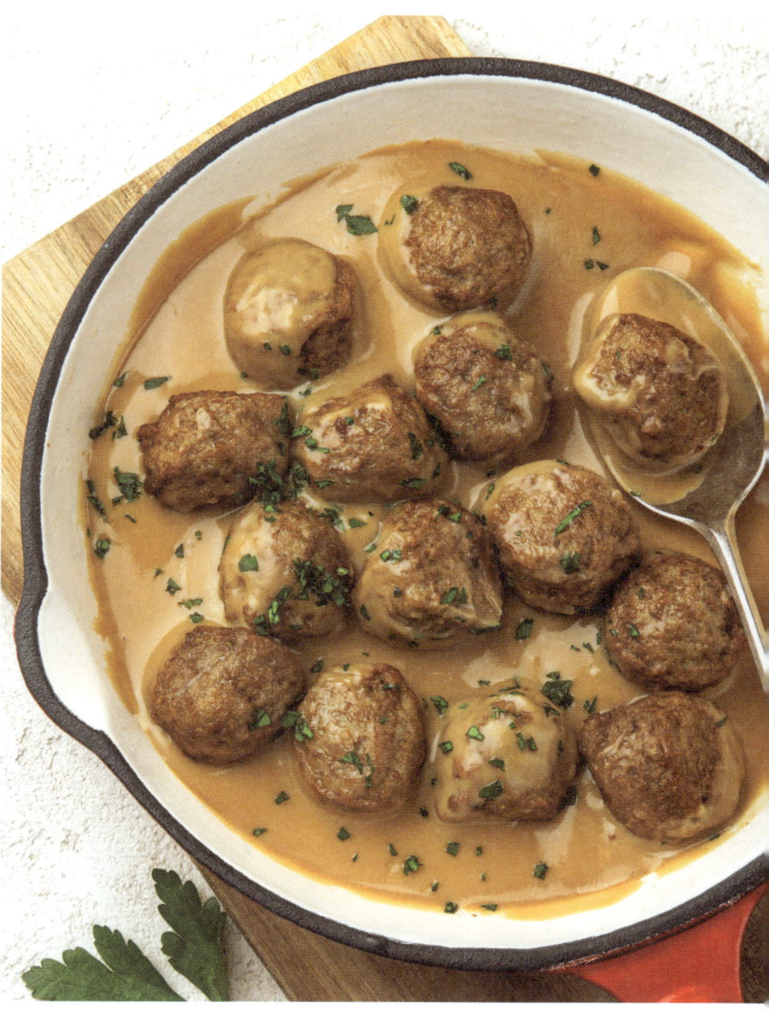

Spicy Steamed Eggplant

SERVES 4

PREP + COOK TIME: 20 MINS

GLUTEN FREE • DAIRY FREE

Swedish Meatballs

SERVES 4

PREP + COOK TIME: 30 MINS

GLUTEN FREE

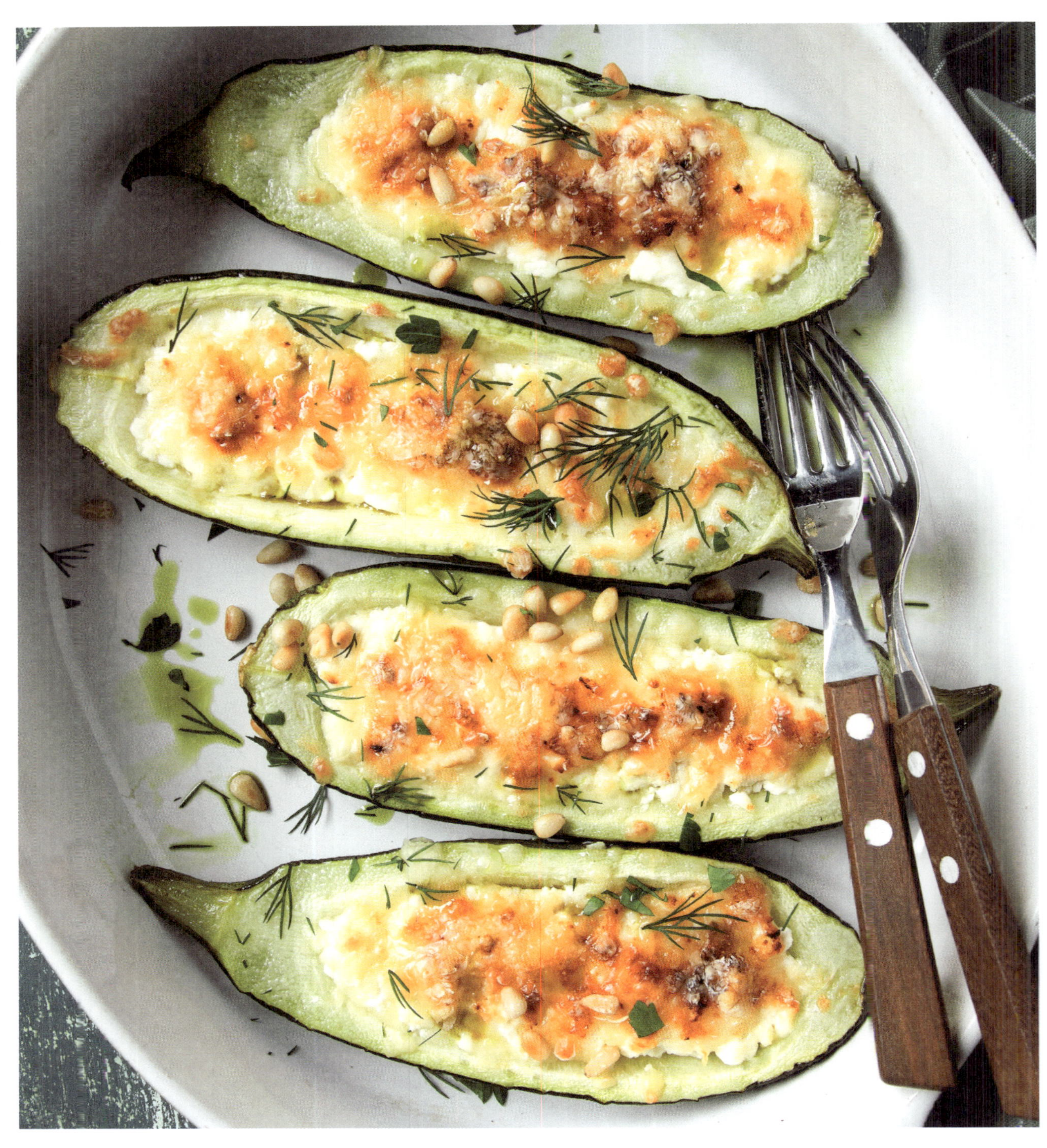

Zucchini Boats

SERVES 4

PREP + COOK TIME: 40 MINS

VEG • GLUTEN FREE

ZUCCHINI BOATS

4 zucchinis
2 tbsps olive oil
Salt and pepper to taste
1 egg
3 tbsps cottage cheese
2 tbsps sour cream
1 tsp garlic powder
⅛ tsp dried chilli flakes
3 tbsps grated Cheddar cheese
¼ cup (25g) grated Parmesan cheese
¼ cup (35g) pine nuts
1 tsp chopped dill to serve
1 tsp chopped parsley to serve

Preheat oven to 180°C. Line a baking tray with greaseproof paper.

Cut the zucchinis lengthways. Use a teaspoon to hollow out the centre of each zucchini, leaving approximately ½cm rim around the edge.

Finely chop the scooped-out zucchini centres and set aside.

Brush the zucchinis with olive oil and season with salt and pepper. Place cut-side up on the prepared baking tray.

In a bowl combine the egg, cottage cheese, sour cream, garlic powder and chilli flakes. Mix well. Add Cheddar cheese, season with salt and pepper and stir to combine.

Add ¼ cup of the reserved zucchini to the mixture and stir well.

Spoon the mixture into the zucchini boats. Transfer to the oven for 20 minutes.

Remove from the oven, sprinkle with Parmesan cheese and scatter with pine nuts. Return to the oven for 5-10 minutes until the cheese is melted and the pine nuts are toasted.

Scatter with dill and parsley to serve.

Mediterranean-Style Salmon

SERVES 4

PREP + COOK TIME: 20 MINS + MARINATING

GLUTEN FREE • DAIRY FREE

2½ tbsps fennel seeds
6 sprigs thyme; 2 finely chopped
3 cloves garlic, crushed
2 small spring onions, finely chopped
1 tsp lemon zest
1 tbsp olive oil
Salt and pepper to taste
4 x 150g salmon fillets

Mix together the fennel seeds, chopped thyme, garlic, spring onion, zest, olive oil and a couple of grinds of salt and pepper.

Brush the salmon with the fennel mixture and let sit for 30 minutes.

Heat a large non-stick frying pan over medium heat. Fry the salmon, skin-side down, for 3 minutes, then cook on the other side for 2 minutes until cooked through.

Serve hot, garnished with the sprigs of thyme.

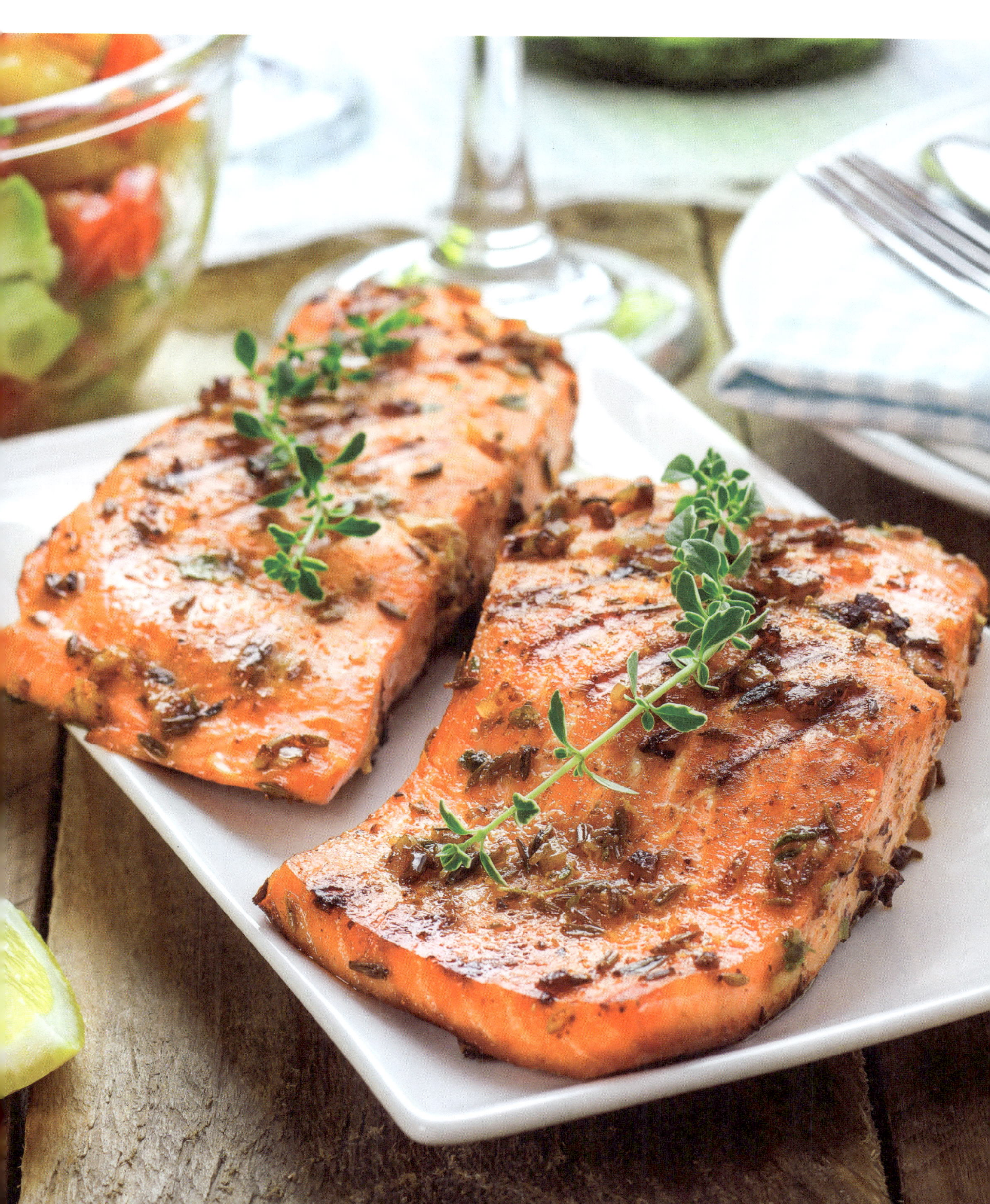

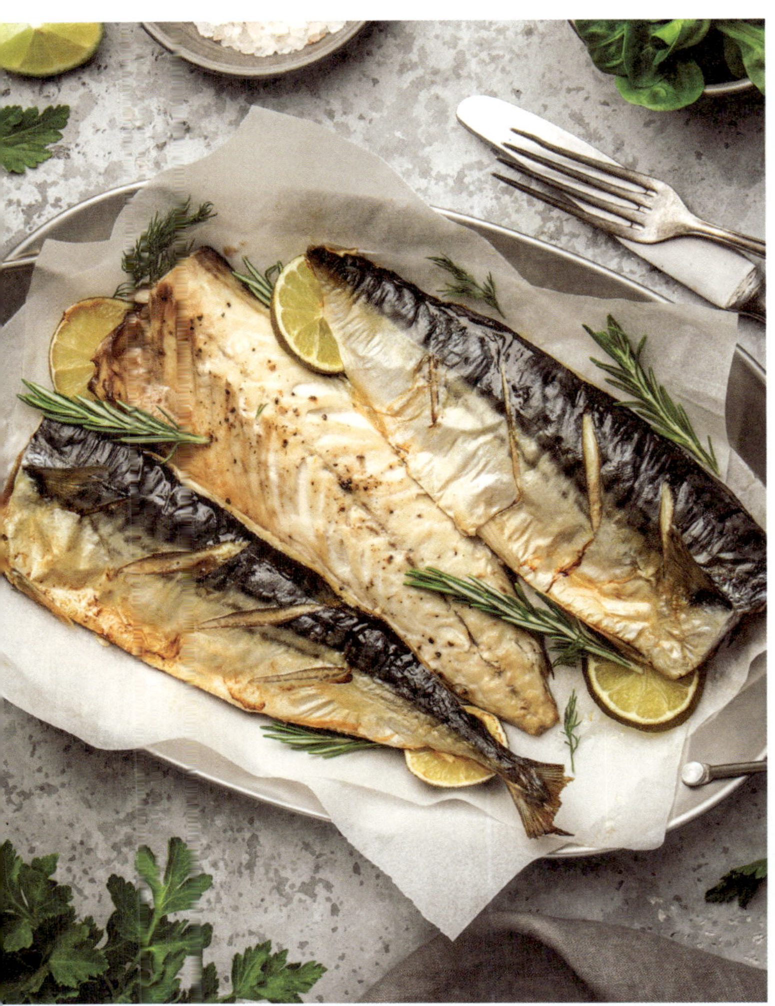

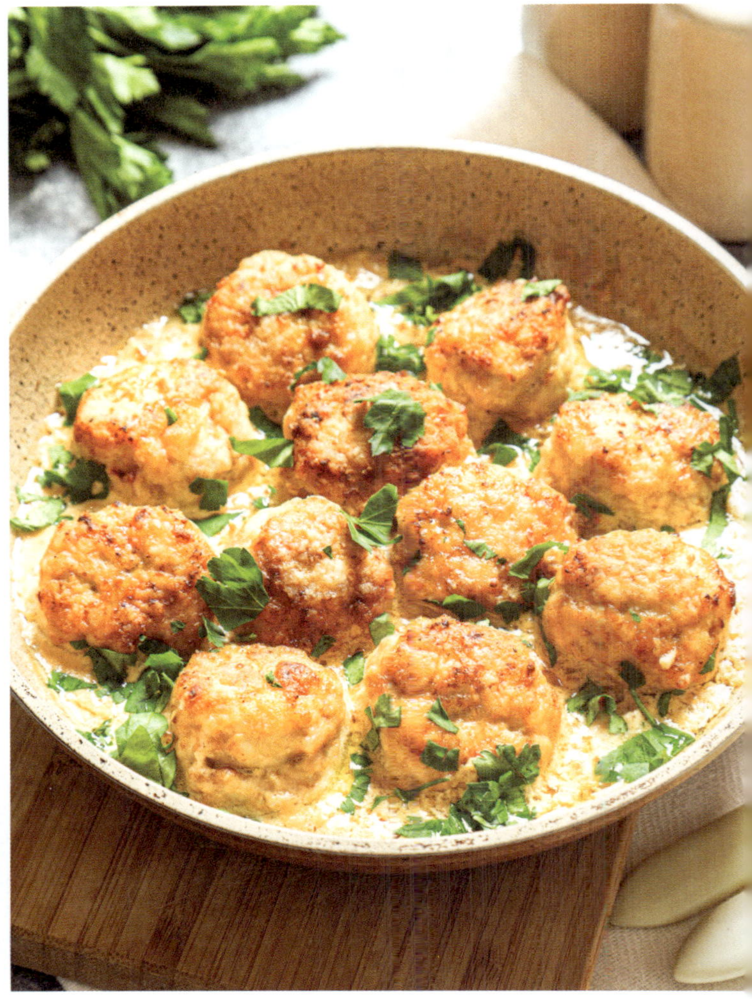

Oven-Baked Mackerel

SERVES 4

PREP + COOK TIME: 15 MINS

GLUTEN FREE • DAIRY FREE

Chicken Meatballs in Garlic Cream Sauce

SERVES 4

PREP + COOK TIME: 35 MINS

GLUTEN FREE

OVEN-BAKED MACKEREL

4 cloves garlic, peeled
2 tsps paprika
1 tbsp finely chopped rosemary
1 tsp salt + more to taste
2 tbsps olive oil
8 mackerel fillets
1 lemon, sliced

Preheat the oven to 200°C. Line a baking tray with greaseproof paper.

Put the garlic, paprika, rosemary and salt into a mortar, and pound to a smooth paste. (Alternatively, mince the garlic and combine with the paprika, rosemary and salt in a small bowl). Add the olive oil, and stir to combine.

Rub the flesh side of the mackerel fillets with the paste and set aside.

Lay the lemon slices on the baking tray then place the mackerel fillets skin-side up on top. Season with salt.

Roast for 8-10 minutes until the fish is cooked through.

CHICKEN MEATBALLS IN GARLIC CREAM SAUCE

MEATBALLS

500g chicken mince
½ cup (60g) almond meal
1 large egg
3 cloves garlic, minced
½ tsp salt
¼ tsp pepper
¼ cup (10g) chopped parsley to serve

SAUCE

2 cups (500ml) cream
2 tbsps chopped fresh rosemary
1 tsp ground paprika
3 cloves garlic, minced
½ tsp salt
Pinch of pepper

Preheat the oven to 220°C. Line a baking tray with greaseproof paper.

Place the chicken mince, almond meal, egg, garlic, salt and pepper into a large bowl. Mix well with your hands then form into golf ball-sized balls and place on prepared baking tray.

Bake for 12-14 minutes, until just cooked through.

Meanwhile make the sauce. Combine all the sauce ingredients in a large pan. Simmer for 10-15 minutes, until thick and reduced in volume by half.

When the meatballs are done add to the sauce and simmer for 1 minute more. Scatter with fresh parsley to serve.

Baked Eggplant with Cheese, Tomato & Chicken

SERVES 4

PREP + COOK TIME: 1 HOUR 20 MINS

GLUTEN FREE

4 medium eggplants

¼ cup (50ml) olive oil

1 medium onion, finely chopped

3 large cloves garlic, crushed

500g chicken breast fillets, cut into 1cm cubes

2 cups (450g) tomato passata

Salt and pepper to taste

1¼ cups (155g) grated Cheddar cheese

Sprigs of parsley, to garnish

Handful of cherry tomatoes, to garnish

Preheat oven to 180°C.

Cut the eggplants lengthways so that you have 1cm thick slices that are still attached at the stem.

Heat 2 tablespoons of the oil in a large frying pan over medium heat. Fry the onion and garlic for 5 minutes. Add the chicken and fry for another 5 minutes.

Stir in the passata and simmer for 10 minutes until the sauce has thickened. Season to taste.

Place the eggplants in a large casserole dish and place spoonfuls of mixture between the slices. Drizzle with the remaining oil, sprinkle with cheese and bake for 50 minutes. Garnish with parsley and cherry tomatoes to serve.

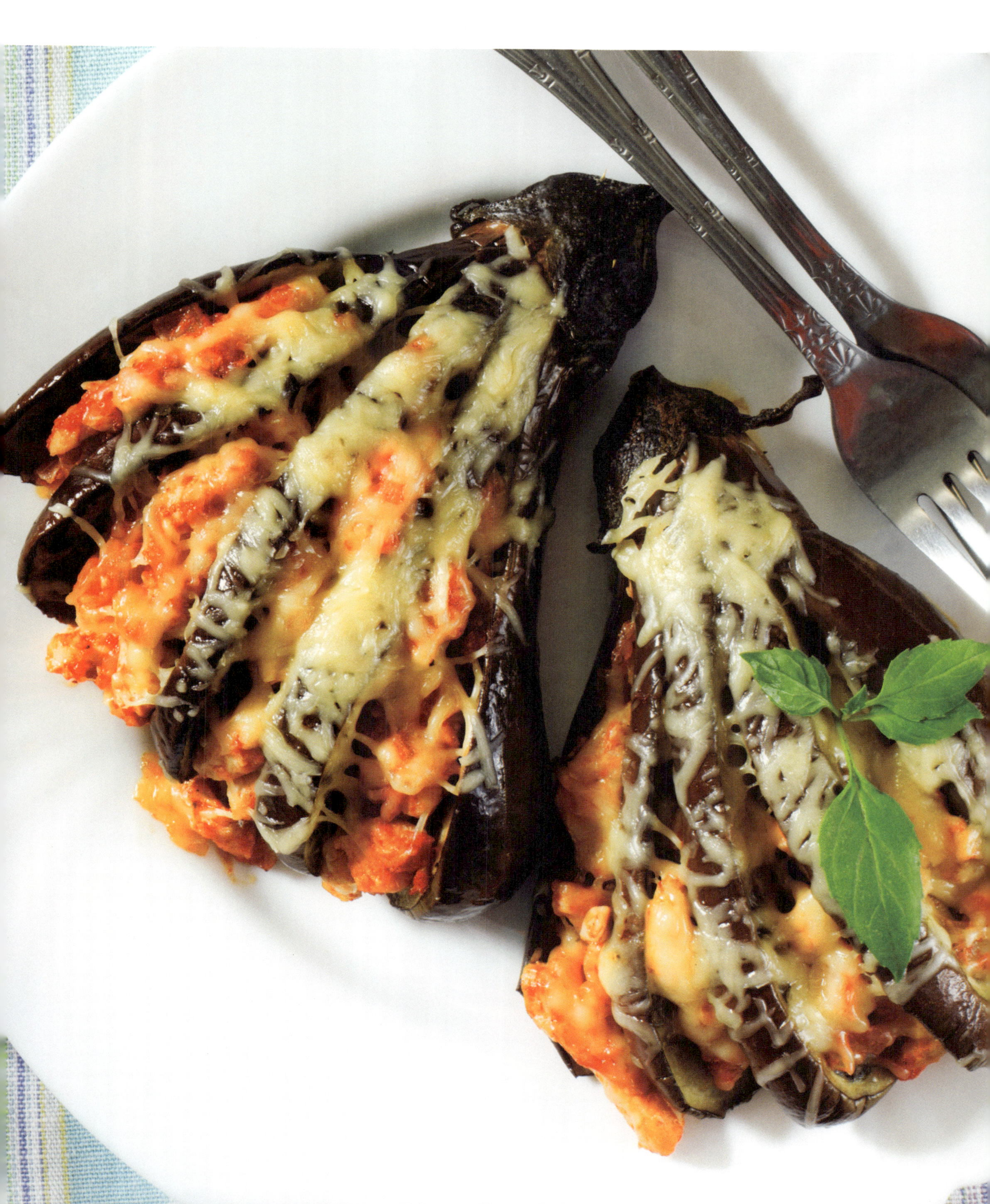

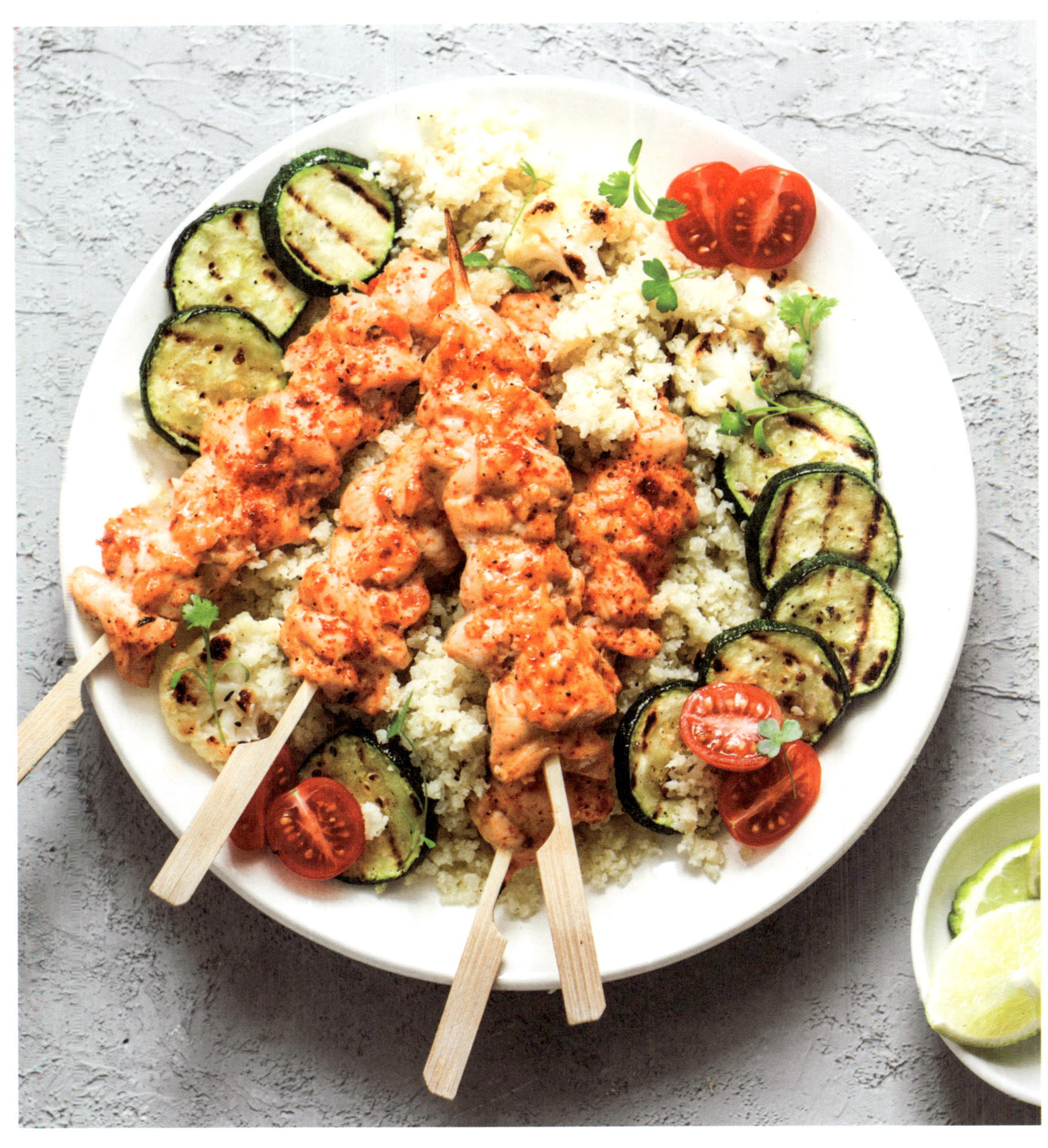

Chicken Kebabs with Cauliflower Couscous & Grilled Zucchini

SERVES 4

PREP + COOK TIME: 40 MINS

GLUTEN FREE

CHICKEN KEBABS WITH CAULIFLOWER COUSCOUS & GRILLED ZUCCHINI

1 large head cauliflower, broken into small florets

30g butter

1½ tbsps coconut oil

Salt and pepper to taste

3 small zucchinis, cut into 5mm slices

1 punnet cherry tomatoes, halved

¼ cup (60ml) olive oil

2 tsps chilli powder

½ tsp Dijon mustard

1kg chicken breast fillets, cut into 2cm chunks

⅓ cup (15g) parsley microgreens, to garnish

If using wooden skewers, soak the skewers in hot water for 30 minutes prior to grilling.

Place the cauliflower into a food processor in batches, pulsing until it resembles couscous grains. To cook, heat half the butter and the coconut oil in a large frying pan over medium heat. Stir-fry for 8 minutes until the cauliflower is cooked. Remove from the heat, fluff with a fork and season to taste.

Heat the remaining butter in the frying pan and fry the zucchini for 5 minutes until cooked through. Remove from the heat and toss with the cauliflower and tomatoes.

Mix together the olive oil, chilli, mustard and 1 teaspoon each of salt and pepper.

Thread the chicken onto the skewers and brush the chicken with the oil mixture.

Heat a grill pan or large frying pan over medium-high heat. Grill the chicken for 10 minutes, turning every 2 minutes, to cook evenly on all sides.

Serve the skewers on top of the couscous, garnished with microgreens.

German Meatloaf

SERVES 10

PREP + COOK TIME: 1 HOUR

GLUTEN FREE • DAIRY FREE

2 tbsps olive oil
1 onion, finely chopped
250g pork mince
250g beef mince
3 tbsps almond meal
½ tsp salt
½ tsp pepper
1 tsp paprika
1 tsp Dijon mustard
1 large egg

FILLING

100g cherry tomatoes, chopped
½ cup (75g) gherkins, sliced into 1cm-thick slices
3 hard boiled eggs, peeled
2 tbsps chopped parsley

Preheat oven to 200°C. Line a 22cm loaf tin with greaseproof paper.

Heat the oil in a frying pan over medium-high heat. Add the onion and cook for 3-5 minutes until soft and translucent. Remove from the heat and set aside.

In a large bowl, combine the pork, beef, almond meal, onion, salt, pepper, paprika and mustard. Add the raw egg and mix together with your hands until the mixture is well combined.

Place slightly less than half of the meat mixture into the bottom of the loaf pan and spread it out with a rubber spatula until smooth.

Scatter the cherry tomatoes and gherkins along the centre of the meat. Slice the boiled eggs into ½cm-thick slices and lay on top of the gherkins. Scatter with parsley leaves.

Add the rest of the meat around and on top of the fillings and press down slightly. Bake the meatloaf in the middle rack of the oven for around 40-45 minutes.

Allow to rest for 5-10 minutes before slicing.

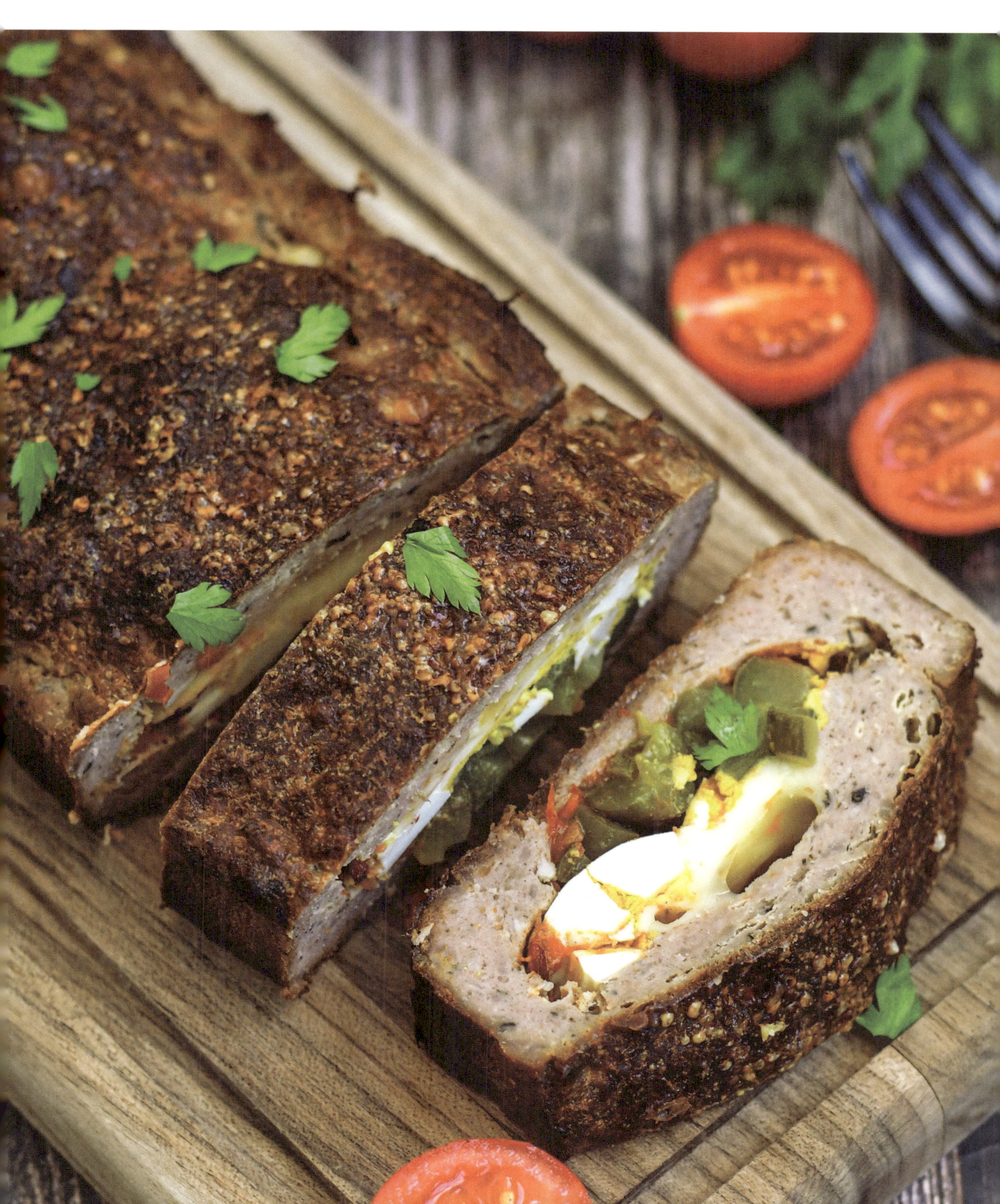

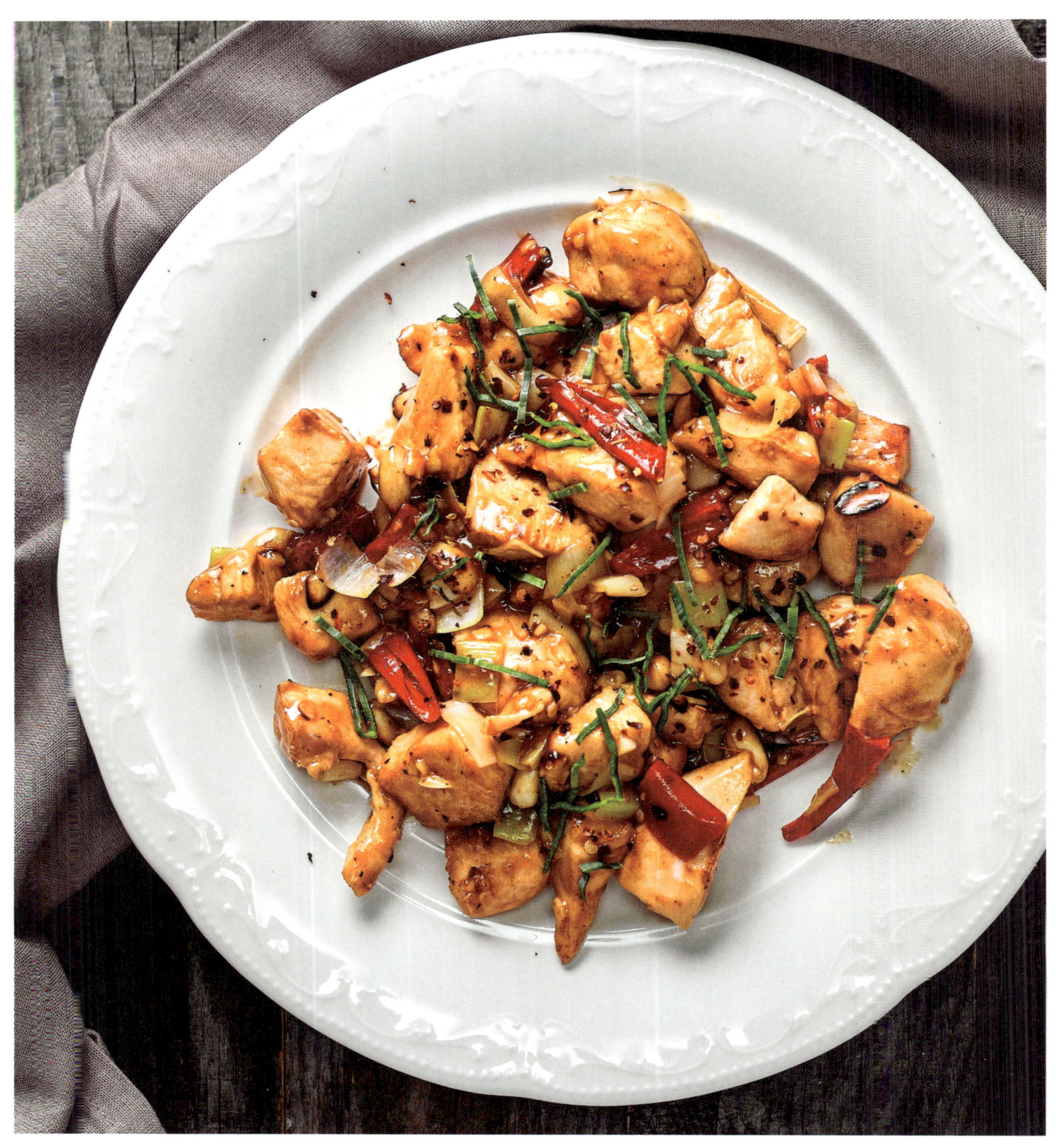

Kung Pao Chicken

SERVES 4

PREP + COOK TIME: 30 MINS

GLUTEN FREE • DAIRY FREE

KUNG PAO CHICKEN

2 tbsps coconut oil

800g chicken thigh fillets, cut into bite-size chunks

3 small cloves garlic, crushed

½ small onion, chopped

1 cup (125g) roasted unsalted peanuts, chopped

4 large red chillies, quartered

2 tbsps chilli flakes

⅓ cup (80ml) tamari

2 tbsps apple cider vinegar

Pinch of stevia powder, or more to taste

⅓ cup (80ml) water

Salt and pepper to taste

2 medium green chillies, seeded and thinly sliced, to garnish (optional)

Heat 1½ tablespoons of the oil in a wok or large saute pan over medium-high heat. Add chicken and saute for 5 minutes, flipping occasionally, or until the chicken is completely cooked through. Remove from the wok and set aside.

Add the rest of the oil and add the garlic and onion and fry for 5 minutes over medium heat until the onion has softened. Add the peanuts and red chillies and cook for a further 2 minutes.

Add the chilli flakes, tamari, vinegar, stevia and water. Bring to a boil, then reduce to a simmer and add the chicken.

Stir-fry for 5 minutes until the sauce has thickened.

Season to taste and serve hot, garnished with green chillies if desired.

Cheese-Stuffed Meatballs

SERVES 4

PREP + COOK TIME: 1 HOUR

GLUTEN FREE

250g beef mince
250g pork mince
1 large egg
½ cup (25g) grated Parmesan cheese
½ small onion, finely chopped
2 cloves garlic, minced
2 tbsps parsley
Salt and pepper to taste
150g mozzarella, cut into 1½ cm cubes

SAUCE

1 tbsp olive oil
1 onion, finely chopped
1 carrot, finely chopped
2 stalks celery, finely chopped
4 cloves garlic, minced
1 tsp dried oregano
2 x 400g cans chopped tomatoes
1 cup (250ml) water
Salt and pepper to taste

Preheat the oven to 200°C. Line a baking tray with foil and grease with olive oil.

Combine the beef, pork, egg, Parmesan, onion, garlic and parsley in a bowl. Season with salt and pepper. Mix well with your hands. Use a medium cookie scoop or spoon to scoop the meat onto the prepared tray. Place a piece of cheese in the centre of each scoop, then wrap the meat around the cheese to form a ball.

Bake uncovered for 15-20 minutes, turning the meatballs halfway through cooking.

Meanwhile heat the olive oil in a large pan over medium heat. Add the onion, carrot and celery. Cover and cook, stirring occasionally, for 10 minutes until the onions are soft and translucent. Add the garlic and oregano and cook for 1 minute until fragrant.

Add the tomatoes and water (pour the water into the empty cans before adding to the pan, to get the last of the tomatoes out of the cans). Season with salt and pepper. Bring to a simmer and simmer gently, uncovered, for 20 minutes. Add the cooked meatballs to the sauce and simmer for 10 minutes before serving.

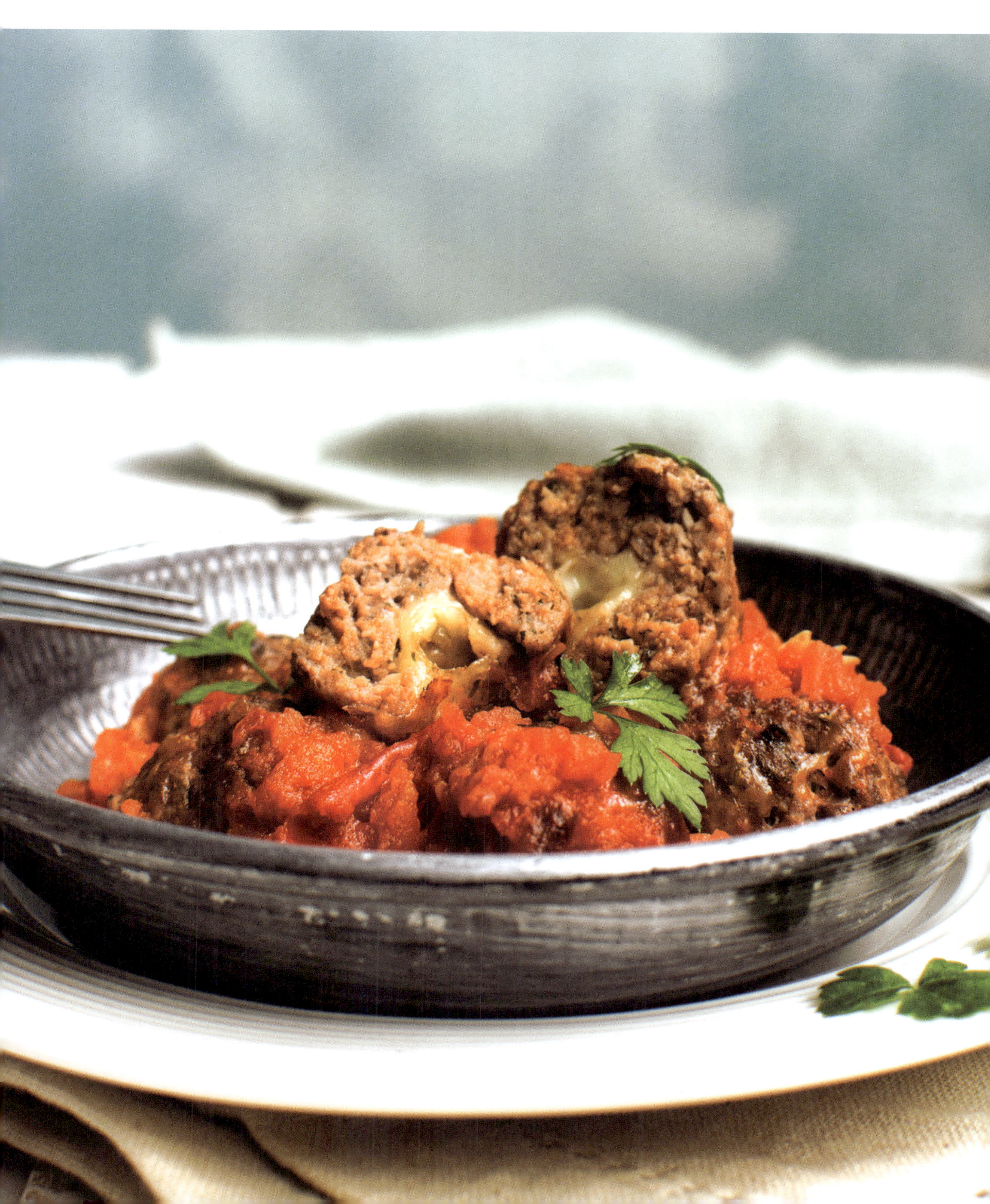

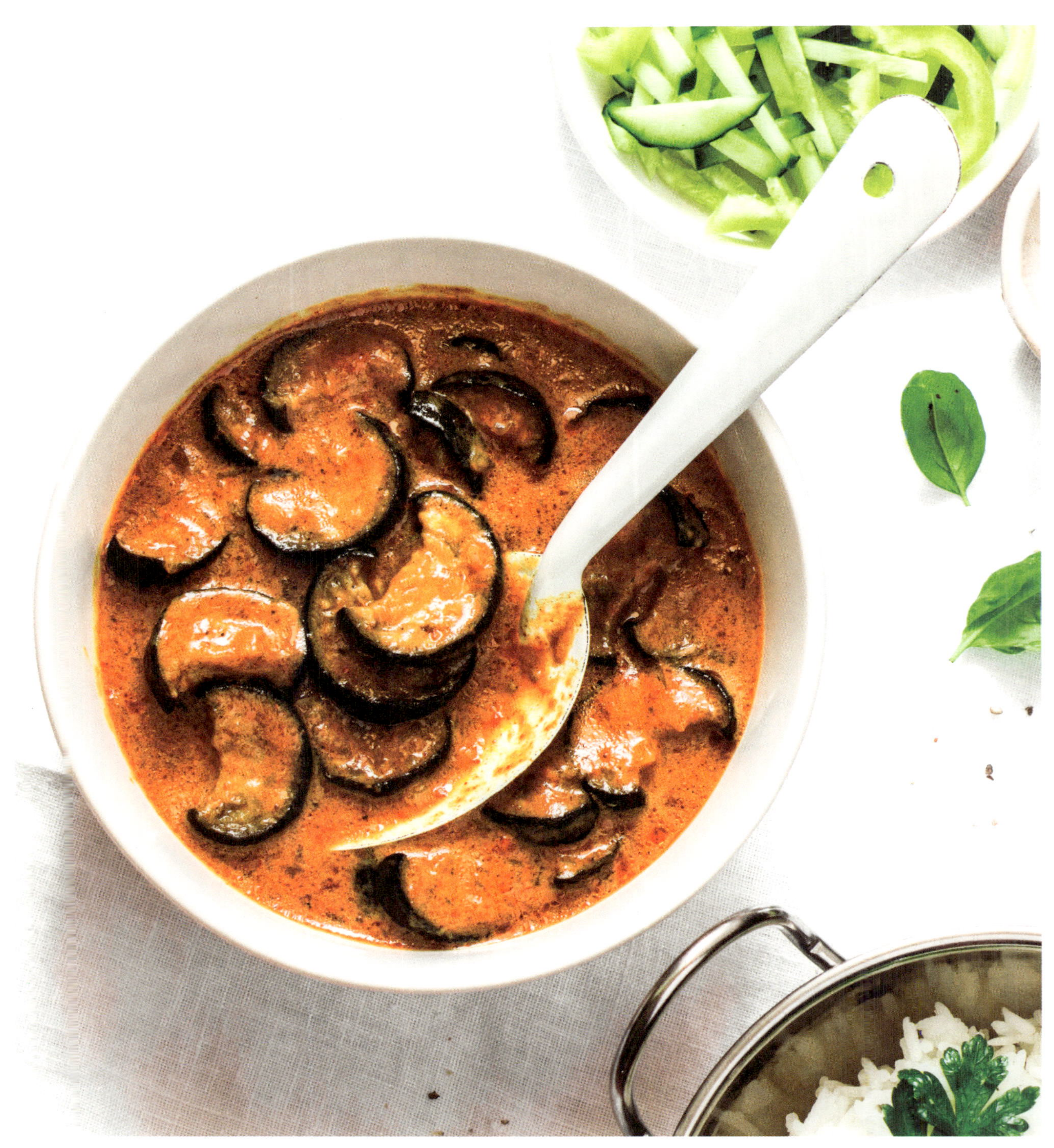

Roast Eggplant Curry

SERVES 4

PREP + COOK TIME: 1 HOUR

VEG • GLUTEN FREE • DAIRY FREE

ROAST EGGPLANT CURRY

4 large Japanese eggplants, cut into 1cm rounds
2 tbsps olive oil
Salt and pepper to taste
2 tbsps coconut oil
2 cloves garlic, crushed
1 tbsp fresh ginger, minced
2½ tbsps Japanese curry powder
3 tbsps coconut flour
2 tbsps tomato paste
¼ cup (60ml) tamari
3 cups (800ml) water
1 cup (250ml) coconut cream

Preheat oven to 180°C and line a large baking tray with baking paper.

Toss the eggplant with the olive oil and a pinch each of salt and pepper. Arrange in a single layer on the baking tray and roast for 30 minutes. Set aside.

Heat the coconut oil in a large saucepan over medium heat. Fry the garlic, ginger and curry powder for 1 minute. Stir in the coconut flour for 1 minute. Stir in the tomato paste for another minute.

Stir in the tamari and water. Bring to a boil, then reduce heat to a simmer and cook for 15 minutes. Stir through the coconut cream and add the eggplant.

Season to taste and serve hot.

Baked Fish with Cheese, Mustard & Cream Crust

SERVES 4

PREP + COOK TIME: 40 MINS

GLUTEN FREE

- 3 tbsps butter
- 3 tbsps coconut flour
- ½ cup (125ml) vegetable stock
- 2 cups (500ml) cream
- 1 cup (125g) grated Cheddar cheese
- ¼ cup (25g) grated Parmesan cheese
- 2½ tbsps seeded mustard
- Salt and pepper to taste
- 800g hoki or mahi mahi fillets, deboned

Preheat oven to 180°C and line a large, flat baking tray with baking paper.

Melt the butter in a medium saucepan over medium heat. Add the coconut flour and fry for 1 minute. Slowly add the stock, stirring the mixture the entire time so it stays smooth.

Next slowly add the cream and stir until just simmering. Turn the heat to low and stir through the cheeses and mustard, along with a couple of grinds of salt and pepper. Cook for another 3 minutes.

Place the fillets in a casserole dish small enough to fit them snugly.

Pour the sauce over the fillets. Bake for 30 minutes until the cheese is golden and bubbling.

Let cool for 5 minutes before serving.

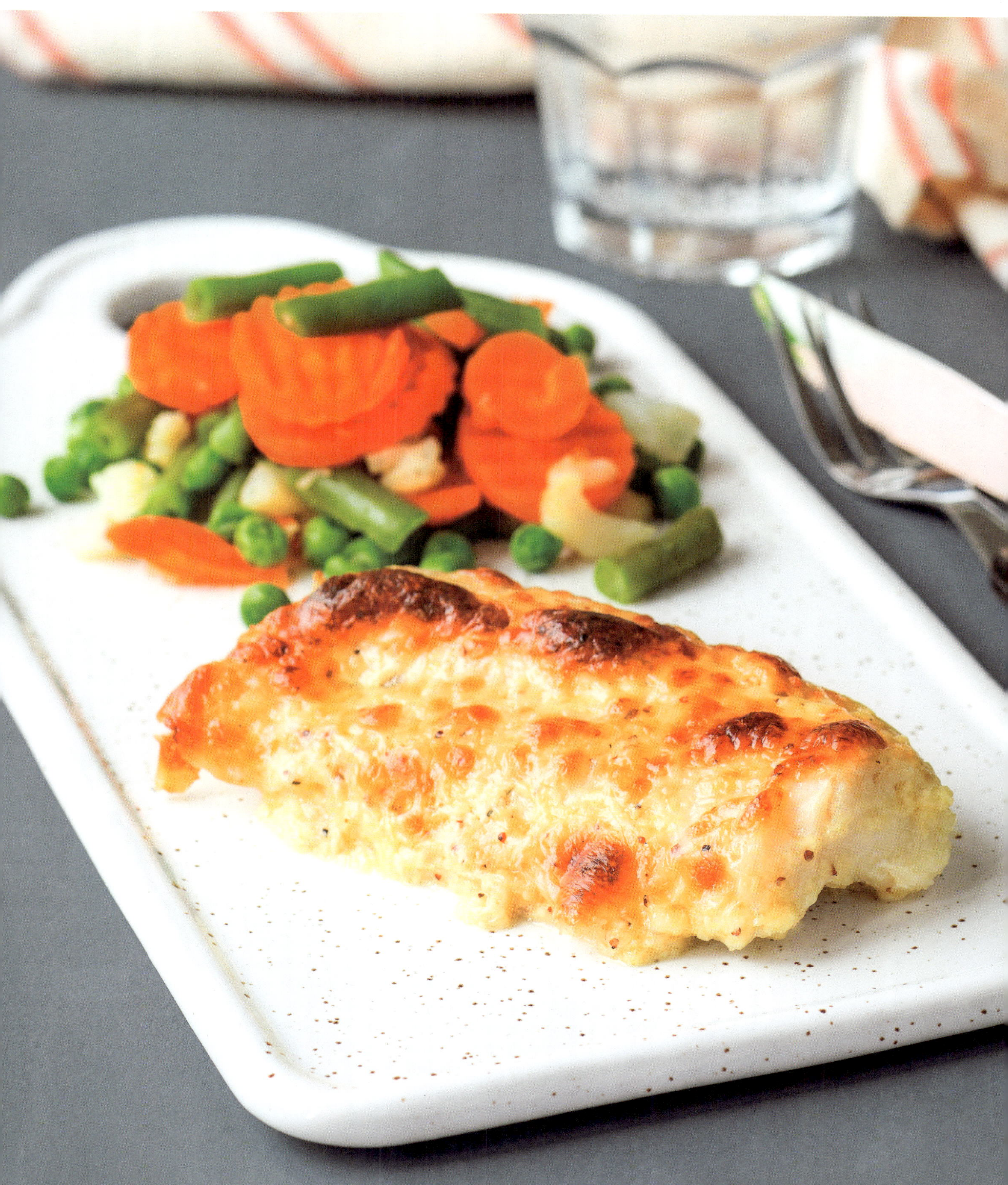

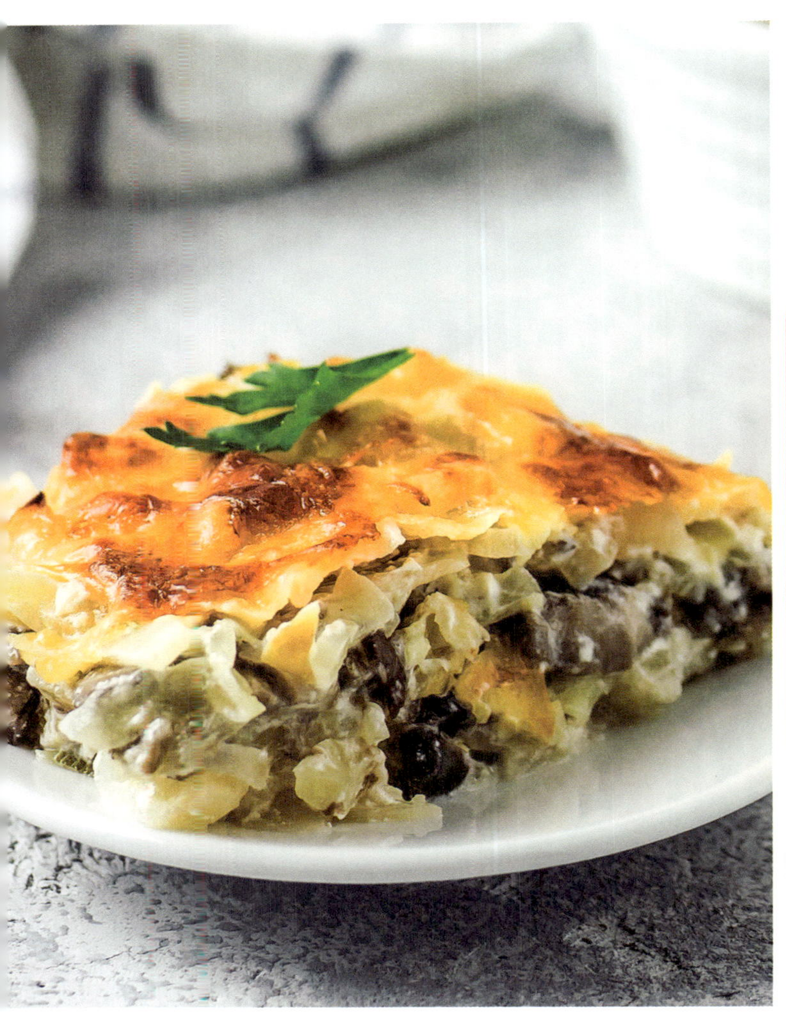

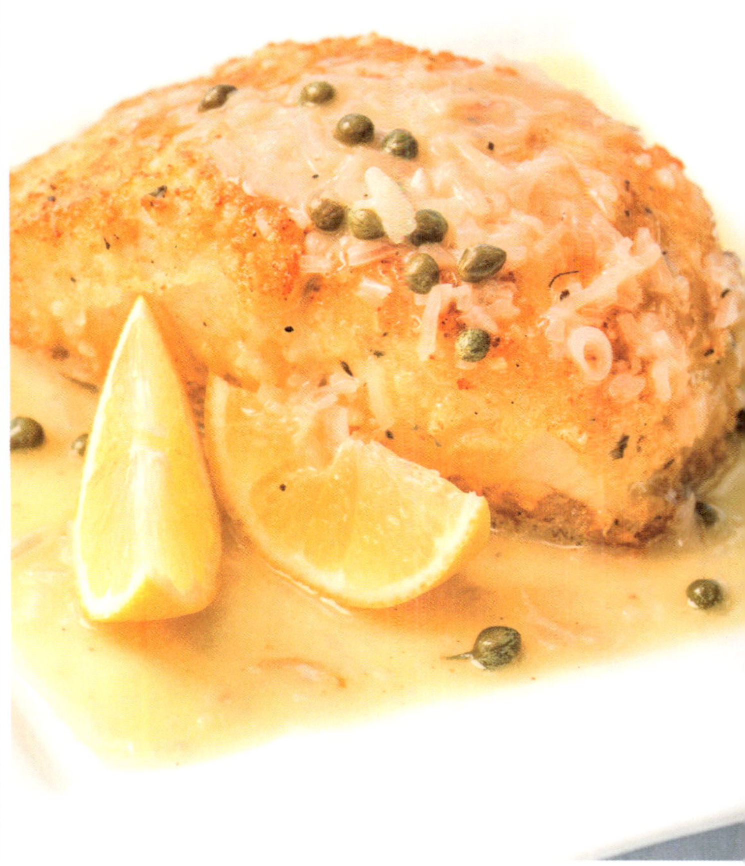

Cabbage Mushroom Bake

SERVES 6

PREP + COOK TIME: 1 HOUR

VEG • GLUTEN FREE

Macadamia Nut Snapper with Caper & Lemon Sauce

SERVES 4

PREP + COOK TIME: 30 MINS

GLUTEN FREE

CABBAGE MUSHROOM BAKE

2 tbsps butter
1 onion, chopped
200g button mushrooms, halved and sliced
500g cabbage, shredded and chopped
100g cream cheese
¼ cup (50ml) thickened cream
Salt and pepper to taste
1 cup (125g) grated tasty cheese

Preheat oven to 180°C.

Heat the butter in a large frying pan over medium heat. Fry the onion for 5 minutes. Add the mushrooms and stir through for 1 minute. Add the cabbage in batches and cook for another 5 minutes.

Whisk together the cream cheese and cream and mix through the cabbage. Season to taste.

Spread out in a casserole dish and sprinkle the cheese over the top.

Bake for 30 minutes until the cheese is golden and bubbling.

MACADAMIA NUT SNAPPER WITH CAPER & LEMON SAUCE

1½ cups (185g) macadamia nuts, processed into meal
2 large cloves garlic, crushed
½ tsp salt
½ tsp pepper
4 x 150g snapper steaks
4 tbsps butter
1 small onion, finely chopped
2 tsps coconut flour
2 large lemons; 1 juiced, 1 cut into wedges
2 tbsps apple cider vinegar
½ cup (130ml) water
⅓ cup (50g) capers, drained
2 tbsps olive oil

Mix the macadamia meal with the garlic, salt and pepper and place in a shallow dish. Dredge the snapper fillets in the mixture then set aside.

Heat the butter in a small saucepan over medium heat. Add the onion and fry for 5 minutes. Stir in the coconut flour for 1 minute. Add the lemon juice, vinegar and water. Simmer for 5 minutes until thickened. Remove from heat and add the capers.

Meanwhile, heat the olive oil in a large frying pan over medium-high heat. Fry the snapper for 3 minutes on one side, then flip and fry for 2 minutes until cooked through and the crust is browned.

Serve the fillets with the lemon sauce and lemon wedges on the side.

Roasted Cauliflower Salad

SERVES 2

PREP + COOK TIME: 35 MINS

VEG • GLUTEN FREE • DAIRY FREE

1 small head cauliflower, cut into small florets

4 tbsps olive oil

1 tsp turmeric

2 tbsps dried oregano

Salt and pepper to taste

3 tbsps balsamic vinegar

SALAD

¾ cup (90g) walnuts, chopped

¼ cup (10g) parsley, finely chopped

3 cups (120g) baby spinach

1 medium red onion, finely chopped

¼ cup (50ml) olive oil

Preheat the oven to 220°C and line a baking tray with baking paper.

Toss the cauliflower with the oil, turmeric and oregano. Spread the florets out evenly on the baking tray and season with salt and pepper.

Roast for 8 minutes, then remove the tray and turn the pieces over. Return to the oven for another 8 minutes.

Sprinkle the vinegar over the cauliflower and bake for 7 minutes. Remove from the oven and let it cool.

Dry fry the walnuts in a small frying pan over medium heat for 2 minutes until just starting to brown. Remove immediately from the pan and set aside.

Toss together the cauliflower with the rest of the salad ingredients, including the olive oil.

Season to taste with salt and pepper and serve.

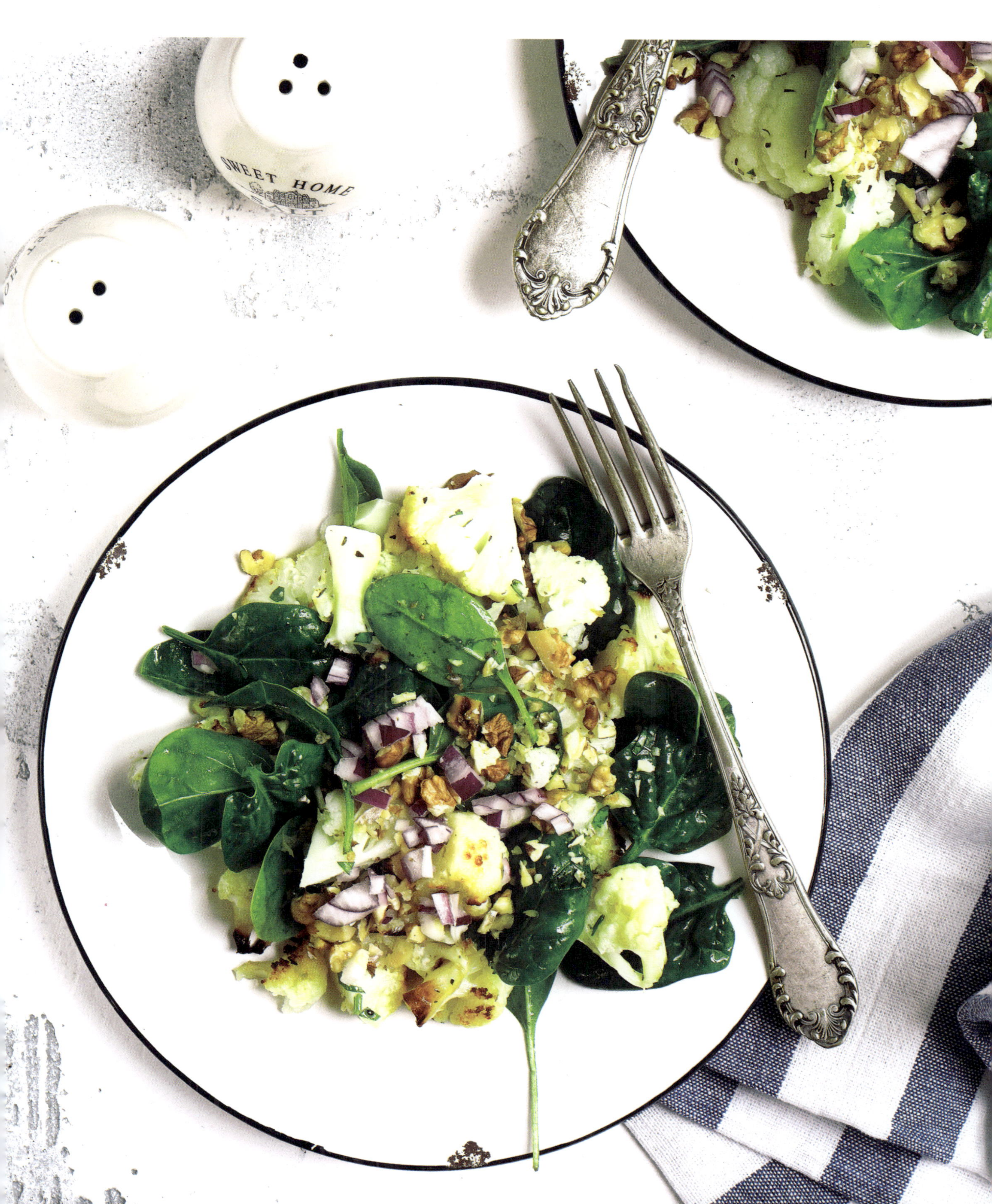
SWEET HOME

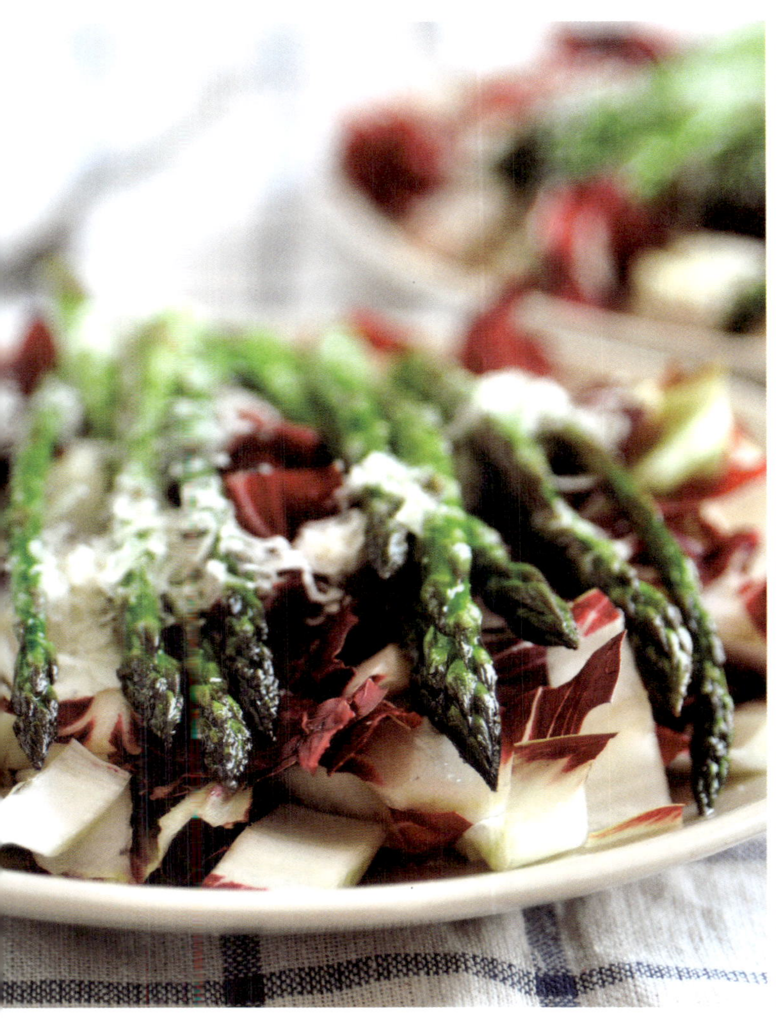

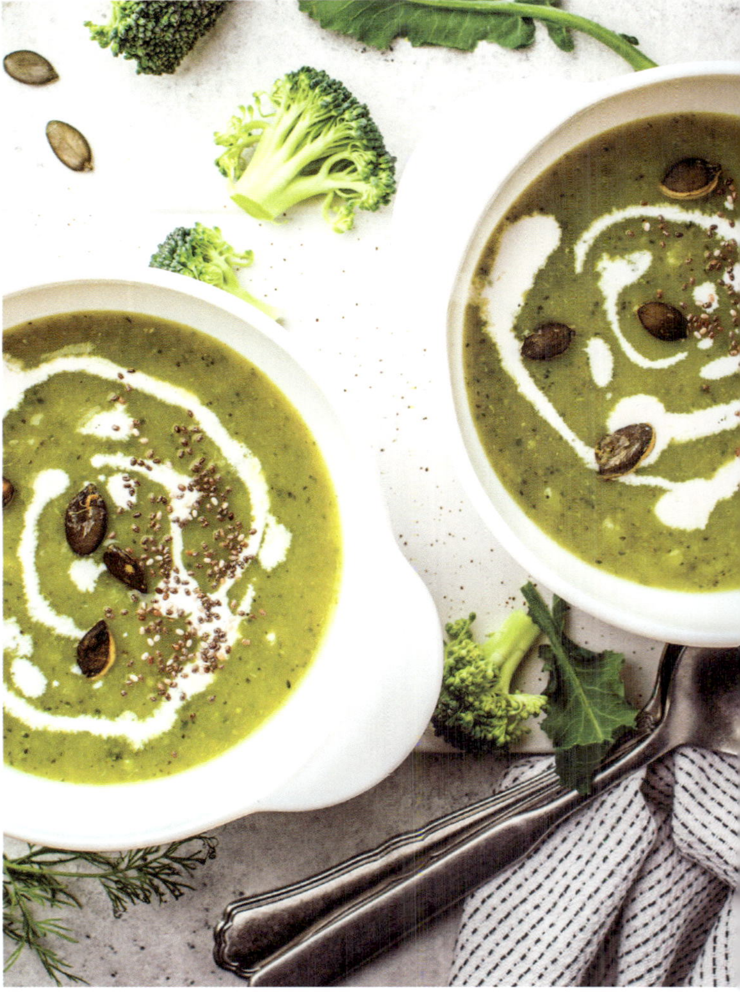

Asparagus Radicchio Salad

SERVES 2

PREP + COOK TIME: 15 MINS

VEG • GLUTEN FREE

Broccoli Coconut Cream Soup

SERVES 4

PREP + COOK TIME: 30 MINS

VEG • GLUTEN FREE

ASPARAGUS RADICCHIO SALAD

½ radicchio
50g butter
2 tbsps olive oil
1 tsp salt
¼ tsp pepper
10 spears asparagus
2 cloves garlic, minced
Juice and zest of ½ lemon
¼ cup (25g) grated Parmesan cheese

Cut the radicchio into 2cm-thick slices and arrange on a plate.

Melt butter in a large frying pan over medium-high heat. Stir in 1 tablespoon olive oil, salt and pepper.

Add the asparagus and cook for 9 minutes, turning asparagus often to ensure even cooking. Add the garlic and cook for 1 minute more until fragrant. Asparagus should be glossy and tender. Remove the asparagus from the pan and lay on top of the radicchio.

Whisk together remaining olive oil, lemon juice and zest. Drizzle over the asparagus.

Top with grated Parmesan to serve.

BROCCOLI COCONUT CREAM SOUP

100g butter
1 large leek, white part only, roughly chopped
2 large cloves garlic, finely chopped
1 tsp ground cumin
½ cup (125ml) + 2 tbsps coconut cream
2 large heads of broccoli, roughly chopped
4 cups (1L) vegetable stock
Salt and pepper to taste
2 tbsps chia seeds, to garnish
¼ cup (30g) pepitas, to garnish

Heat the butter in a large pot over medium heat. Add the leek, garlic and cumin and saute for 5 minutes. Stir through ½ cup of coconut cream then add the broccoli and stock.

Bring to a boil, reduce to low and simmer for 10 minutes until the broccoli is cooked through.

Place the soup in a blender in batches or use a stick blender to puree the soup.

Reheat for 3 minutes and season to taste.

Serve hot garnished with the extra cream and garnished with chia seeds and pepitas if desired.

Italian Wedding Soup with Spinach & Meatballs

SERVES 4
PREP + COOK TIME: 1 HOUR + CHILLING
GLUTEN FREE

800g chicken mince
2 small onions; 1 finely chopped, 1 roughly chopped (see tip)
300g baby spinach, roughly chopped
⅔ cup (65g) roughly grated Parmesan cheese
2 small eggs, lightly beaten
¼ cup (25g) almond flour
Salt and pepper to taste
¼ cup (60ml) olive oil
2 medium carrots, chopped
1 cup (100g) celery, chopped
4 cups (1L) chicken stock

Place the mince, the finely chopped onion, ½ cup of the spinach, half the Parmesan, the eggs, almond flour and 1 teaspoon each of salt and pepper in a large bowl and mix thoroughly.

Shape the mixture into small meatballs and place in the refrigerator for at least 1 hour to chill.

Heat half the oil in a large pot over medium heat. Fry the meatballs in batches for 10 minutes, turning every 2 minutes to cook thoroughly. Remove from the pot and set aside.

Heat the rest of the oil and fry the rest of the onion along with the carrot and celery for 8 minutes until softened.

Add the stock and bring to a boil. Reduce heat and simmer for 15 minutes. Return the meatballs to the pot along with the rest of the spinach and heat through for 3 minutes.

Season to taste and top with the rest of the Parmesan.

Tip:

Omit the onion to further reduce carbs, if required.

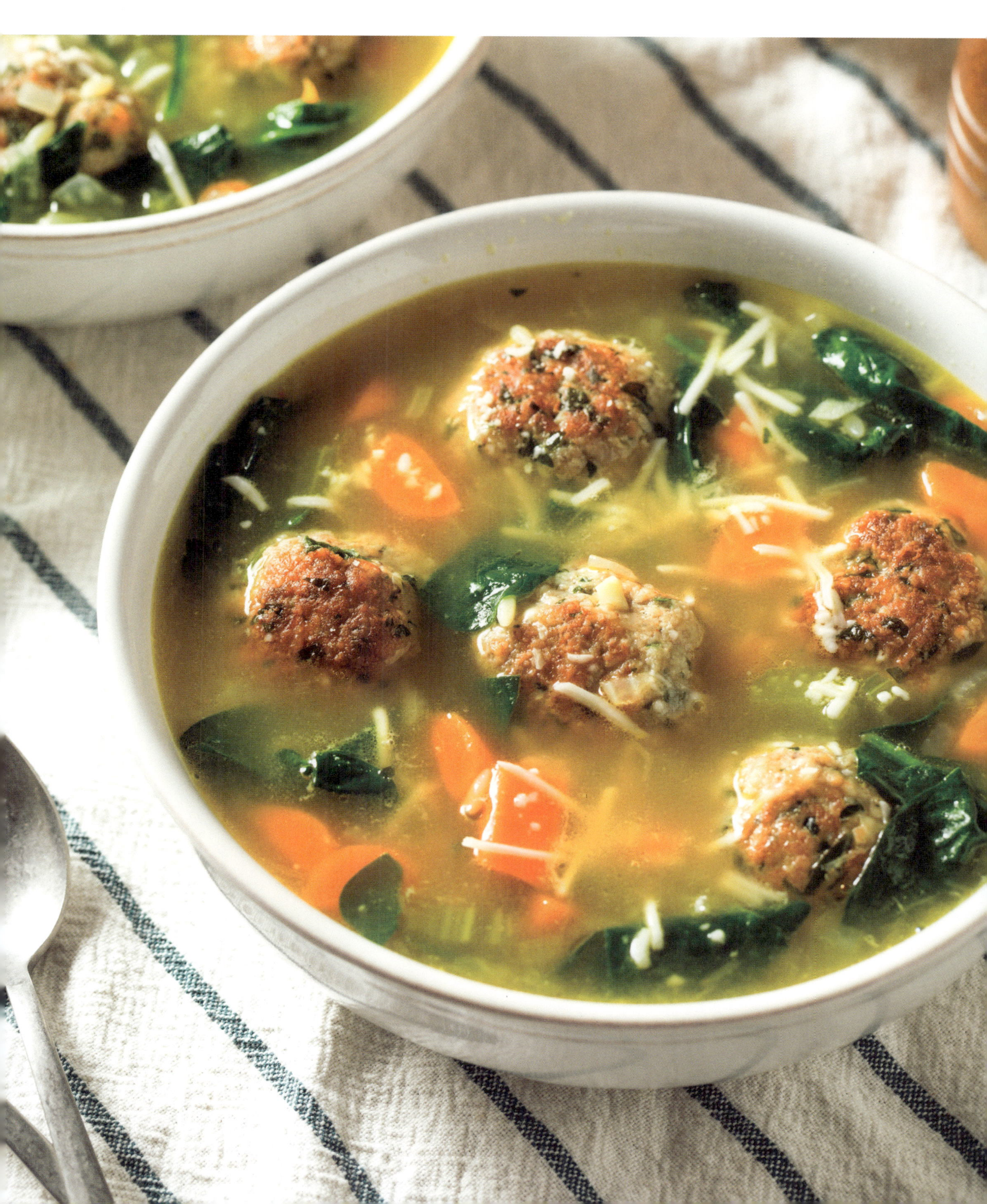

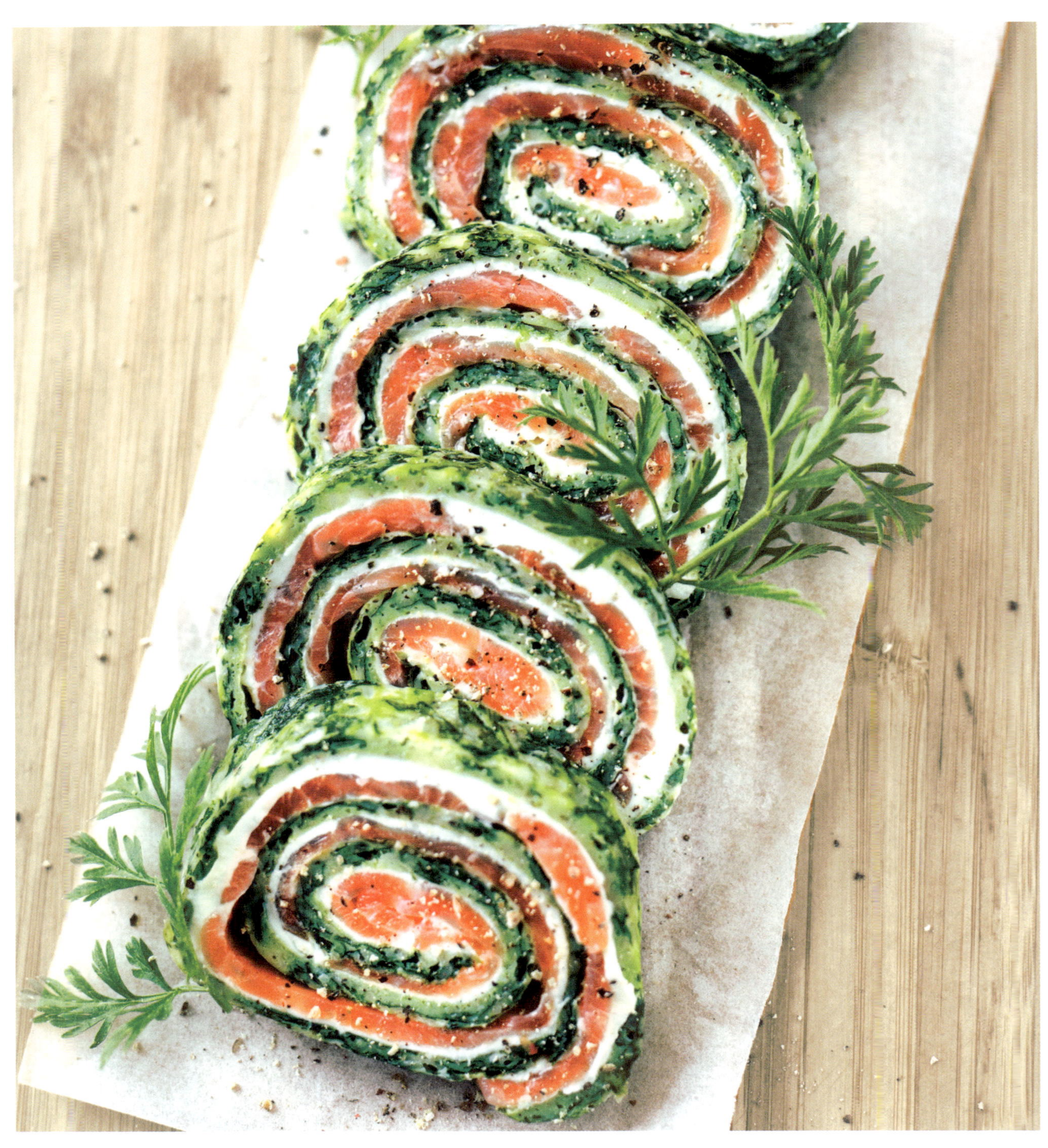

Smoked Salmon, Cream Cheese & Spinach Roulade

SERVES 2

PREP + COOK TIME: 30 MINS

GLUTEN FREE

SMOKED SALMON, CREAM CHEESE & SPINACH ROULADE

4 cups (120g) fresh spinach leaves, finely chopped
¼ cup (10g) parsley, roughly chopped
½ tsp psyllium husk powder
¼ tsp xanthan gum
4 large eggs, room temperature
Salt and pepper to taste
1 tbsp olive oil
200g cream cheese
200g smoked salmon slices

Place the spinach, parsley, psyllium powder, xanthan gum, eggs and a pinch each of salt and pepper in a large bowl and whisk thoroughly to combine.

Heat half the oil in a large non-stick frying pan over medium heat.

Pour half the egg mixture into the pan and swirl to coat the bottom completely.

Cook for 3 minutes, then flip and cook for another 2 minutes. Remove and let cool completely. Repeat with the rest of the egg mixture.

Spread half the cream cheese over each cooked spinach and egg base and spread the salmon out over both. Roll them up carefully to form your roulade and cut into 1cm thick slices.

Baked Salmon & Spring Veg

SERVES 4
PREP + COOK TIME: 25 MINS
GLUTEN FREE • DAIRY FREE

4 x 175g salmon fillets
4 baby bok choy, cut in halves lengthwise
150g Swiss brown mushrooms, quartered
500g cherry tomatoes on the vine
1 bunch asparagus
4 tbsps olive oil
2 tbsps lemon juice
2 cloves garlic, minced
1 tsp chopped fresh rosemary
Salt and pepper to taste
2 spring onions, chopped, to serve

Preheat the oven to 180°C. Line two baking trays with greaseproof paper.

Arrange the salmon, bok choy, mushrooms, tomatoes and asparagus in one layer on the baking trays.

Mix olive oil, lemon juice, garlic and rosemary together in a small bowl. Season well with salt and pepper. Spoon the mixture over the fish and vegetables and turn to coat all sides.

Transfer to the oven and bake for 10 minutes until the salmon is almost cooked. Then grill for 3 minutes to brown.

Divide the salmon and vegetables between four plates and scatter with spring onions to serve.

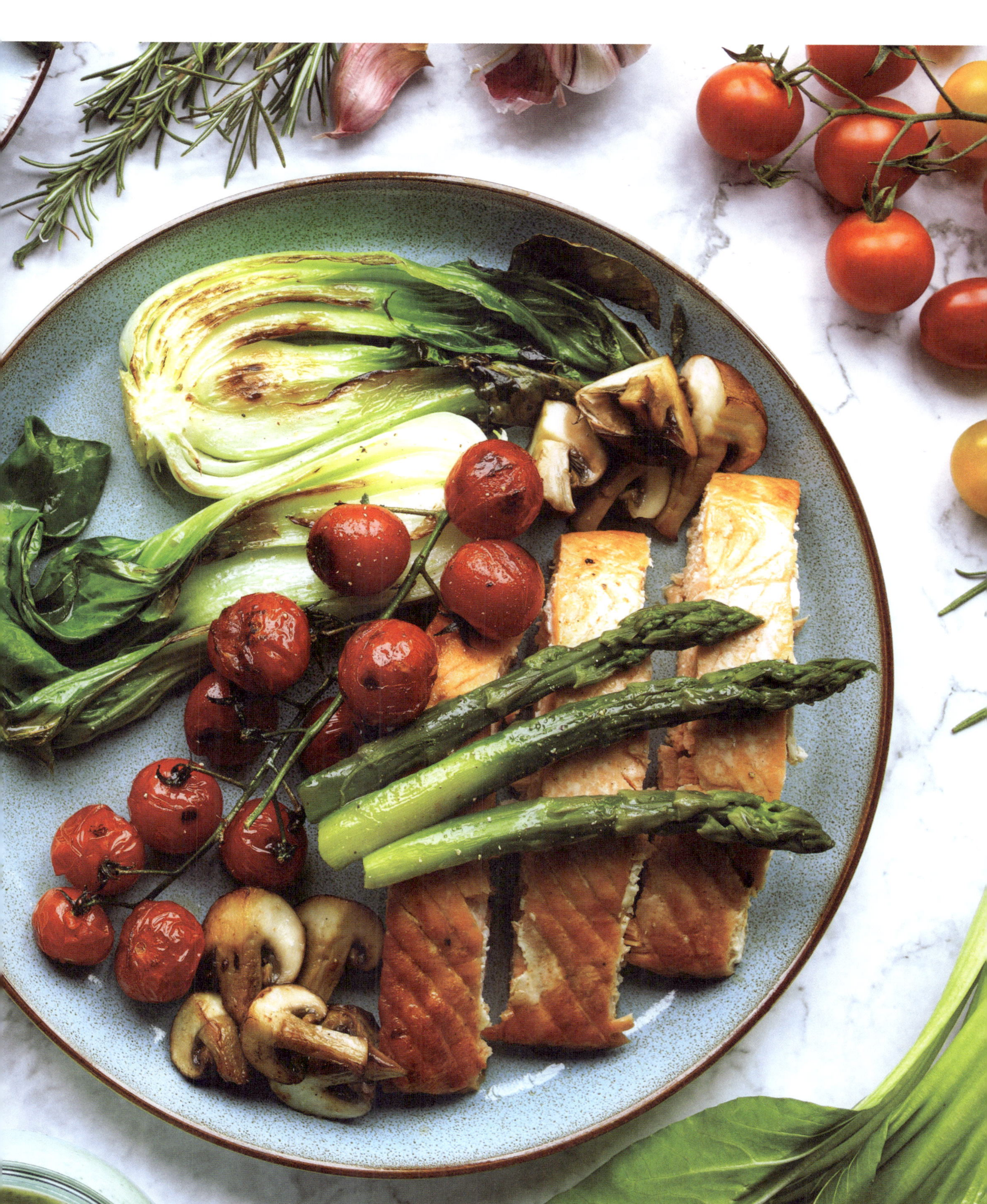

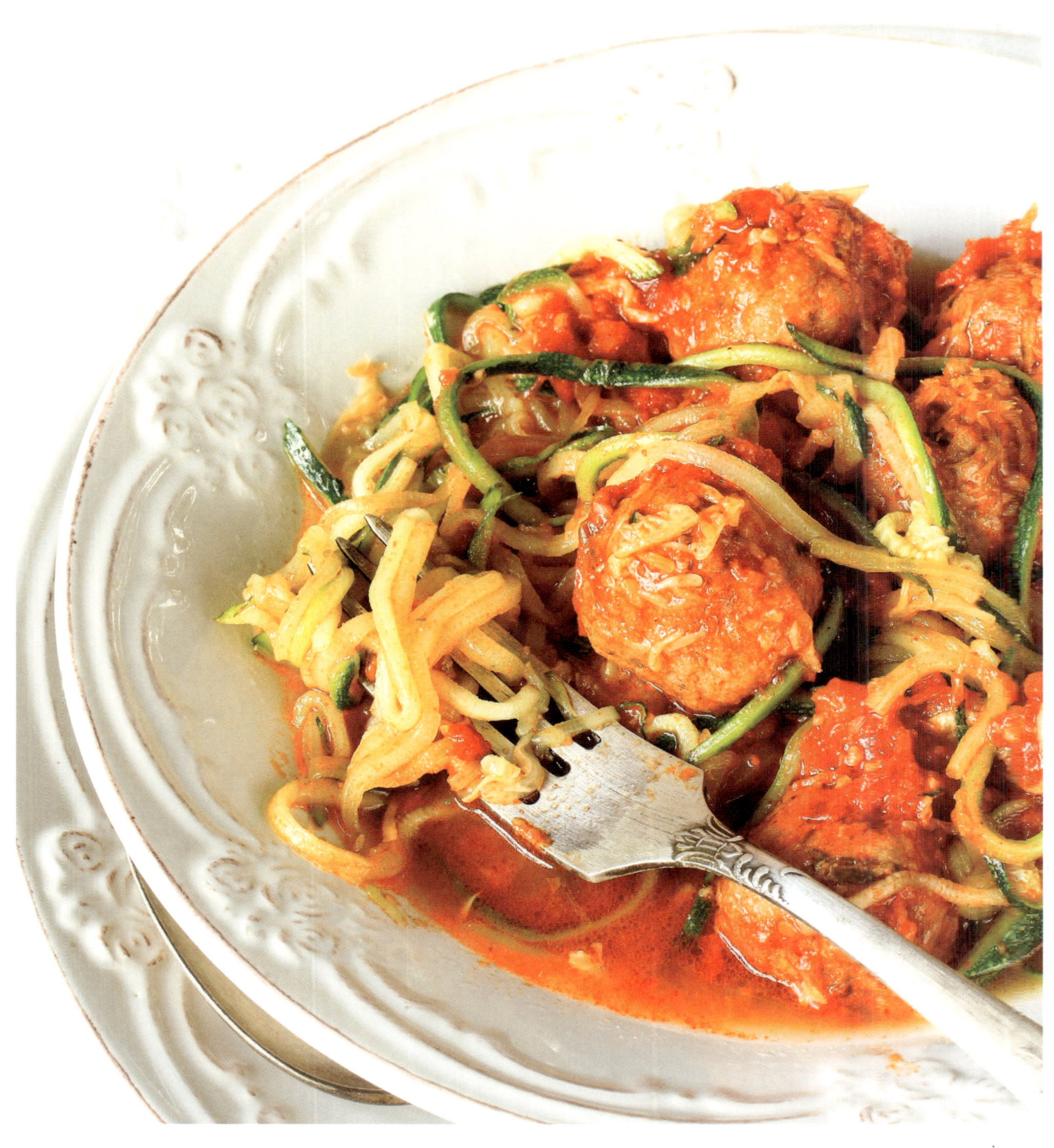

Italian Pork Meatballs with Zoodles

SERVES 4

PREP + COOK TIME: 1 HOUR + CHILLING

GLUTEN FREE

ITALIAN PORK MEATBALLS WITH ZOODLES

700g pork mince
3 large cloves garlic, finely chopped
½ small onion, finely chopped
½ cup (50g) grated Parmesan cheese
3 tbsps almond flour
1 large egg, beaten
Salt and pepper to taste
2 tbsps olive oil
2 cups (450g) tomato passata
½ cup (125ml) water
5 large zucchinis, cut into spaghetti strips

Place the mince, garlic, onion, ¼ cup cheese, almond flour, egg and a couple of grinds of salt and pepper in a large bowl and mix together thoroughly.

Form the mince into 24 meatballs and chill in the refrigerator for at least 1 hour.

Heat the oil in a large frying pan over medium heat. Fry the meatballs in batches for 10 minutes, turning every 2 minutes.

Pour the tomato passata and the water over the meatballs. Bring to a boil, then reduce the heat to low and simmer for 20 minutes.

Bring a large pot of salted water to a boil and cook the zucchini noodles for 2 minutes, then drain.

Serve the zoodles with the meatballs, sauce and remaining Parmesan.

Avocado Cream Soup

SERVES 2
PREP + COOK TIME: 10 MINS
VEG • GLUTEN FREE

1 avocado
2 cups (60g) spinach
¾ cucumber
1 stalk celery
1 tbsp lime juice
1 bunch fresh coriander
2 tsps cumin
1 tsp ground coriander
1 tsp onion powder
½ tsp salt
1 tsp tamari
1 cup (250ml) water
½ cup (125ml) sour cream + 1 tbsp to serve

Scoop the avocado flesh into a high-speed blender along with all the remaining ingredients. Blend until completely smooth.

Pour into bowls and swirl with extra sour cream to serve.

Serve cold.

Tip:

For a vegan or dairy-free version of this soup use coconut cream instead of sour cream.

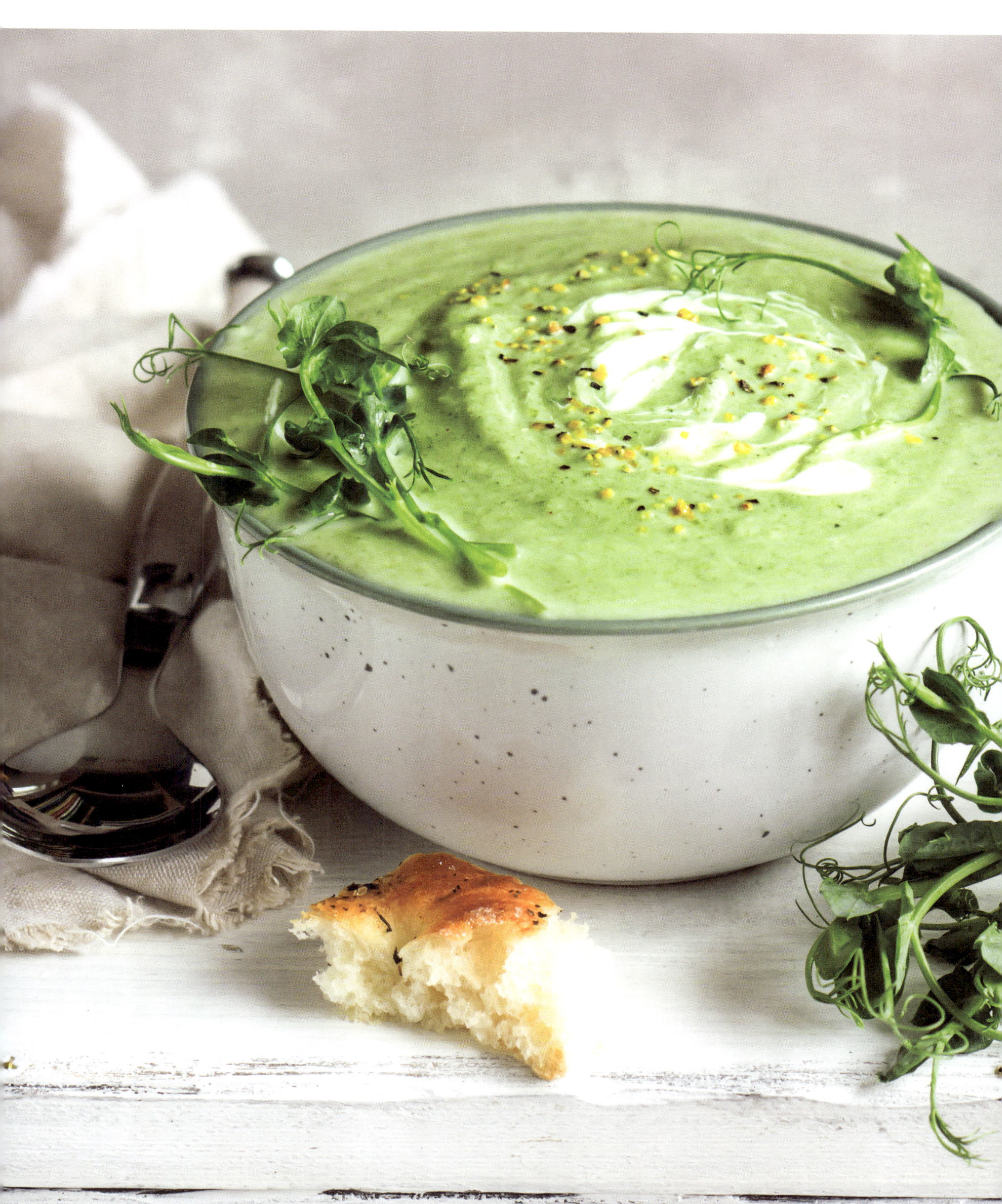

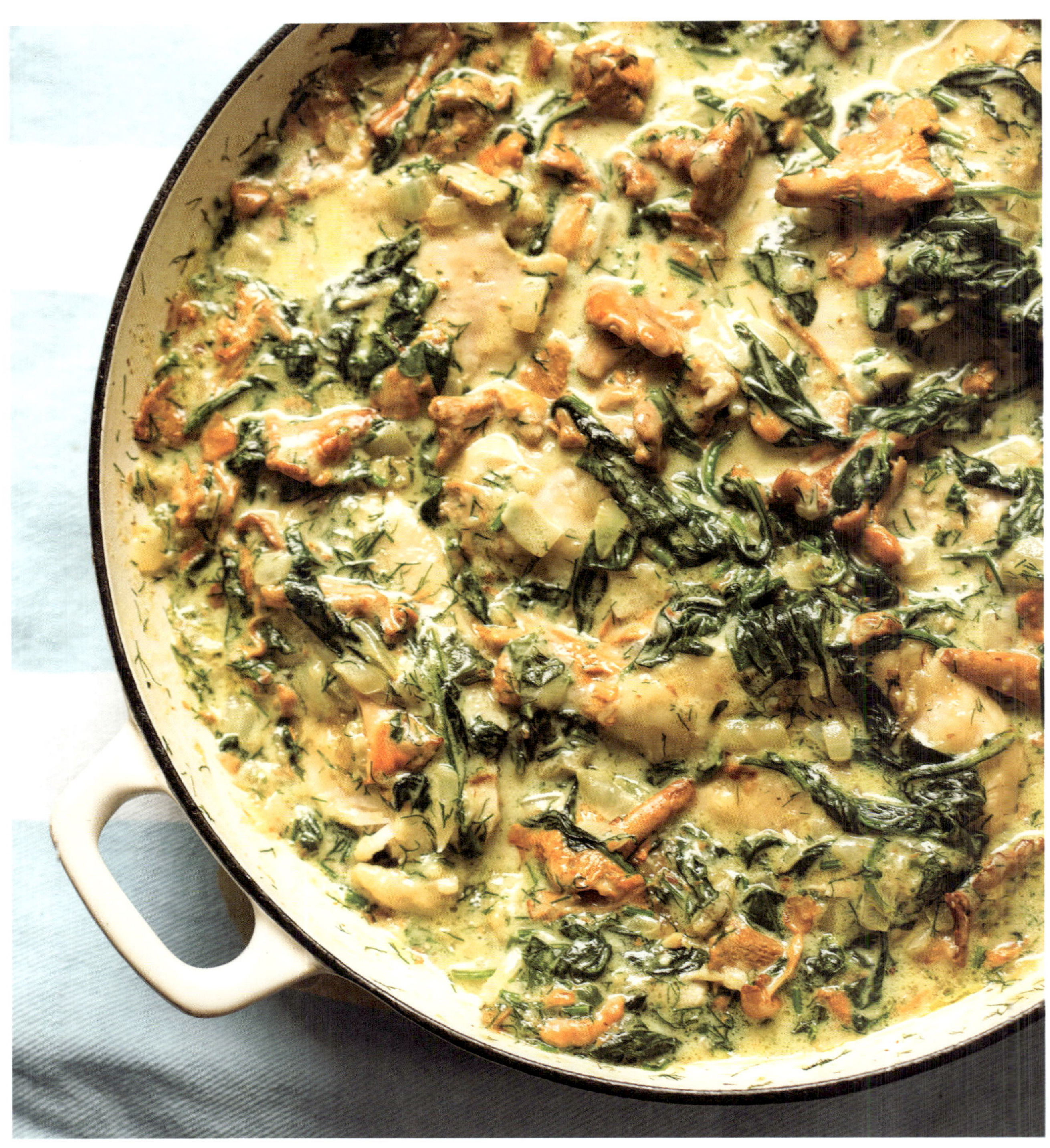

Chicken & Dill Cream Casserole

SERVES 6

PREP + COOK TIME: 30 MINS

GLUTEN FREE

CHICKEN & DILL CREAM CASSEROLE

- 4 chicken breasts, halved crosswise
- Salt and pepper to taste
- 2 tbsps olive oil
- 4 tbsps butter
- 1 medium onion, chopped
- 280g cremini (or preferred) mushrooms, sliced
- 4 cloves garlic, minced
- 2½ tbsps unflavoured whey protein isolate
- 1 cup (250ml) chicken stock
- 1 cup (250ml) thickened cream
- ½ cup (50g) finely grated Parmesan cheese
- 1 cup (30g) spinach
- ½ cup (10g) fresh dill, chopped

Season the chicken with salt and pepper. Heat 1 tablespoon of olive oil in a large frying pan over medium-high heat. Cook the chicken breasts for 4 minutes on each side undisturbed. Remove from the heat, cover loosely with foil and set aside to rest.

Add 1 tablespoon each of oil and butter to the hot pan and swirl around to deglaze. Add the onion and cook, stirring, for 3 minutes until soft. Add the mushrooms, and saute for 5 minutes until tender. Remove from the pan and set aside.

Add the remaining 3 tablespoons of butter to the pan. When melted add the garlic and cook, stirring, for 1 minute. Add the whey protein and stir well to form a paste. Slowly add the chicken stock and cream, stirring constantly. Bring to a gentle simmer. Add Parmesan, salt and pepper and stir well until thickened. Stir through the spinach and dill.

Return the chicken and mushrooms to the pan and heat through for a few minutes before serving.

Chapter Five

Sweet

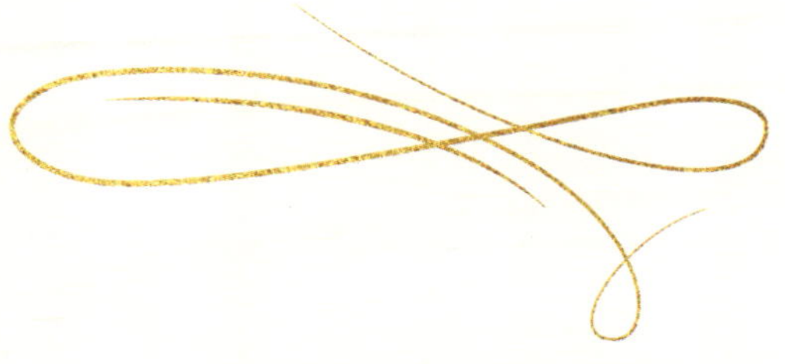

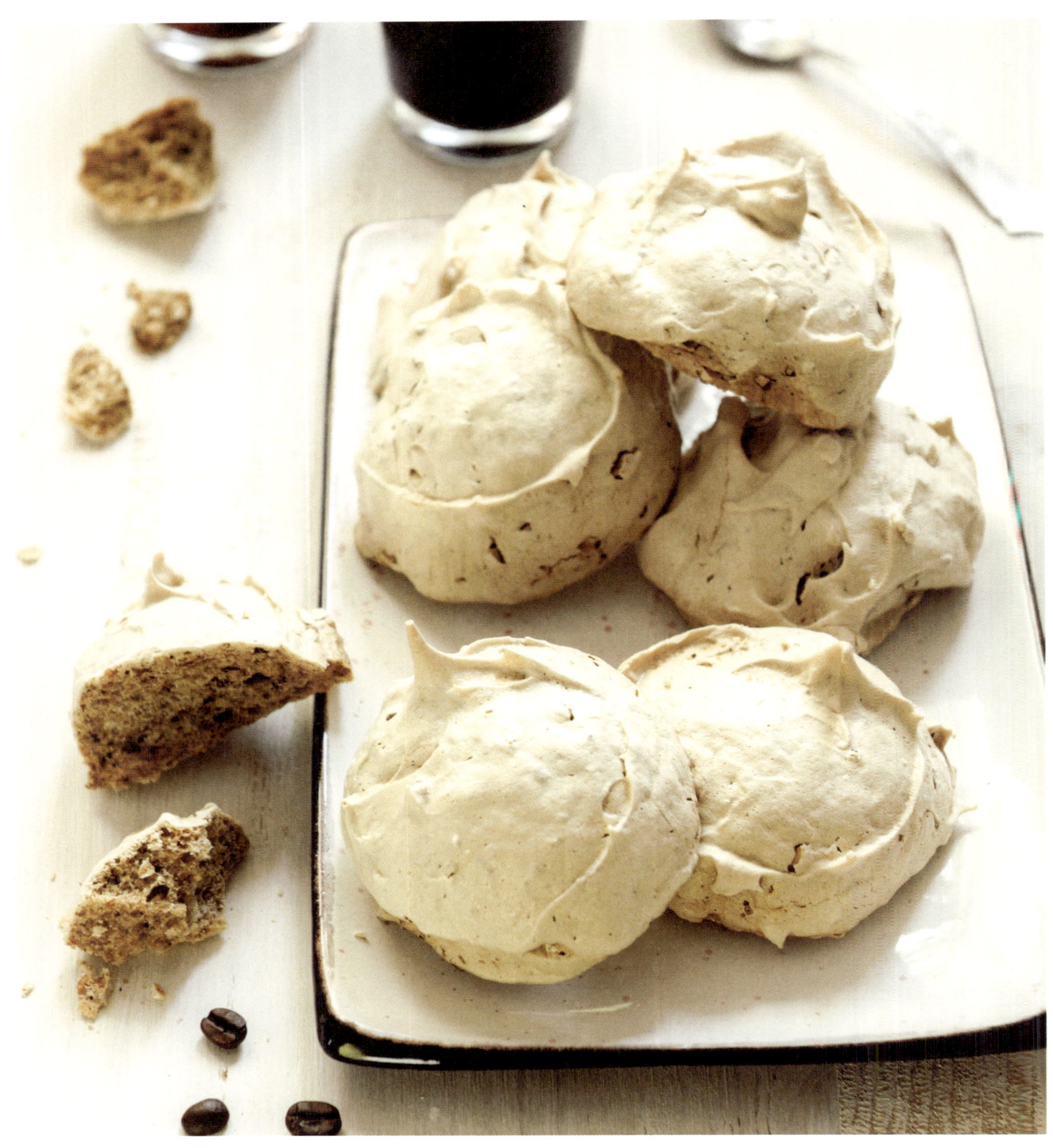

Mini Hazelnut Pavs

MAKES 20

PREP + COOK TIME: 2 HOURS 55 MINS

VEG • GLUTEN FREE • DAIRY FREE

MINI HAZELNUT PAVS

4 egg whites, room temperature
6 tbsps powdered erythritol
¼ tsp cream of tartar
⅛ tsp salt
2 tsps instant coffee granules
2 tsps hot water
½ cup (60g) roasted hazelnuts

Preheat oven to 120°C and line two baking trays with greaseproof paper.

Arrange oven racks in second lowest and second highest positions.

In clean glass or metal bowl, combine egg whites, erythritol, cream of tartar and salt. Beat with an electric hand mixer on medium-high until medium-stiff peaks form and mixture becomes somewhat glossy. Do not beat until stiff.

Dissolve coffee in the water in a small jug. Fold coffee mixture into egg white mixture.

Pulse the hazelnuts in a food processor until finely chopped. Fold hazelnuts into egg white mixture.

Spoon or pipe mixture into 20-24 large meringues.

Bake for 18-20 minutes. Then reduce oven temperature to 95°C and continue to bake for another 18-20 minutes, until crisp.

Turn off oven, but leave the meringues inside the oven for at least 2 hours.

Remove from the oven and carefully peel off the greaseproof paper and serve.

Raw Chocolate Coconut Bites

MAKES 20 BALLS

PREP + COOK TIME: 40 MINS + CHILLING

VEG • GLUTEN FREE • DAIRY FREE

1½ cups (130g) desiccated coconut
¼ cup (60ml) almond milk
½ cup (50g) almond flour
½ tsp stevia
2 tbsps coconut oil
235g sugar-free dark cooking chocolate, roughly chopped

Place all the ingredients except the chocolate in a large bowl and mix to combine into a sticky mixture.

Form into approximately 20 small balls and place in the refrigerator for 1 hour to chill.

Gently heat the chocolate in a heatproof bowl placed over a pan of simmering water until melted.

Line a large, flat baking tray with greaseproof paper.

Dip the balls into the chocolate to coat completely. Place on the greaseproof paper after each is coated. Once finished, use a small spoon to drizzle the remaining melted chocolate over the top of the balls. Chill in the refrigerator for another hour before serving.

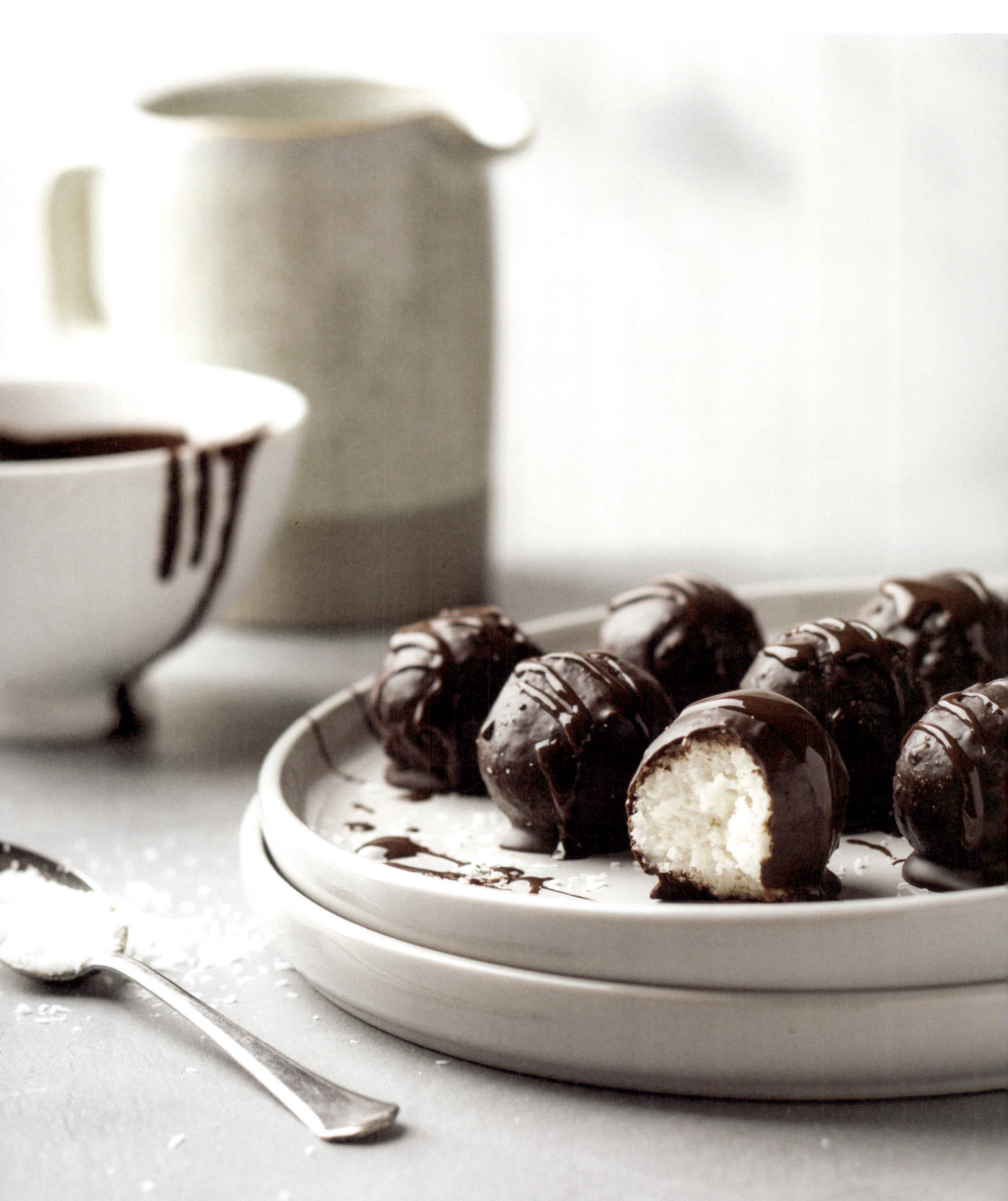

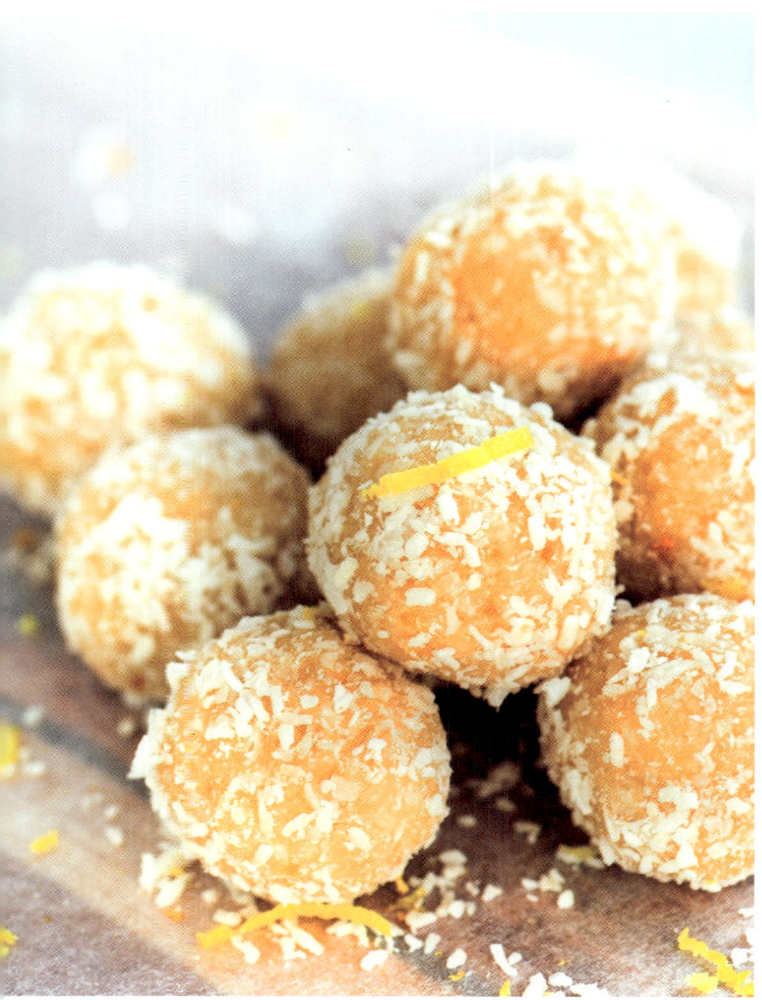

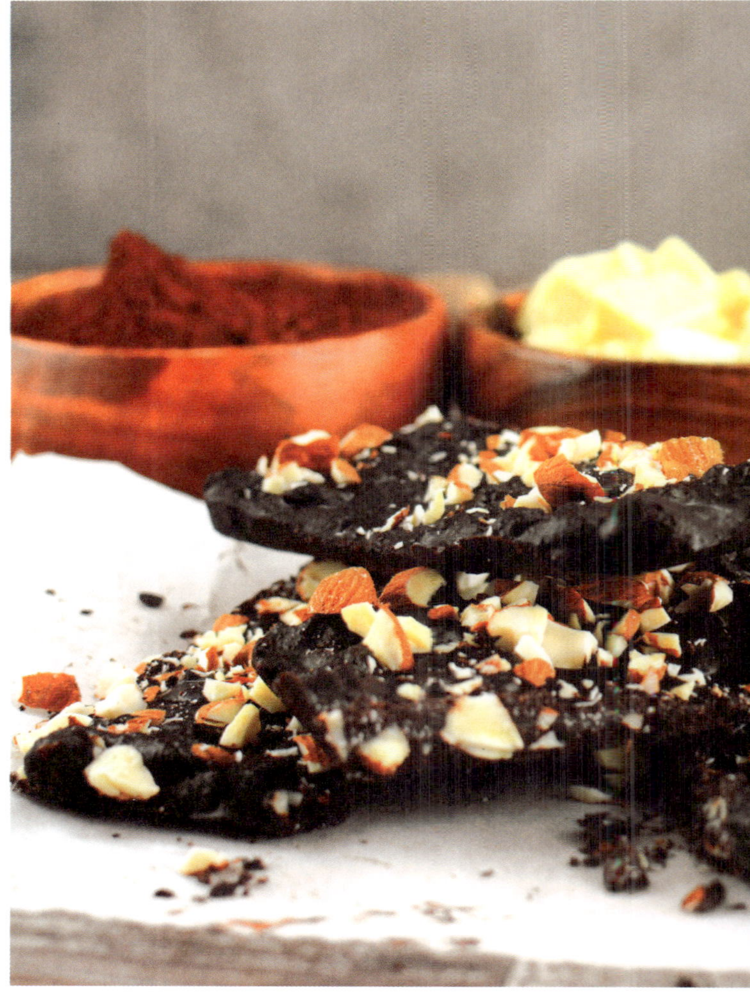

Coconut & Lemon Truffles

SERVES 4

PREP + COOK TIME: 30 MINS + CHILLING

VEG • GLUTEN FREE

Dark Choc-Almond Bark

SERVES 4

PREP + COOK TIME: 15 MINS + CHILLING

VEG • GLUTEN FREE

COCONUT & LEMON TRUFFLES

70g cream cheese
1 tbsp sour cream
1 lemon, to make 1 tbsp lemon zest + 2 tsps lemon juice
½ cup (40g) almond flour
½ cup (40g) coconut flour
¼ tsp liquid stevia
½ tsp vanilla essence
¼ tsp salt
1 cup (90g) desiccated coconut

Mix together all the ingredients, except the desiccated coconut, in a large bowl.

Form into a large ball and flatten into a disc. Wrap in plastic and chill in the refrigerator for at least 30 minutes.

Form the mixture into round truffle balls and roll in the coconut to coat.

Chill the truffles for 30 minutes before serving.

DARK CHOC-ALMOND BARK

3¼ cups (500g) sugar-free dark chocolate chips
½ tsp salt
½ cup (60g) almonds, chopped

Line a baking tray with baking paper.

Place the chocolate chips in a heatproof bowl over a pan of simmering water on medium-low heat. Stir for 3-5 minutes until all the chocolate is melted, ensuring no water gets into the bowl.

Add the salt to the melted chocolate and stir.

Pour the chocolate mixture in a thin layer about 1cm thick on the prepared baking tray. Sprinkle with the chopped almonds and place in the fridge for 20 minutes or until the chocolate is hard.

Peel the paper from the chocolate and break into pieces. Store in the refrigerator.

Avocado Chocolate Mousse

SERVES 4

PREP + COOK TIME: 5 MINS + CHILLING

VEG • GLUTEN FREE • DAIRY FREE

1 large avocado

¼ cup (30g) unsweetened cocoa powder

⅓ cup (60g) erythritol

1¼ cups (310ml) canned coconut cream

1 tsp vanilla extract

OPTIONAL TOPPINGS

Flaked chocolate, mint leaves and berries

Scoop the flesh of the avocado into a blender along with cocoa powder, sweetener, coconut cream and vanilla extract.

Blend for 1 minute until smooth.

Transfer the chocolate mousse into small bowls, glasses or ramekins and refrigerate for at least 1 hour.

Serve with chocolate flakes, mint leaves and berries or the toppings of your choice.

Tip:

This mousse can be stored in the fridge for up to 2 days if kept covered.

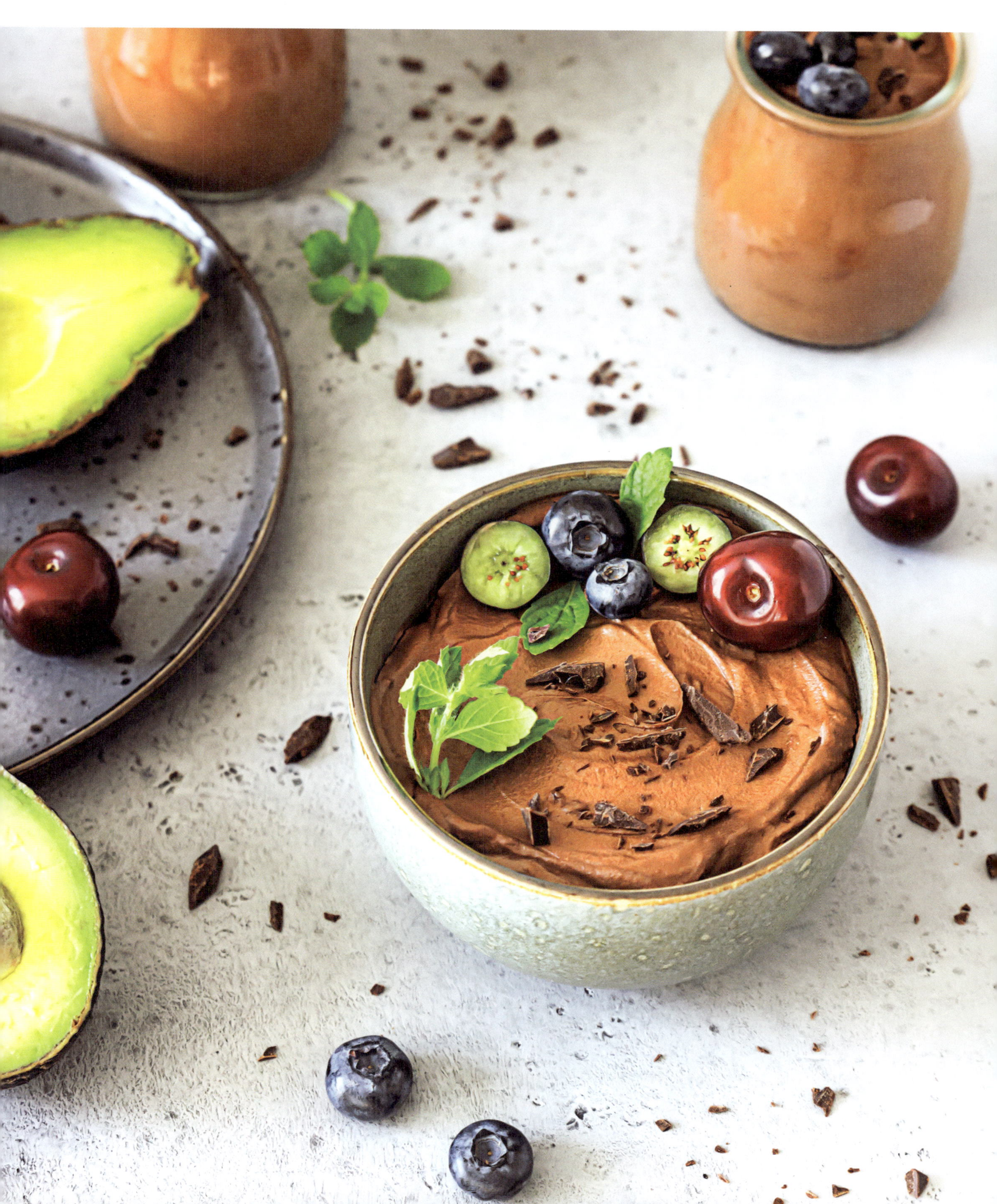

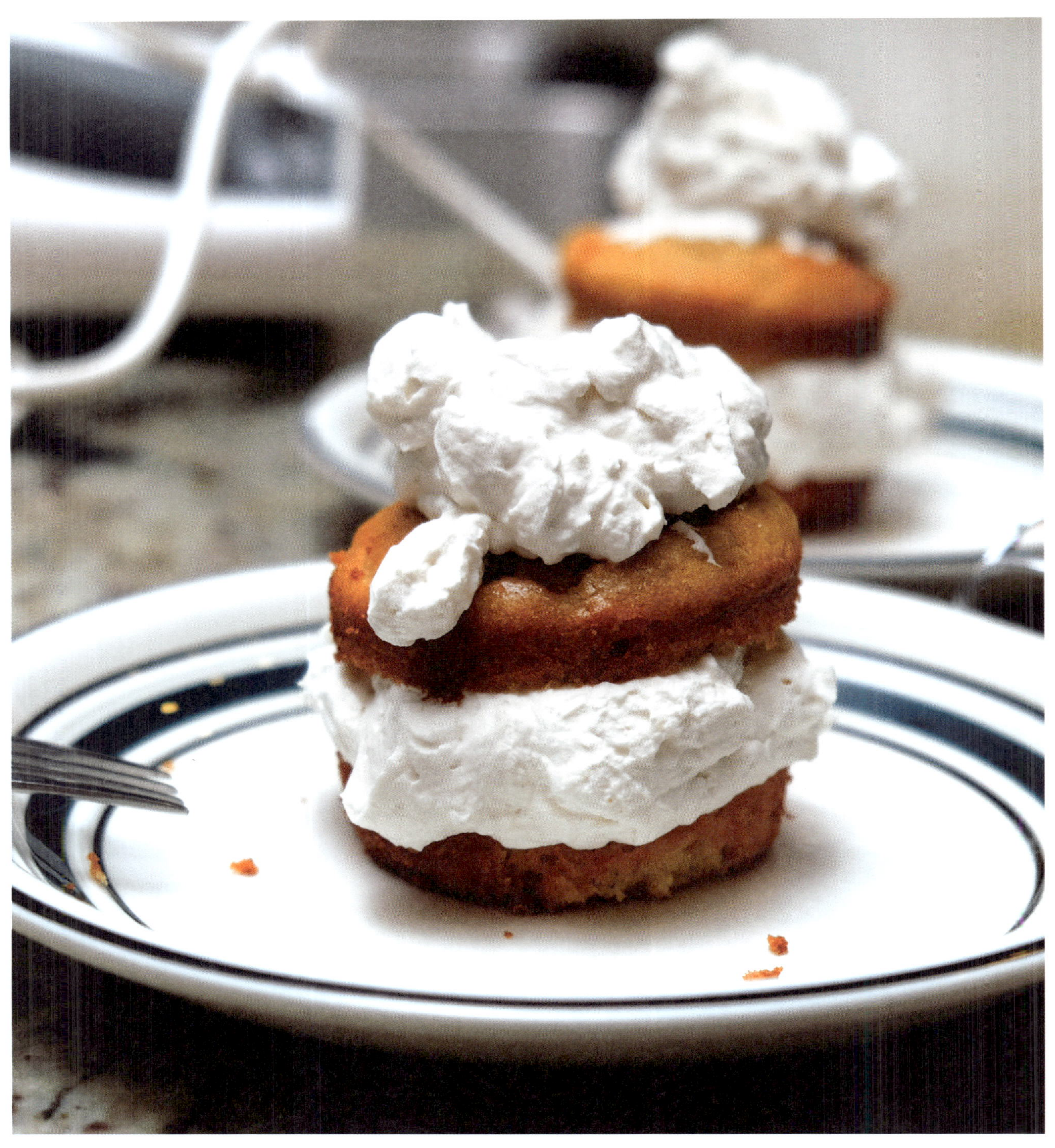

Cupcakes with Whipped Cream

MAKES 12

PREP + COOK TIME: 30 MINS + COOLING

VEG • GLUTEN FREE

CUPCAKES WITH WHIPPED CREAM

1⅔ cups (165g) almond flour
1 tsp baking powder
½ tsp bicarbonate of soda
2 tbsps butter
1 tsp vanilla essence
1 tbsp molasses
¼ cup (55g) erythritol
3 medium eggs, room temperature
1¼ cups (300ml) thickened cream
1 cup (250ml) coconut cream

Preheat oven to 190°C and grease two six-hole cupcake tins.

Sift together the almond flour, baking powder and bicarb.

Beat together the butter, vanilla essence, molasses and 3 tablespoons of the erythritol until mixed through. Mix through the eggs, one at a time, until fully combined.

Add the dry ingredients, a third at a time, until just combined.

Spoon the mixture into the cupcake holes and bake for 18 minutes or until a skewer inserted in the middle of them comes out clean. Remove from the holes and cool on a wire rack to room temperature.

Whip the cream with the remaining erythritol until stiff peaks form. Add the coconut cream and whip until mixed thoroughly.

Cut the cupcakes in half, place a tablespoon of cream on each bottom half, replace the top halves of the cakes, then top with another tablespoon of cream.

Raspberry Mousse

SERVES 6

PREP + COOK TIME: 20 MINS

GLUTEN FREE

- 1 tbsp gelatin
- 2 tbsps cold water
- 3 tbsps boiling water
- 2 cups (250g) fresh or frozen raspberries
- ⅓ cup (60g) erythritol or low-carb sugar substitute
- ⅛ tsp stevia
- 1½ cups (375ml) thickened cream
- 1 tsp vanilla extract
- Fresh raspberries and mint leaves, to garnish

In small cup, sprinkle gelatin over the cold water. Stand for 2 minutes to soften. Add 3 tablespoons boiling water and stir until gelatin is completely dissolved and mixture is clear. Allow to cool slightly.

Cook raspberries, erythritol and stevia in a small pan over medium-low heat for 5 minutes, stirring regularly, until sweeteners are dissolved. Cool, then remove seeds by pressing mixture through a sieve with a spoon. Stir in the gelatin and set aside.

Whip cream with vanilla extract until soft peaks form. Gently fold raspberry mixture through the cream. Spoon into six dessert cups.

Top with fresh raspberries and mint leaves to serve.

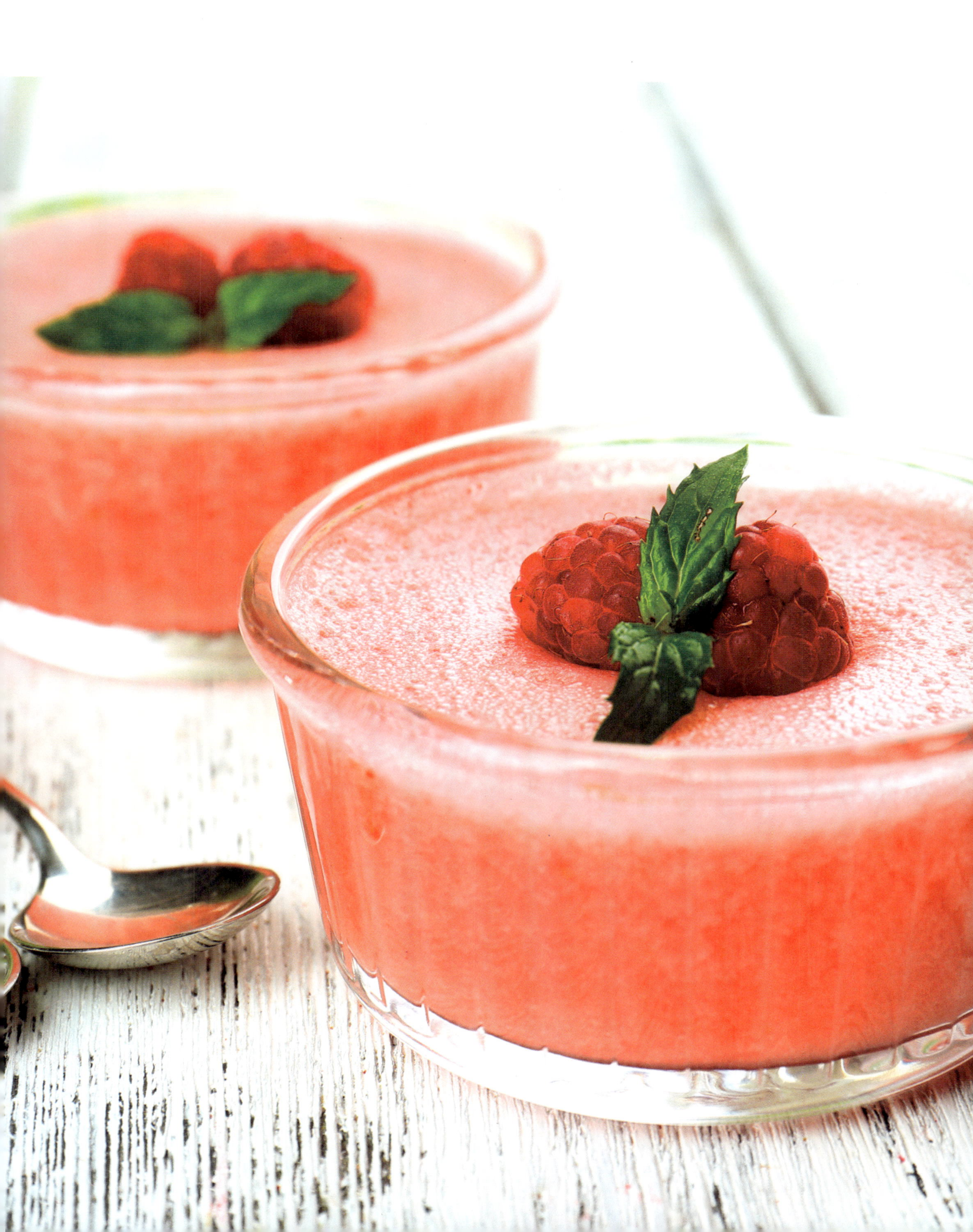

HAZELNUT MUFFINS

2 cups (225g) finely ground hazelnut meal
1 tsp baking powder
¼ tsp salt
115g butter, melted
4 eggs
¼ cup (50g) erythritol or sugar substitute

TOPPINGS

100g dark chocolate (minimum 80% cocoa solids), melted
¼ cup (30g) chopped hazelnuts

Preheat the oven to 180°C. Line a muffin tin with eight paper liners.

Whisk together hazelnut meal, baking powder and salt.

In another bowl mix the melted butter, eggs and erythritol until combined.

Combine the wet and dry ingredients together, and stir well.

Pour the mixture into the muffin tin. Bake for 20-23 minutes until firm.

Allow to cool completely before topping with melted chocolate, chocolate icing or coffee icing. Scatter with chopped hazelnuts to serve.

STRAWBERRY FROZEN YOGHURT BARK

2 cups (500ml) Greek yoghurt
¼ cup (60ml) thickened cream
¼ cup (50g) granulated erythritol
2 tsps vanilla extract
½ cup (100g) strawberries, roughly chopped
⅓ cup (60g) low-sugar, low-carb granola

Line a baking tray with greaseproof paper.

Place the yoghurt, cream, erythritol and vanilla extract into a large mixing bowl and stir to combine well. Fold through the chopped strawberries.

Pour the mixture onto the prepared baking tray and smooth into an even layer. Top with the granola.

Freeze for 2 hours, or until firm. Remove 15 minutes before serving. Cut into pieces. Store in the freezer.

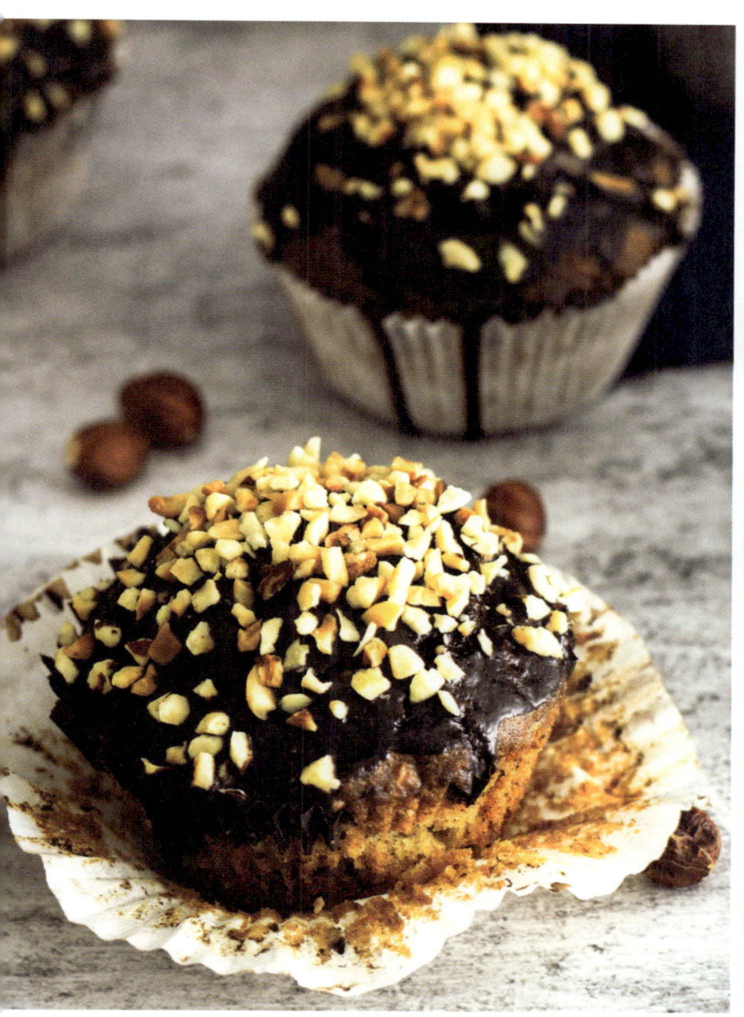

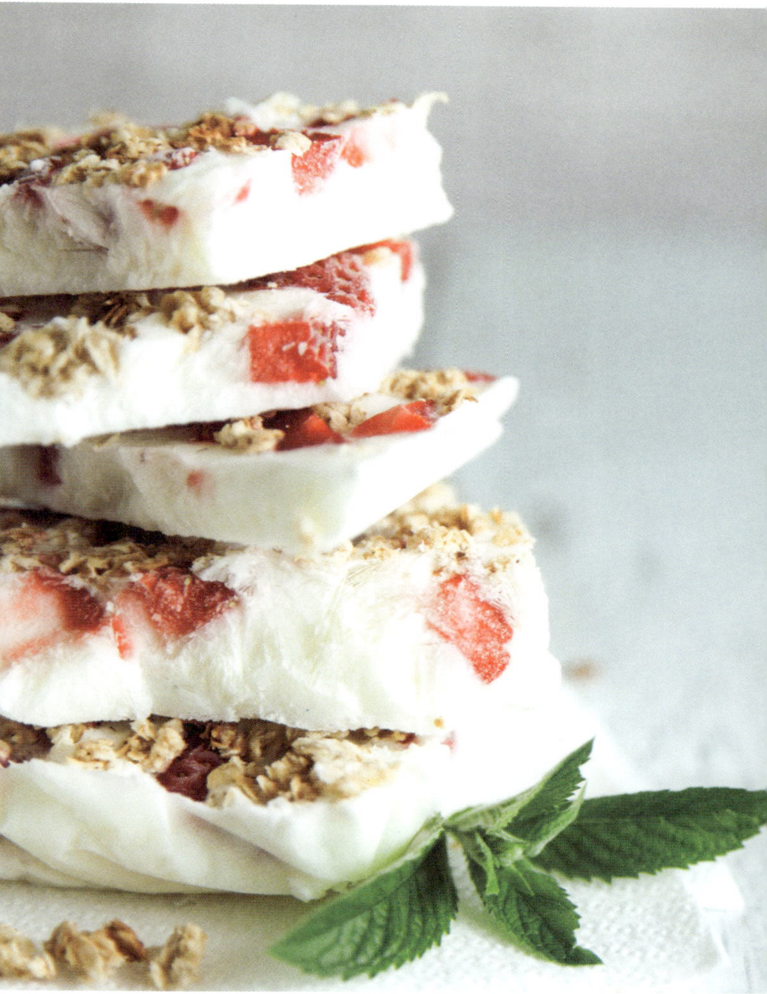

Hazelnut Muffins

MAKES 8

PREP + COOK TIME: 35 MINS

VEG • GLUTEN FREE

Strawberry Frozen Yoghurt Bark

MAKES 12

PREP + COOK TIME: 15 MINS + CHILLING

VEG • GLUTEN FREE

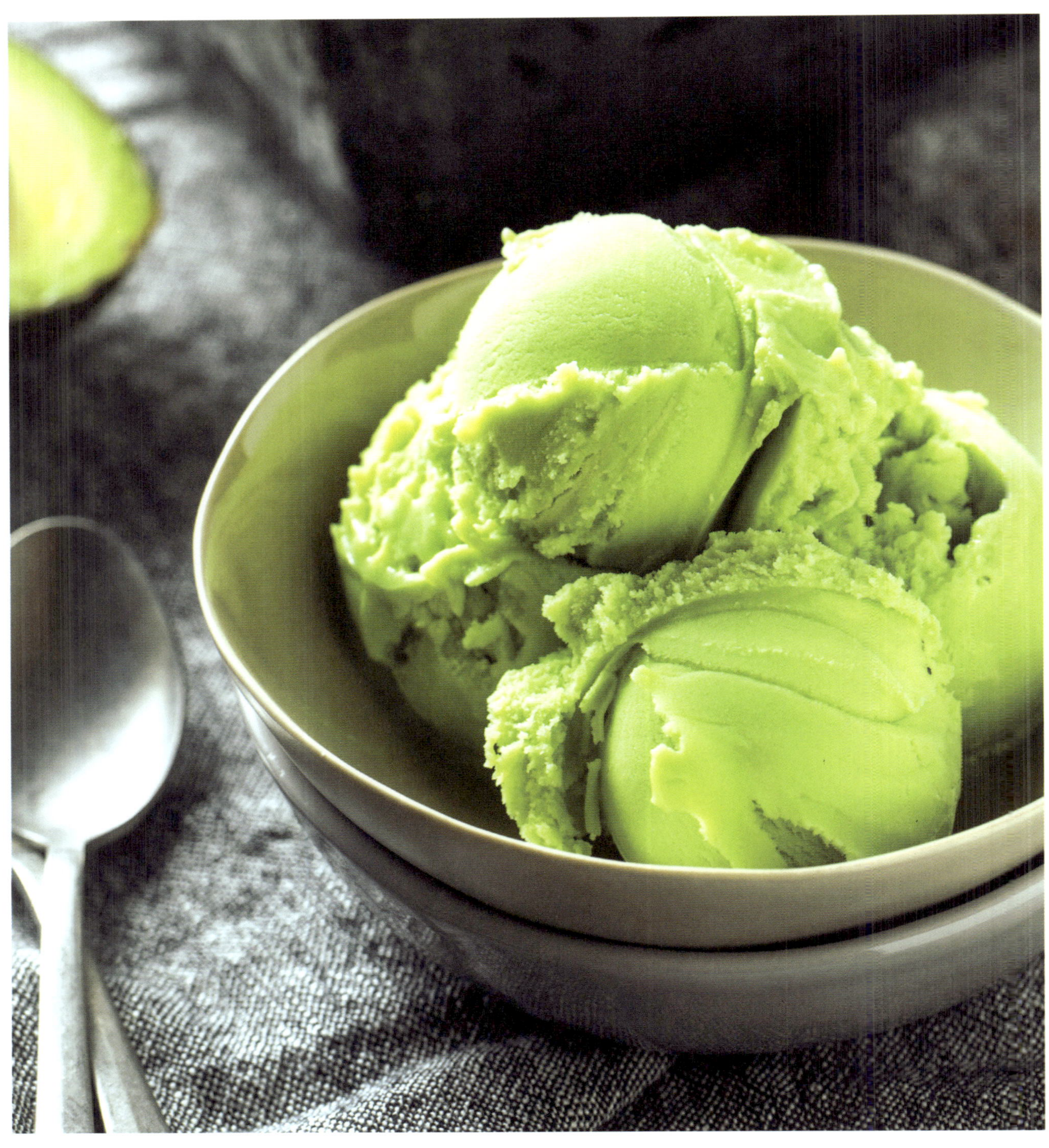

Avocado Ice Cream

SERVES 8

PREP + COOK TIME: 20 MINS + CHILLING AND FREEZING

VEG • GLUTEN FREE

AVOCADO ICE CREAM

2 large avocados
1½ cups (375ml) canned coconut milk
¾ cup (150g) granulated allulose or monkfruit sweetener
1 cup (15g) fresh mint
1 cup (250ml) thickened cream

Scoop the avocado flesh into a high-speed blender along with all the remaining ingredients. Blend until completely smooth.

Transfer into a bowl and refrigerate for 3 hours, to thicken and chill.

Place the chilled avocado ice-cream mixture into an ice-cream maker and churn as per the instructions.

Alternatively, you can transfer the mixture to a freezer-friendly container and place in the freezer for 4 hours. Mix every 30 minutes, to break up the ice crystals.

Let the frozen ice cream sit at room temperature for 15 minutes before serving.

Sponge Cake with Berries & Cream

SERVES 8
PREP + COOK TIME: 1 HOUR
GLUTEN FREE

- 1 cup (120g) almond meal
- ¼ cup (25g) coconut flour
- 1 tsp baking powder
- ¼ tsp salt
- ½ cup (95g) granulated erythritol
- 5 eggs, separated
- ¼ cup (60ml) thickened cream
- 100g butter, melted
- 1 tsp vanilla extract
- 1 tbsp powdered gelatin
- 1 tbsp warm water

TOPPING

- 2½ cups (600ml) thickened cream
- 4 tbsps powdered erythritol
- 1 tsp vanilla extract
- ½ cup (60g) fresh raspberries

Preheat oven to 180°C. Line a 20cm cake tin with greaseproof paper.

In a medium bowl combine the almond meal, coconut flour, baking powder, salt and erythritol. Stir to combine. Set aside.

In a large bowl whisk the egg whites until soft peaks form.

In another medium bowl whisk together the egg yolks, cream, melted butter and vanilla extract. Set aside.

In a small bowl combine the gelatin and warm water. Whisk until all of the gelatin is dissolved. Add to the cream mixture and whisk to combine.

Gently fold the cream mixture into the egg white until well incorporated. Add the flour mixture and gently fold through.

Pour into the cake tin and bake for 45 minutes or until an inserted skewer comes out clean. Set aside to cool.

Whisk together the cream, 3 tablespoons of erythritol and vanilla extract. Smooth over the top of the cooled cake. Top with raspberries then sift over the remaining erythritol to serve.

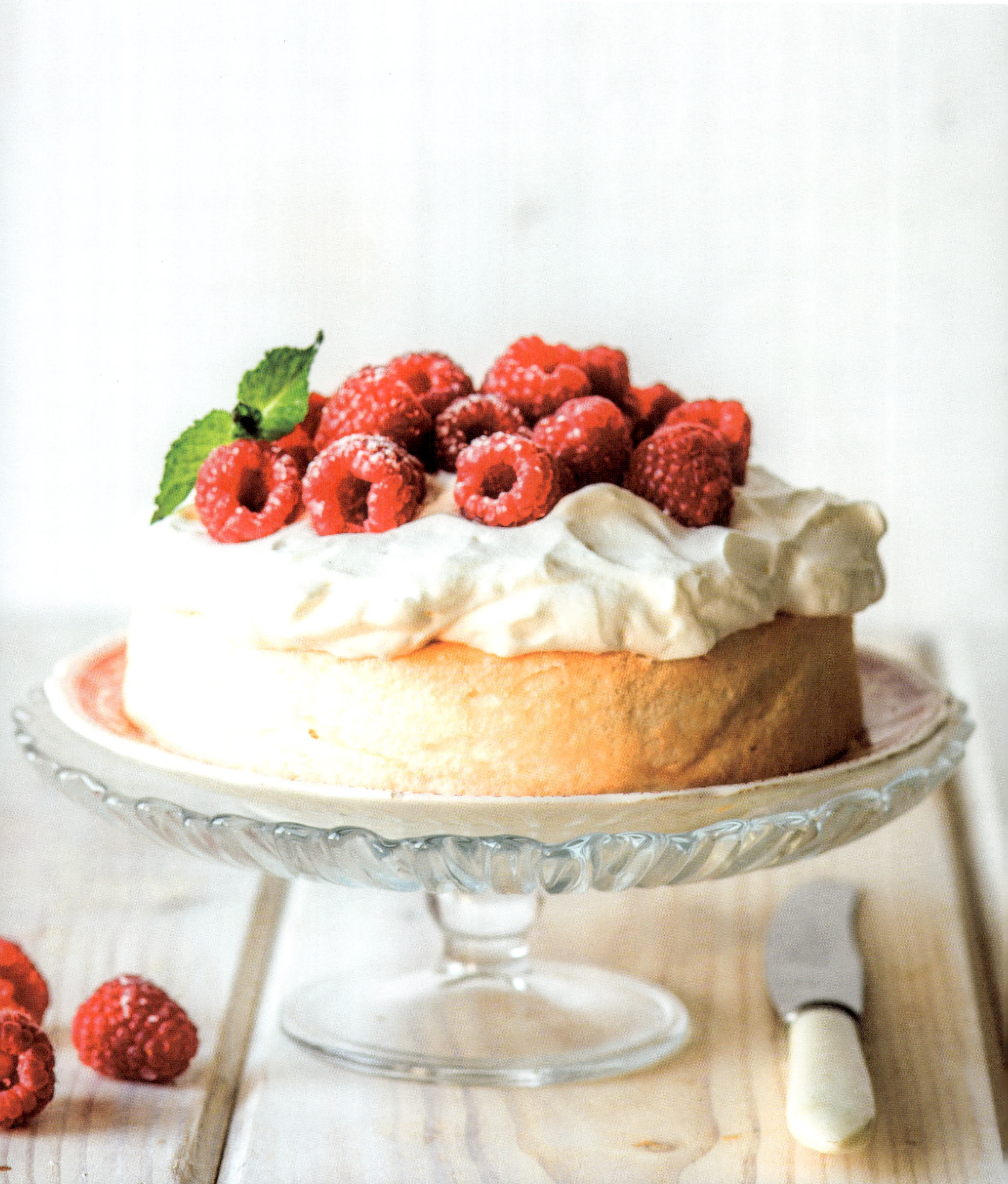

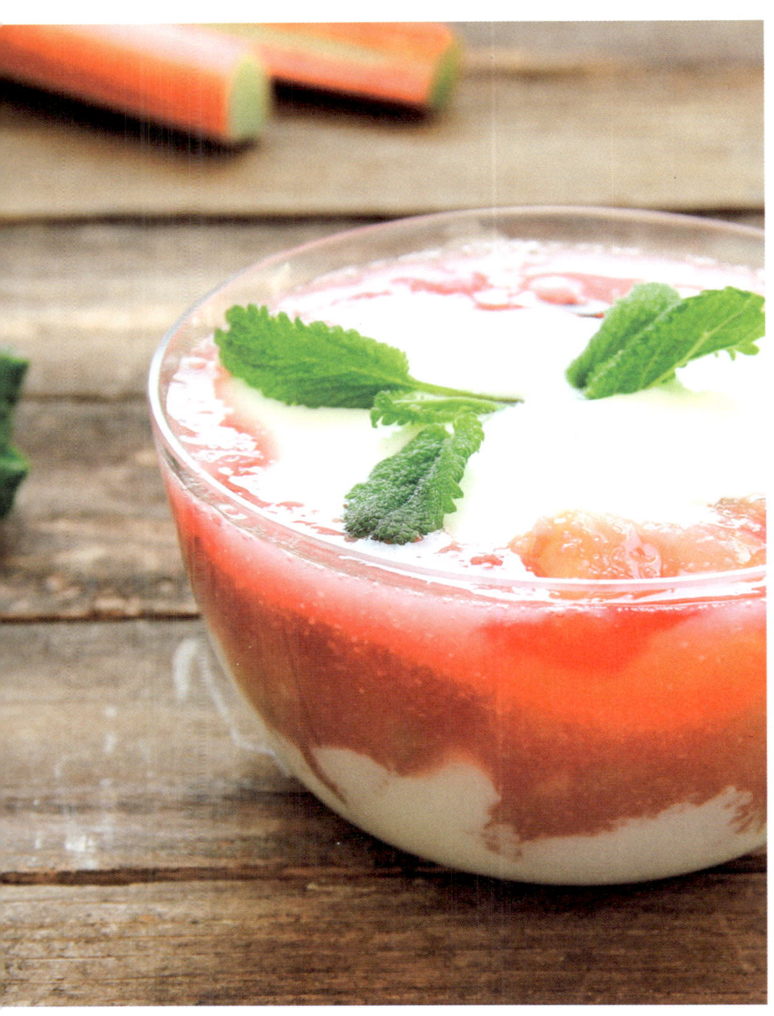

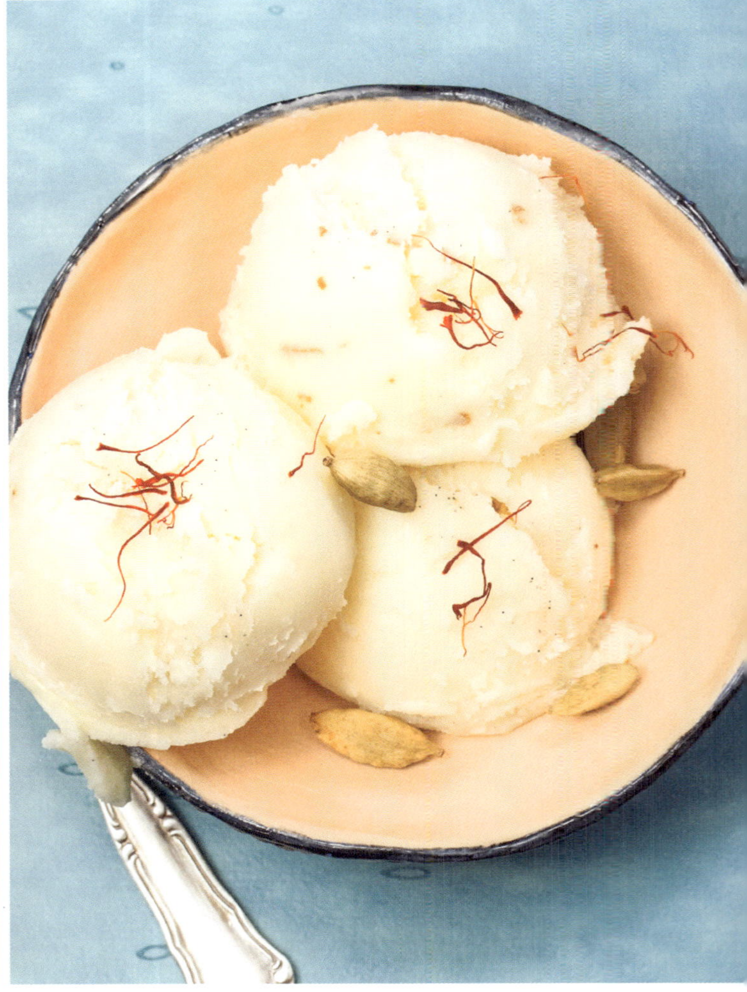

Rhubarb Cream Dessert

SERVES 4

PREP + COOK TIME: 10 MINS + CHILLING

VEG • GLUTEN FREE

Cardamom & Saffron Ice Cream

SERVES 4

PREP TIME: 1 HOUR + CHILLING

VEG • GLUTEN FREE • DAIRY FREE

RHUBARB CREAM DESSERT

3⅓ cups (400g) rhubarb, chopped
⅓ cup (80ml) water
½ cup (95g) erythritol or monkfruit powder
15 drops liquid stevia
½ tsp vanilla bean powder or 1 tsp vanilla extract
1 cup (250ml) thickened cream
½ tsp cinnamon
Mint leaves, to garnish

Place the rhubarb and water in a saucepan and bring to a boil over a medium-high heat. When it starts to simmer, lower the heat to medium and cook for 4-5 minutes until tender. Add sweeteners and vanilla. Mix well until the sweeteners dissolve.

Set aside to cool, then place in the fridge to chill for at least an 30 minutes.

In a large bowl, whisk the thickened cream until soft peaks form. Stir in the cinnamon.

Spoon half of the cream into serving bowls. Spoon in the chilled rhubarb, then top with the remaining cream.

Decorate with mint leaves to serve.

CARDAMOM & SAFFRON ICE CREAM

8 saffron strands
3 tbsps hot water
1 x 400ml can coconut cream
1 x 400ml can coconut milk
1 tsp ground cardamom
¾ cup (165g) erythritol
1 tbsp coconut oil
Cardamom pods for garnish

Place the saffron strands in the hot water for 20 minutes. Remove the strands (reserve for garnish) and retain the water.

Heat the coconut cream, coconut milk, ground cardamom, erythritol, coconut oil and saffron water in a saucepan over medium heat. Once it begins to simmer, remove from heat and let cool for 20 minutes. Strain the mixture into a large bowl and chill in the refrigerator for 1 hour.

Pour into an ice-cream maker and mix according to the maker directions.

Transfer the mixture to an ice-cream container and chill for at least 4 hours, preferably overnight.

Serve chilled, garnished with a couple of strands of saffron and cardamom pods.

Churros

MAKES 15-20
PREP + COOK TIME: 40 MINS
VEG • GLUTEN FREE

⅔ cup (80g) finely ground almond meal
¼ cup (25g) coconut flour
1 tbsp ground psyllium husk
1 tsp xanthan gum
1 cup (250ml) water
60g butter
2 tbsps erythritol or xylitol
¼ tsp salt
2 eggs, lightly beaten
1 tsp vanilla extract
¼ cup (30g) shredded mozzarella cheese
Coconut oil or lard for frying
¼ cup (50g) monkfruit brown sugar substitute
2 tsps ground cinnamon

CHOCOLATE SAUCE

25g unsalted butter
180g sugar-free dark chocolate
½ tsp vanilla extract
⅔ cup (160ml) thickened cream
3 tbsps keto-friendly brown sugar substitute

In a medium bowl whisk together almond meal, coconut flour, psyllium husk and xanthan gum. Set aside.

Heat water, butter, sweetener and salt in a large pan over medium heat until simmering. Reduce heat to low and add in flour mixture, stirring constantly to incorporate. Continue to cook for 2-3 minutes until the dough pulls away from the sides. Transfer back to the bowl and allow to cool for 5 minutes.

Add in one egg at a time, mixing well between each addition. Mix in vanilla extract and mozzarella.

Allow the dough to rest for 10 minutes then spoon into a piping bag with a star nozzle.

Heat 3cm oil in a heavy-bottomed pan until hot (180°C). Working in batches so as not to overcrowd the pan, pipe out a strips of dough into the hot oil, snipping off the ends with kitchen scissors.

Fry for 2-3 minutes on each side until golden, then transfer to a plate lined with paper towel.

Combine the monkfruit sweetener and cinnamon in a bowl and toss the churros in the mix to coat while still warm.

To make the chocolate sauce place a heatproof bowl over a pan of simmering water and add the butter and chocolate. Stir until almost melted then mix through the vanilla, cream and sweetener. Stir well to combine.

Remove from the heat and serve warm with the warm churros.

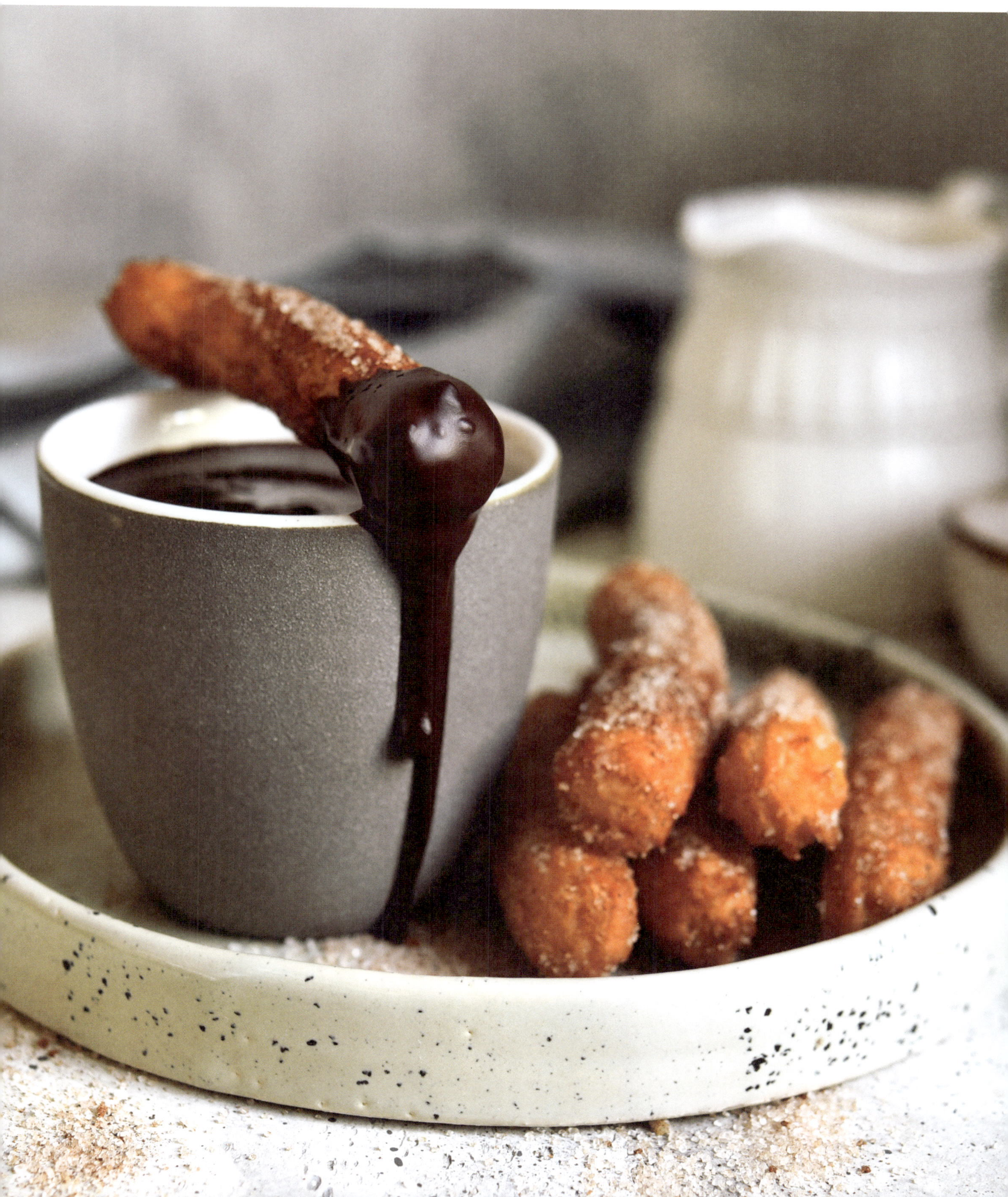

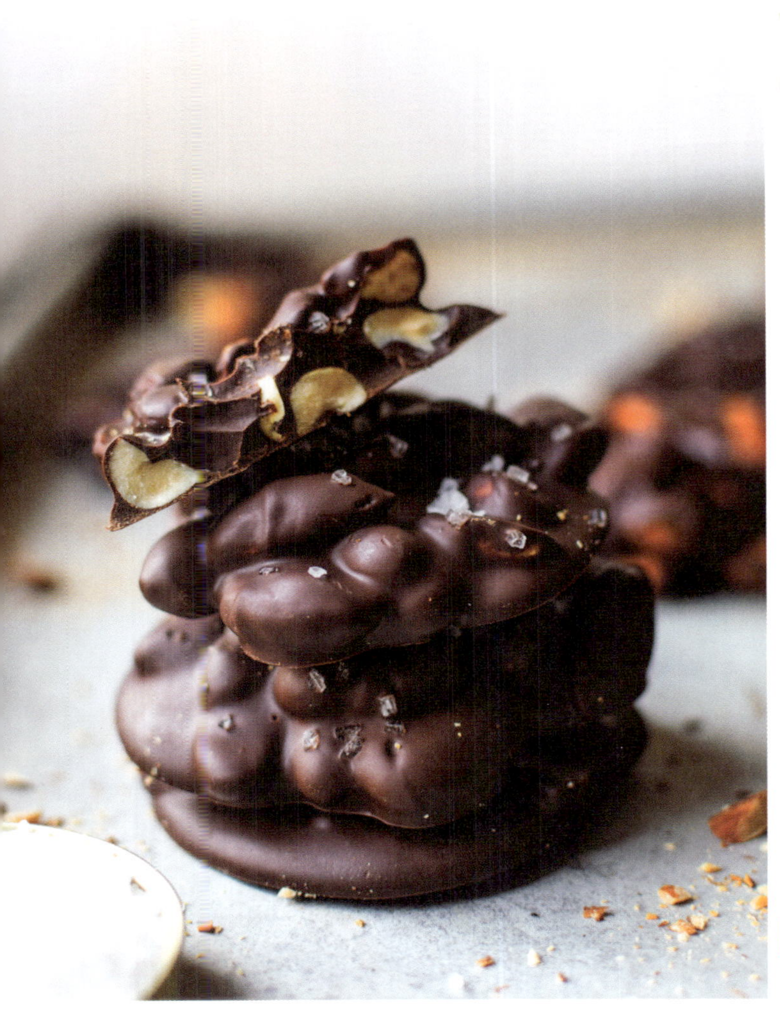

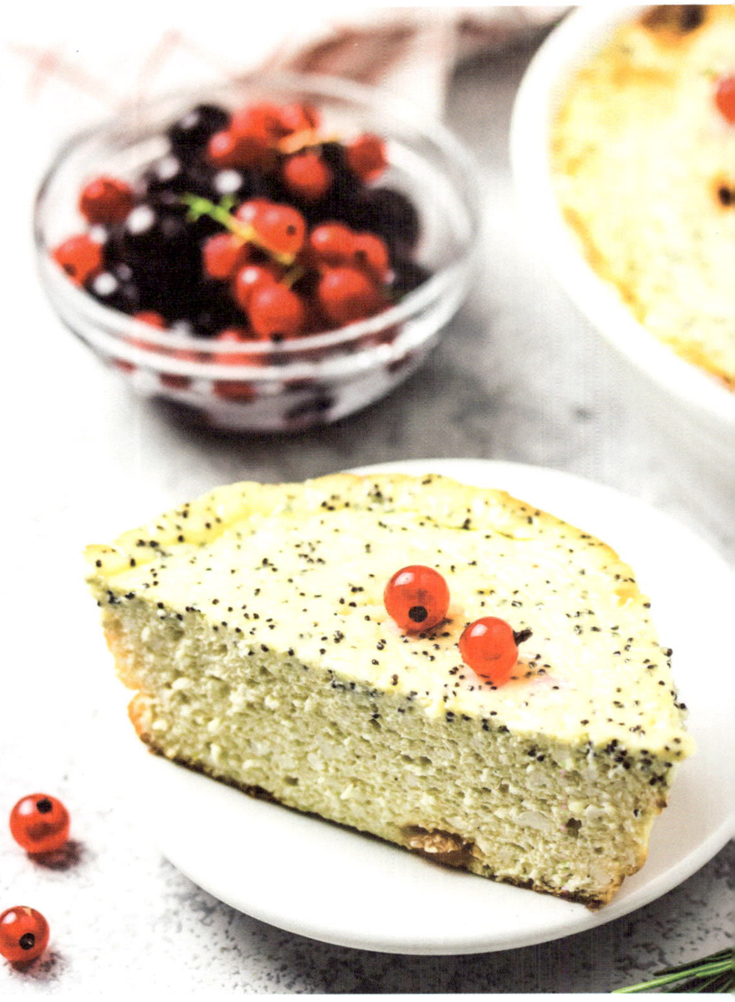

Chocolate Hazelnut Clusters

SERVES 4

PREP + COOK TIME: 15 MINS + CHILLING

VEG • GLUTEN FREE

Cottage Cheese Poppyseed Cake

SERVES 2

PREP + COOK TIME: 1 HOUR

VEG • GLUTEN FREE

CHOCOLATE HAZELNUT CLUSTERS

3¼ cups (500g) sugar-free chocolate chips
½ tsp salt
½ cup (60g) hazelnuts, roughly chopped

Line a baking tray with greaseproof paper.

Place chocolate chips in a heatproof bowl over a pan of simmering water on medium-low heat. Stir for 3-5 minutes until all the chocolate is melted, ensuring no water gets into the bowl. Add the salt and stir.

Spread the hazelnuts on the prepared tray and dollop the chocolate mixture on top. Place in the fridge for 20 minutes or until the chocolate is hard.

Peel the paper from the chocolate and break into pieces if necessary. Store in the refrigerator.

COTTAGE CHEESE POPPYSEED CAKE

500g cottage cheese
230g cream cheese, room temperature
¾ cup (165g) erythritol
¼ cup (25g) almond flour
1 tsp vanilla essence
6 medium eggs, room temperature
¼ cup (35g) poppyseeds
Berries, to garnish

Preheat oven to 180°C and lightly grease two six-hole muffin tins.

Use a stand mixer to mix together the cottage cheese and cream cheese until smooth. Add the erythritol, almond flour and vanilla and roughly mix through.

Add the eggs one at a time, mixing through before adding the next one.

Reserve ⅔ cup of the mixture and divide the rest between the muffin holes.

Mix the poppy seeds into the reserved mixture then divide that between the 12 cakes.

Bake for 30 minutes or until a skewer inserted in the middle comes out clean.

Let the cakes cool to room temperature before removing from the tins and serve garnished with your favourite keto-friendly berries.

Walnut Orange Balls

MAKES 16

PREP + COOK TIME: 15 MINS + CHILLING

VEG • GLUTEN FREE • DAIRY FREE

2 cups (250g) walnuts

⅔ cup (170g) almond butter

½ cup (50g) coconut flour

2 oranges, zested and juiced, to make 1 tbsp orange zest and ¼ cup (60ml) orange juice

2 tbsps xylitol

½ tsp vanilla extract

Pinch of salt

Blitz the walnuts in a food processor until finely processed.

Place all the ingredients in a mixing bowl and stir to combine until a rough batter forms.

Make balls by rolling the dough in clean hands.

Freeze or chill for 10 minutes to firm up before serving. Store in a sealed container in the fridge.

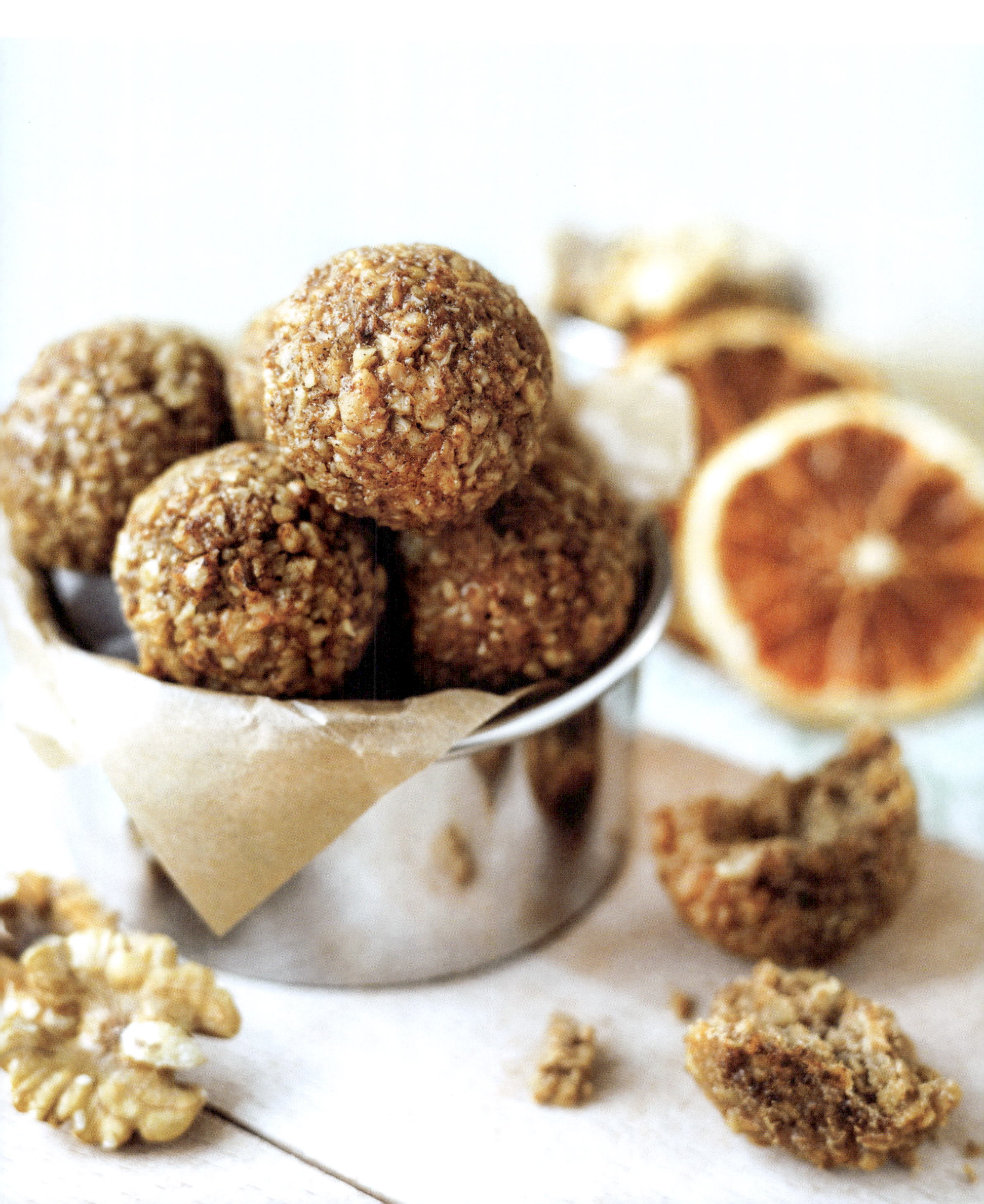

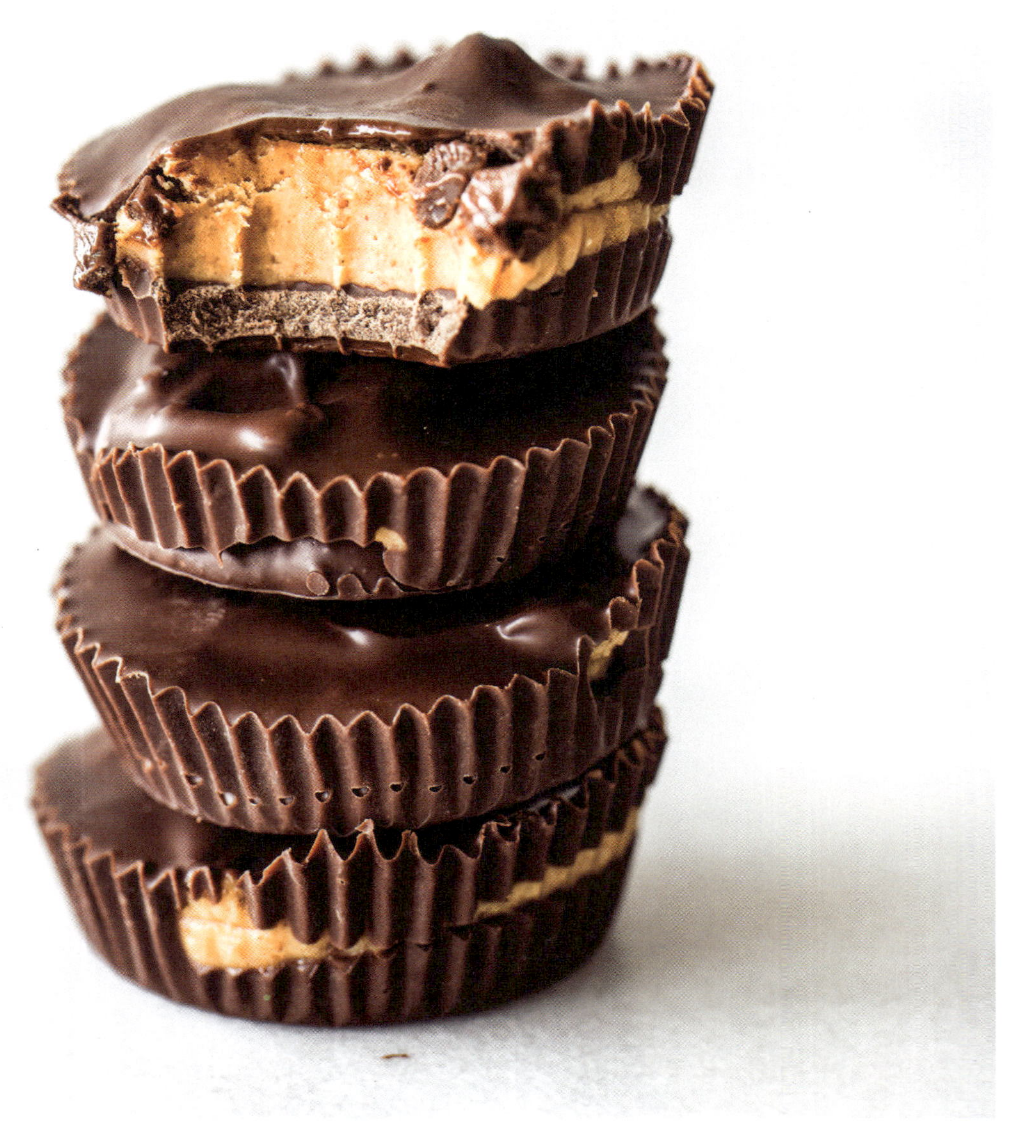

Peanut Butter Dark Choc Bites

MAKES 12

PREP + COOK TIME: 1 HOUR 5 MINS

VEG • GLUTEN FREE • DAIRY FREE

PEANUT BUTTER DARK CHOC BITES

CHOCOLATE LAYERS

290g sugar-free dark chocolate (minimum 85% cocoa solids)

5 tbsps coconut oil

½ tsp vanilla extract

PEANUT BUTTER LAYER

3½ tbsps peanut butter

2 tsps coconut oil

4 tsps powdered erythritol

1½ tsps peanut flour or powdered peanut butter

⅛ tsp vanilla extract

Pinch of salt

Line a 12-hole muffin tin with paper liners.

For the bottom chocolate layer, heat half of the chocolate and half of the coconut oil in a heatproof bowl over a pan of simmering water until melted, or melt in the microwave in 30-second bursts. Stir in ¼ teaspoon vanilla.

Fill the bottom of the paper liners evenly with chocolate mixture. Freeze for 10 minutes.

Meanwhile, for the peanut butter layer, heat the peanut butter and coconut oil in a heatproof bowl over a pan of simmering water until melted, or melt in the microwave in 30-second bursts. Stir in the sweetener, peanut flour, vanilla and salt until smooth.

Spoon a teaspoon of the peanut butter mixture into the centre of each cup over the chocolate layer. Freeze for another 10 minutes.

Meanwhile, make the top chocolate layer. Heat the remaining chocolate and coconut oil in a heatproof bowl over a pan of simmering water until melted, or melt in the microwave in 30-second bursts. Stir in ¼ teaspoon vanilla.

Pour the chocolate into the cups, over and around the peanut butter layer.

Return to the freezer for at least 20-30 minutes, until completely firm. Store in the fridge.

Tip:

You can replace the peanut butter in this recipe with other nut butters if desired.

Easy Lemon Mousse

SERVES 8

PREP TIME: 20 MINS + CHILLING

VEG • GLUTEN FREE

1⅓ cups (340ml) thickened cream

225g cream cheese, room temperature

1-2 lemons, to make 4 tsps lemon zest + 2 tbsps lemon juice

½ cup (110g) erythritol

OPTIONAL TOPPINGS

Mint leaves, to garnish

1 small lemon, thinly sliced, to garnish

Whip the cream until stiff peaks form. Set aside.

Beat together the remaining ingredients until smooth and light.

Beat the cream into the cream cheese mixture and add more lemon or erythritol to taste.

Divide between eight serving bowls and chill for at least 2 hours.

Serve garnished with mint leaves and lemon slices if desired.

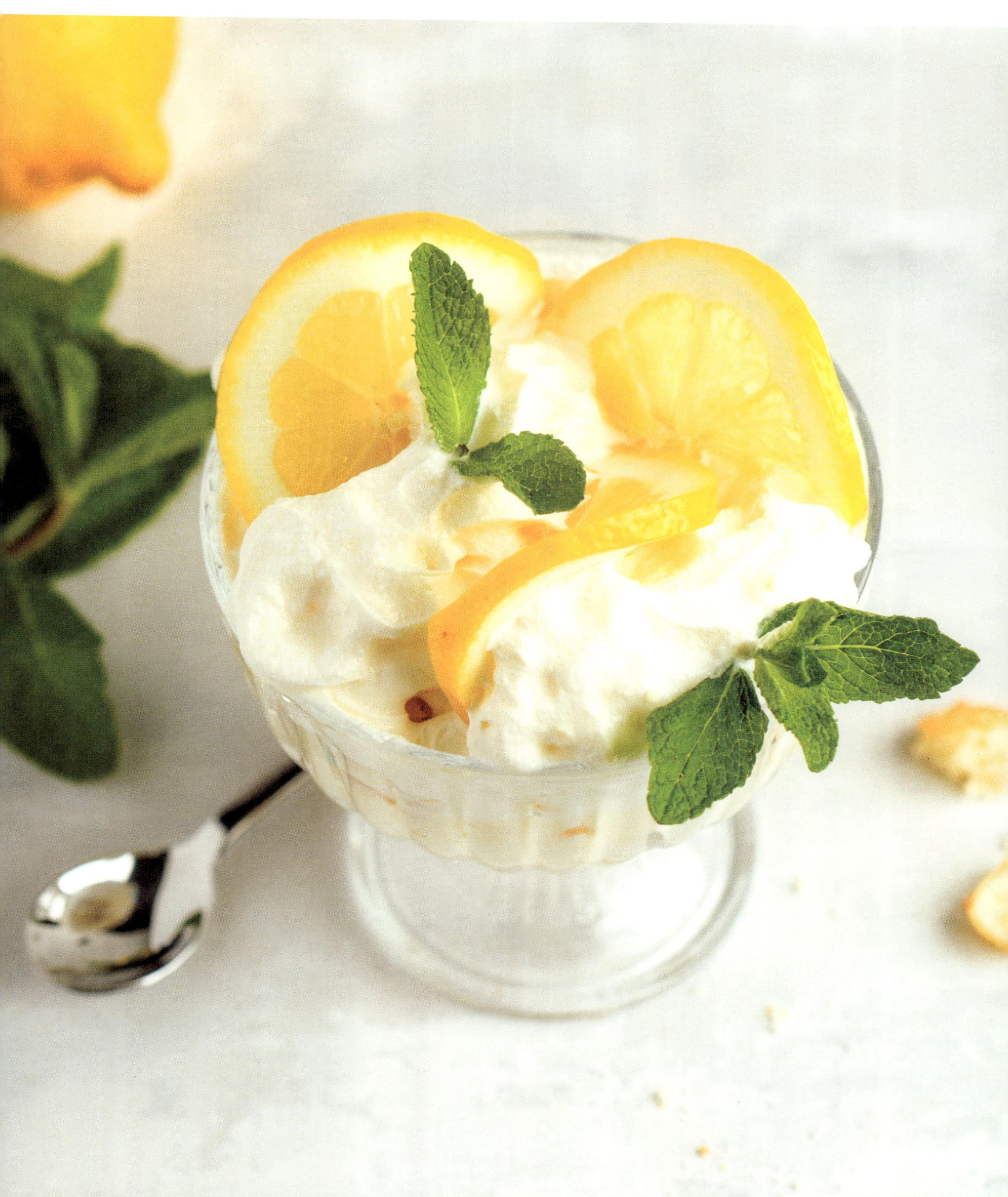

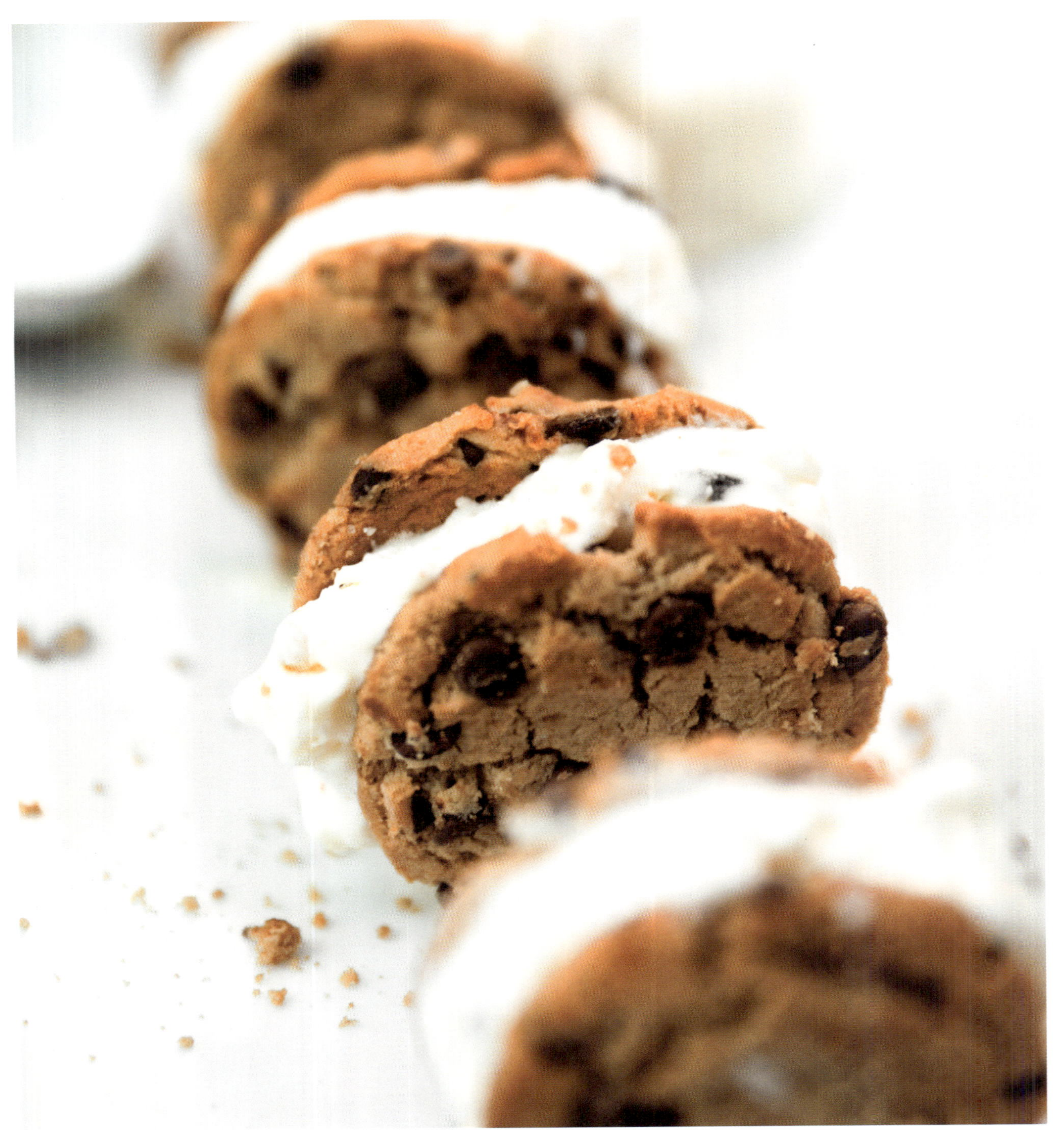

Chocolate-Chip Cookie Ice-Cream Sandwiches

MAKES 10

PREP + COOK TIME: 40 MINS + COOLING

VEG • GLUTEN FREE

CHOCOLATE-CHIP COOKIE ICE-CREAM SANDWICHES

90g butter, room temperature
½ tsp stevia or ½ cup (110g) erythritol
1 large egg, room temperature
1 tsp molasses
1 tsp vanilla essence
2½ cups (250g) almond flour
½ cup (80g) sugar-free dark chocolate chips
2 cups (500ml) keto-friendly vanilla ice cream

Preheat oven to 180°C and lightly grease and line two large, flat baking trays with baking paper.

Beat the butter and sweetener together until it resembles whipped cream. Beat the egg into the mixture until thoroughly combined.

Mix through the molasses and vanilla then add the flour, one-third at a time.

Fold through the chocolate chips. Form the mixture into a roll and cut into 20 segments.

Roll into flattened discs and place on the baking trays. Bake for 14 minutes until browned. Let cool completely to room temperature.

To form the sandwiches, place 1 large dessertspoon of ice cream each on half the cookies. Place the remaining cookies on top and gently press together. Serve immediately.

Green Coconut Bites

MAKES 12

PREP + COOK TIME: 45 MINS

VEG • GLUTEN FREE

BASE

½ cup (125g) almond butter

2 tbsps coconut oil

⅓ cup (30g) desiccated coconut

1 tbsp cocoa powder

¼ cup (40g) chia seeds

2 tbsps granulated erythritol

1 tsp ground cinnamon

1 tsp coconut flour

CENTRE

⅔ cup (65g) almond flour or almond meal

⅔ cup (60g) desiccated coconut

¼ cup (40g) powdered erythritol

1 tsp lemon juice

Zest of 1 lemon

70g cream cheese, softened

1 tsp vanilla essence

TOP LAYER

2 scoops low-carb vanilla protein powder

1 cup (30g) baby spinach

1 avocado

⅔ cup (170g) coconut butter, softened

1 tbsp desiccated coconut

Combine all the ingredients for the base in a food processor and blend until smooth.

Press the mixture into the base of a 12-hole silicone mini-cupcake mould. Place the mould in the freezer while you prepare the centre.

In a large bowl, mix together the almond flour, coconut and sweetener.

Add the lemon juice and zest, cream cheese and vanilla and mix into a thick dough.

Spoon the mixture on top of the bases and press down with a spoon. Return the mould to the freezer while you prepare the topping.

Prepare the top layer by adding the protein powder, spinach, avocado and coconut butter to a high-speed blender and blending until smooth.

Remove the mould from the freezer. Spoon the final layer on top and press down with the back of a spoon. Return to the freezer for 30 minutes.

Remove from the mould and sprinkle with desiccated coconut to serve.

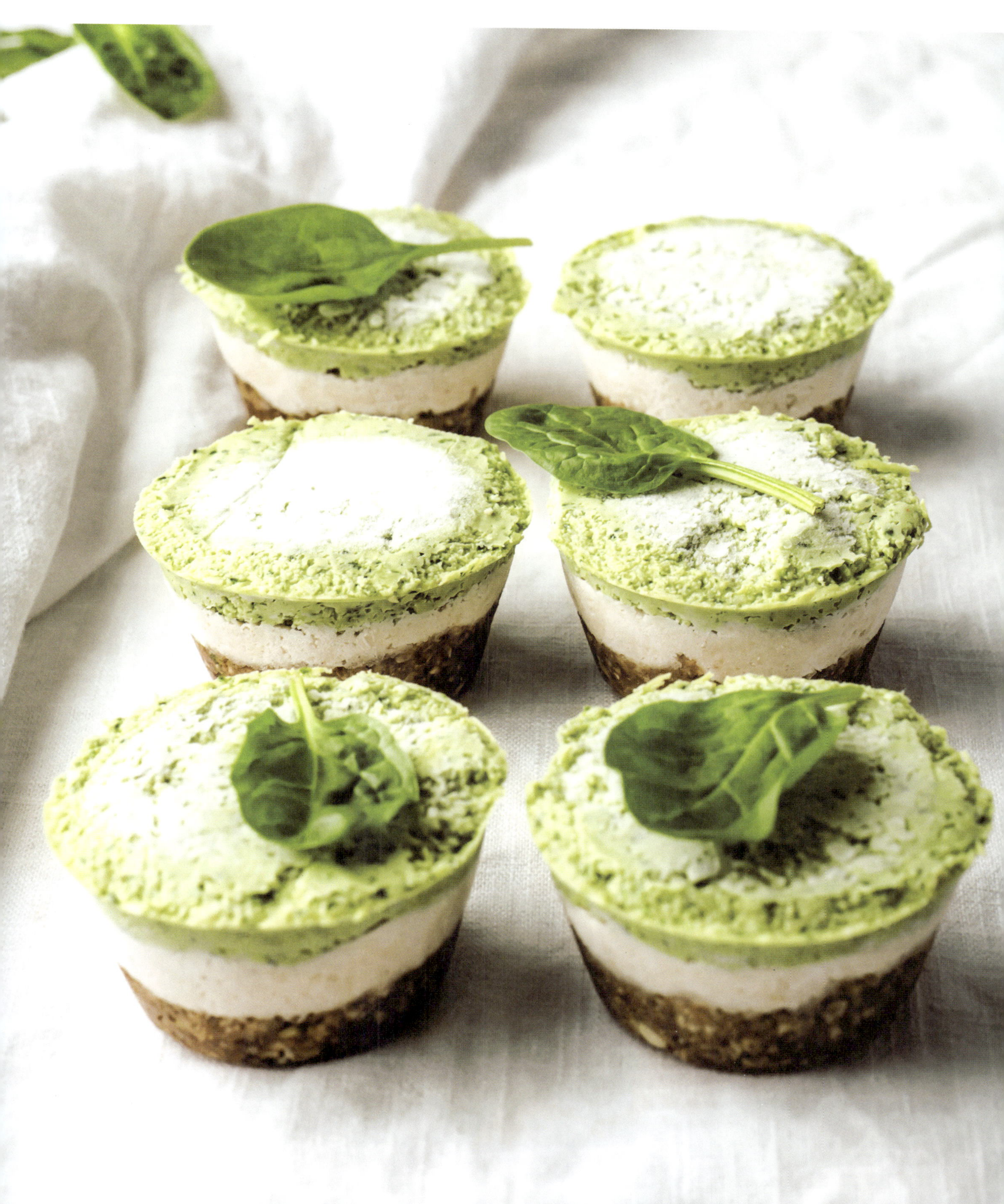

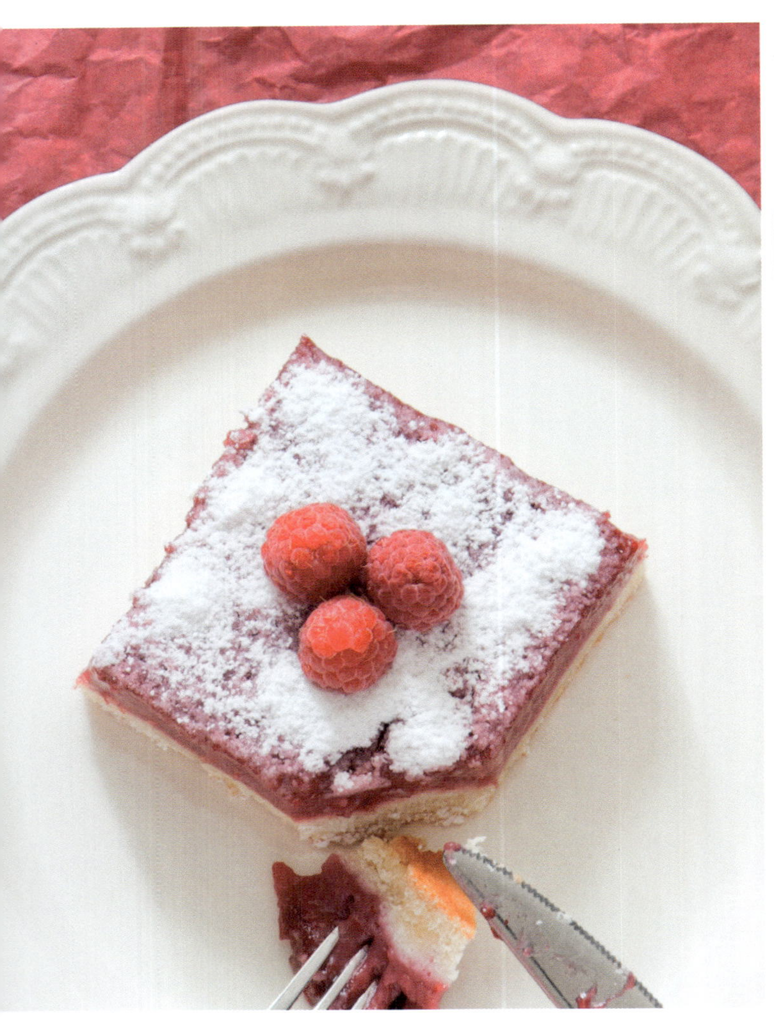

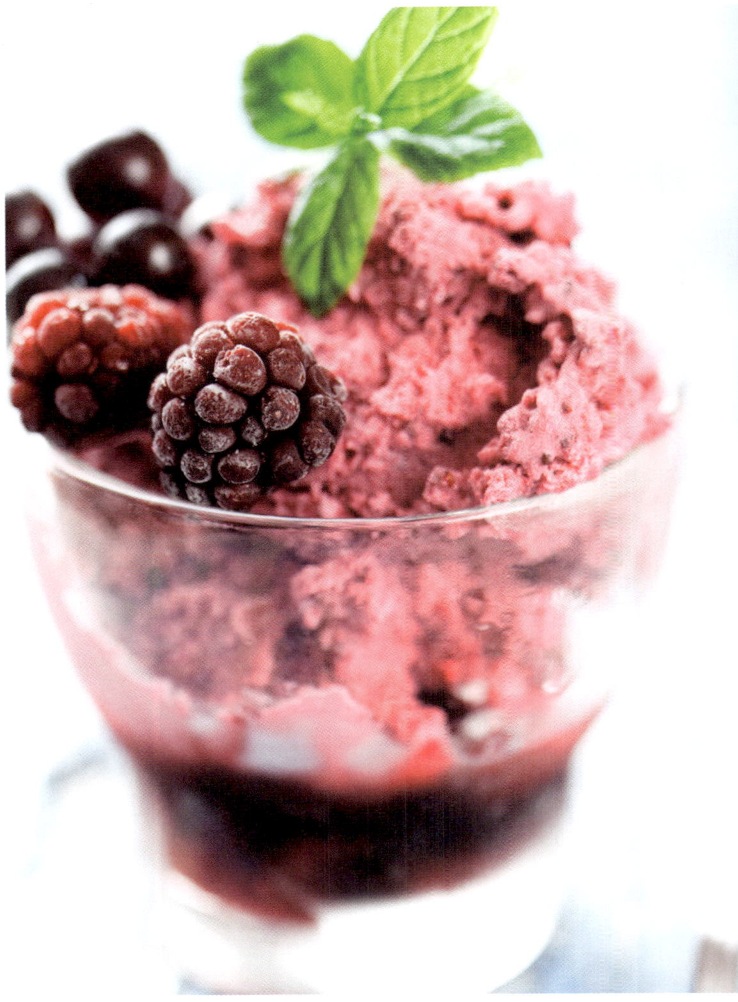

Raspberry Bars

SERVES 4

PREP + COOK TIME: 30 MINS + CHILLING

VEG • GLUTEN FREE

Quick Berry Ice Cream

SERVES 2

PREP + COOK TIME: 10 MINS

VEG • GLUTEN FREE

RASPBERRY BARS

BASE

¼ cup (30g) almond meal
½ cup (125ml) coconut oil
Pinch of salt
¼ tsp liquid stevia
1 cup (100g) coconut flour

TOP LAYER

1 tsp lemon zest
3 cups (375g) fresh or frozen raspberries
450g cream cheese, room temperature
½ cup (120ml) sour cream
⅓ cup (100ml) double cream
2 tsps liquid stevia
⅓ cup (50g) coconut flour, reserve 2 tbsps for dusting

Preheat oven to 180°C and grease and line a 15 x 20cm slice tin with baking paper.

To make the crust, combine almond meal, coconut oil, salt and liquid stevia. Mix through coconut flour. Press into the bottom of the slice tin and bake for 12 minutes until slightly browned on top. Remove from the oven and let cool while making the topping.

Place the lemon zest, raspberries, cream cheese, sour cream, double cream, liquid stevia and coconut flour in a mixer and mix until thoroughly combined. Spoon in an even layer over the base and chill in the refrigerator for at least 2 hours.

Dust with the reserved coconut flour and cut into serving squares.

QUICK BERRY ICE CREAM

1½ cups (185g) frozen berries + more to garnish
½ cup (125ml) double cream or coconut cream, chilled
⅛ tsp stevia powder or monkfruit powder
Mint leaves, to garnish

Place ½ cup of frozen berries in a small pan over medium heat. Heat gently, stirring regularly for 3-5 minutes until soft. Spoon into the base of two serving glasses.

Add the remaining frozen berries to a food processor or high-speed blender. Blend for a few seconds until the berries are broken into pieces.

Add the cream and sweetener and process for 20-30 more seconds until the ice cream is nice and smooth. Scrape down the sides as needed.

Spoon into the glasses, top with mint leaves and additional frozen berries and serve immediately.

Chocolate Caramel Fudge

SERVES 8

PREP + COOK TIME: 50 MINS

VEG • GLUTEN FREE

FUDGE

- 75g + 1 tbsp unsalted butter
- 100g dark chocolate (minimum 85% cocoa solids)
- ¾ cup (190g) crunchy peanut butter
- 2 tbsps powdered monkfruit sweetener or erythritol
- 1 tsp vanilla extract

CARAMEL

- 1 cup (90g) shredded coconut
- 1 cup (250g) macadamia butter
- 35g cacao butter
- 1 tbsp monkfruit sweetener
- 1 tsp vanilla extract
- ½ tsp salt

Melt the butter and chocolate in a heatproof bowl over a pan of simmering water, or in the microwave in 30-second bursts.

When melted, remove from the heat or microwave and stir in the peanut butter, sweetener and vanilla.

Pour into a square baking tin lined with greaseproof paper.

Place in the freezer for 30 minutes to set.

Meanwhile place the shredded coconut into a high-speed blender and blend for 2-3 minutes until broken down and starting to clump.

Add macadamia butter, cacao butter, sweetener, vanilla and salt. Blend until smooth.

Remove the fudge from the freezer, pour the caramel over the top of the fudge, then return to the freezer for 10 more minutes.

Cut into squares and serve.

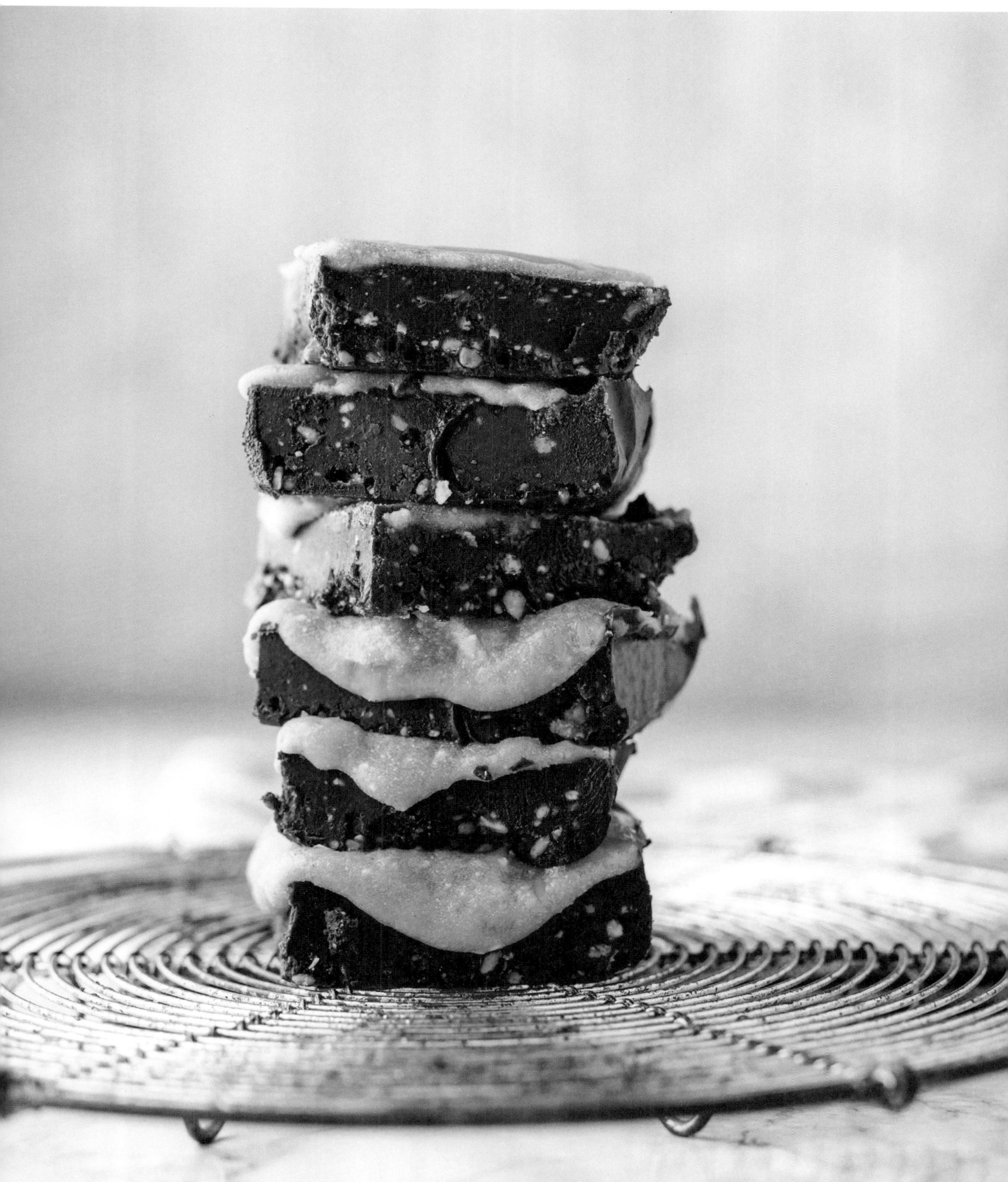

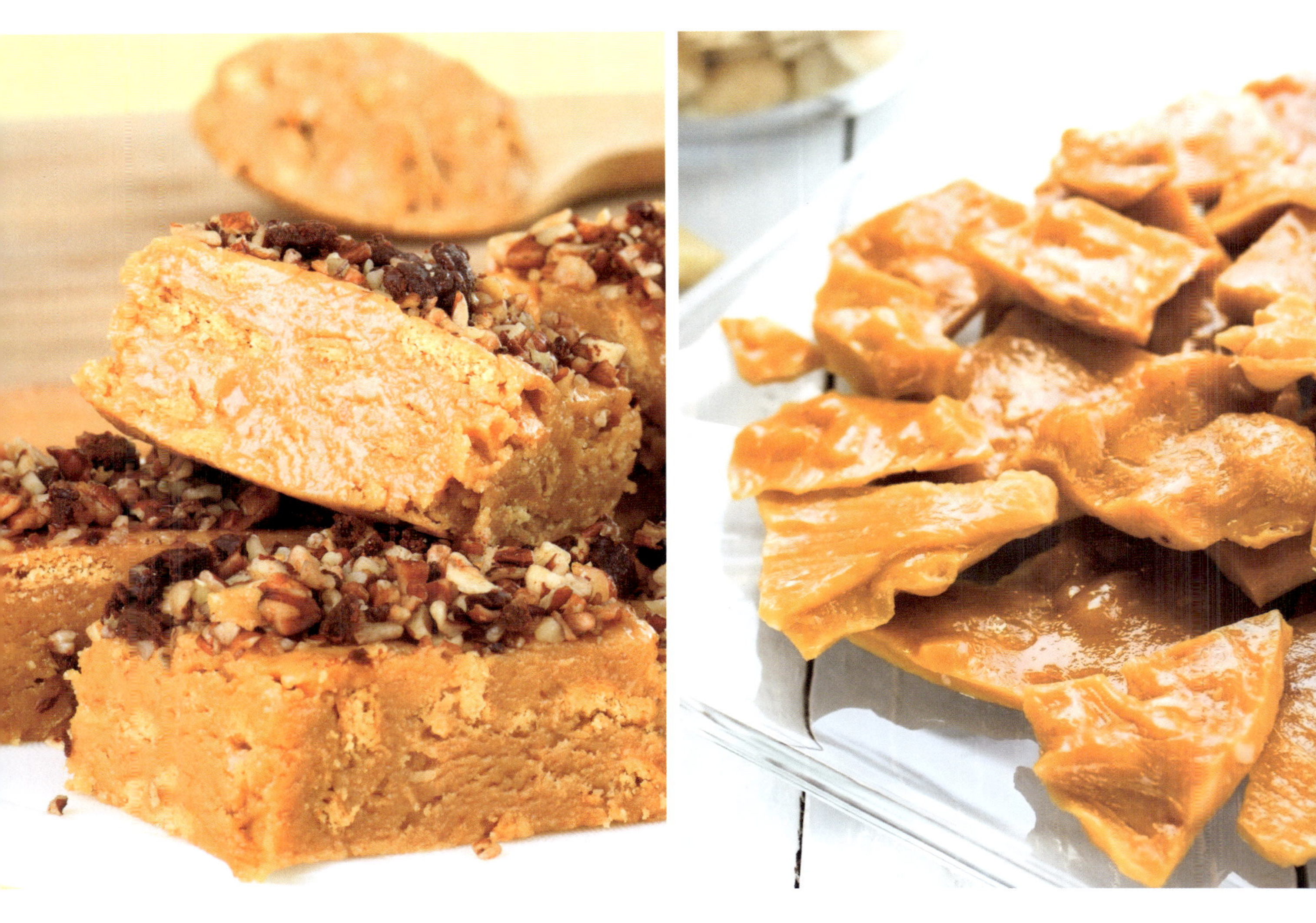

Peanut Butter Bars

SERVES 8

PREP + COOK TIME: 20 MINS + CHILLING

VEG • GLUTEN FREE

Macadamia Nut Brittle

SERVES 4

PREP + COOK TIME: 15 MINS + COOLING

VEG • GLUTEN FREE

PEANUT BUTTER BARS

1¼ cups (300g) peanut butter

120g butter

¼ tsp stevia, more to taste

1¼ cups (130g) almond flour

1 tsp vanilla essence

1 cup (155g) sugar-free chocolate chips, roughly chopped

1 cup (125g) pecans, roughly chopped

Mix together the peanut butter, butter, stevia, almond flour and vanilla essence until completely combined. Taste and adjust sweetness if needed.

Press into a small slice pan.

Mix together the chocolate chips and pecans and press into the top of the peanut butter mix.

Chill in the refrigerator for at least 4 hours, preferably overnight.

Once firm, cut into desired serving sizes.

MACADAMIA NUT BRITTLE

¼ cup (55g) erythritol

75g butter

1 tsp vanilla essence

¼ tsp bicarbonate of soda

1¼ cups (155g) roasted and salted macadamia nuts, roughly chopped

Line and grease a large, flat baking tray with baking paper.

Place all the ingredients except the macadamia nuts in a large saucepan over medium-high heat.

Keep at a simmer until the mixture turns golden brown.

Stir in the macadamias and then spread over the baking sheet in a thin layer.

Let cool, break into bite-size pieces and serve.

Tip:

Erythritol will work better than stevia in this recipe as it behaves more similarly to sugar.

Avocado & Coconut No-Bake Cheesecake

SERVES 8

PREP + COOK TIME: 20 MINS + CHILLING OVERNIGHT

VEG • GLUTEN FREE

BASE

1 cup (120g) almond meal

½ cup (45g) desiccated coconut

1 tbsp coconut oil

½ tbsp butter

3 tbsps xylitol

TOPPING

⅓ cup (70g) xylitol

1 avocado

300g cream cheese

Juice and zest of ½ lime

¾ cup (185ml) double cream or coconut cream

TO SERVE

2 tbsps desiccated coconut

¼ cup (60ml) cream or coconut cream

Line a rectangular cake tin with greaseproof paper. Use a piece of greaseproof paper large enough to hang beyond the edges of the tin, to help with easy removal.

To create the cheesecake base, add the almond meal, coconut, coconut oil, butter and xylitol to a food processor and pulse to form a chunky crumb.

Tip the crumb mixture into the cake tin and press firmly into the base, creating an even layer. Transfer to the fridge to set while you prepare the filling.

Add the xylitol to a food processor and blend to a fine powder.

Scoop the avocado flesh into the food processor along with the cream cheese and blend until smooth.

Add the lime juice and zest and cream. Blend until thick and creamy.

Spoon the filling on top of the base and level with a spatula. Transfer to the fridge to set overnight.

Run a knife under hot water, then cut into bars. Scatter with desiccated coconut and drizzle with cream or coconut cream to serve.

Tip:

Use coconut cream instead of cream (and add an extra half a tablespoon of coconut oil in place of the butter in the base) if you want to make this recipe vegan and dairy free.

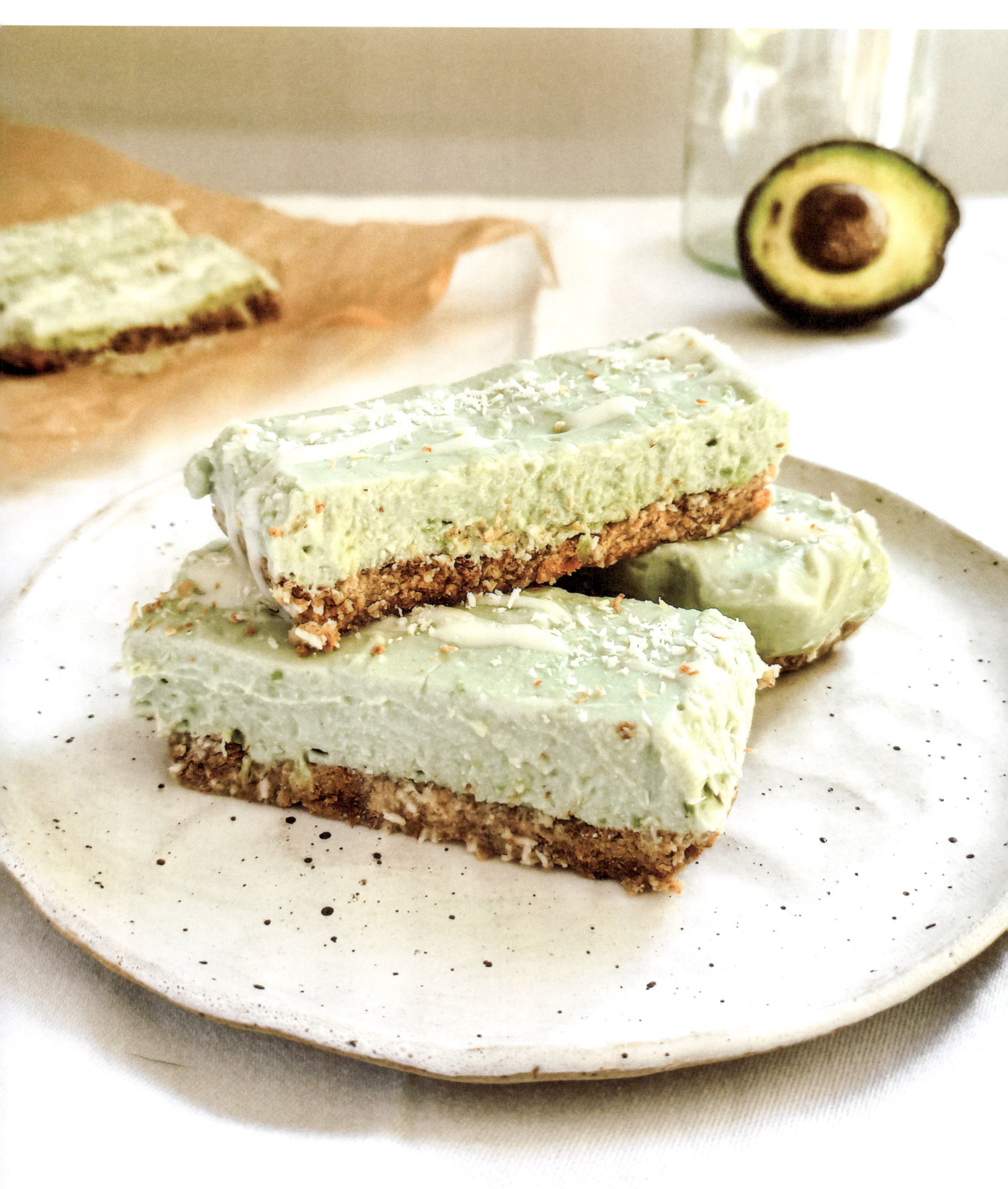

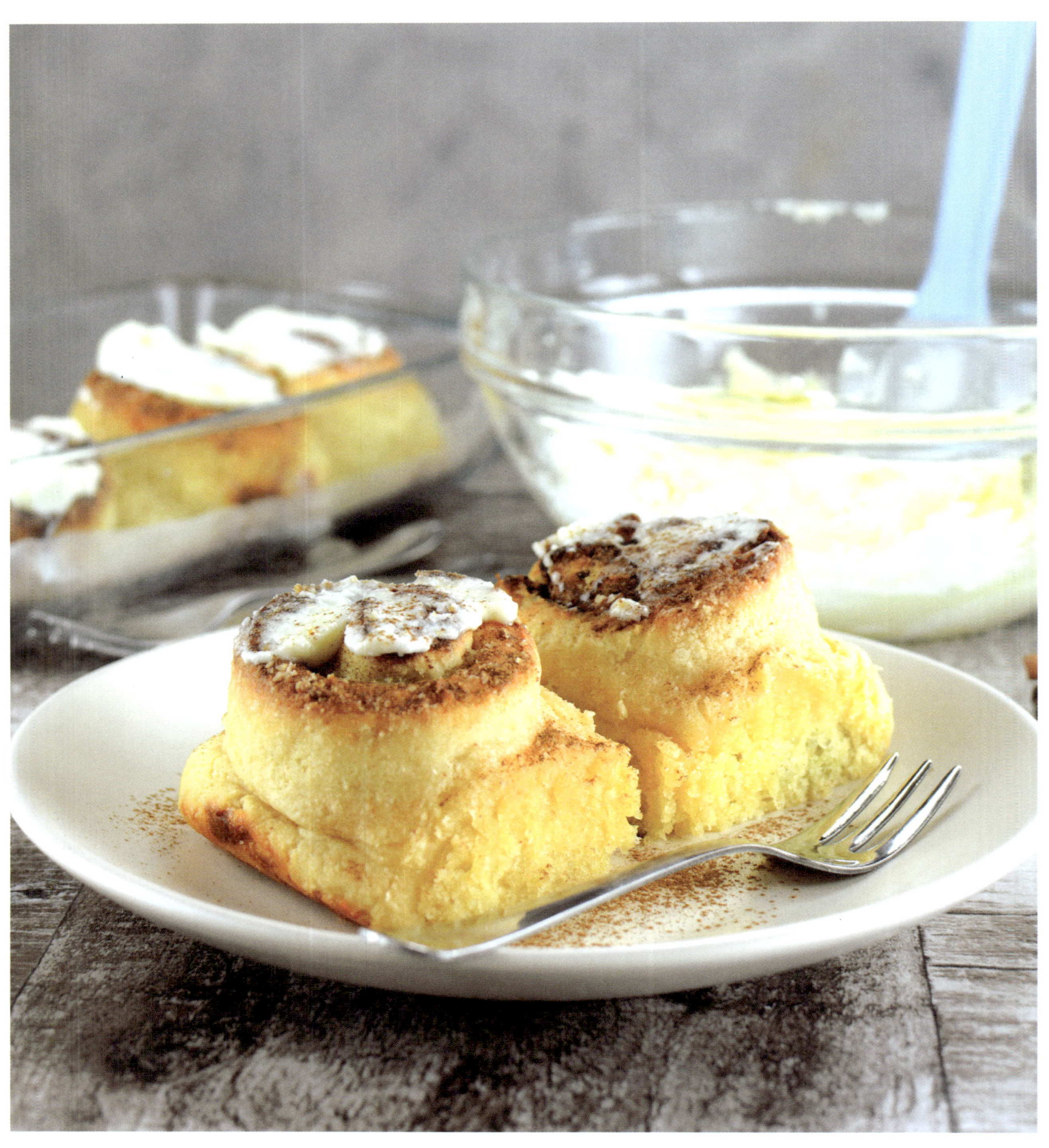

Cinnamon Scrolls

MAKES 12

PREP + COOK TIME: 1 HOUR 20 MINS

VEG • GLUTEN FREE

CINNAMON SCROLLS

2 cups (240g) finely ground almond meal

2 tbsps coconut flour

¼ cup (50g) keto-friendly granulated sweetener

1 tbsp gluten-free baking powder

2 large eggs

2 tsps vanilla extract

2 cups (250g) shredded mozzarella cheese

125g cream cheese

3 tbsps butter, melted

⅓ cup (50g) keto-friendly brown sugar substitute

1 tbsp ground cinnamon

Cream cheese icing (see recipe page 324)

Preheat the oven to 190°C. Line a 20cm square baking dish with greaseproof paper and grease with butter.

In a large bowl, whisk together the almond meal, coconut flour, granulated sweetener and baking powder. In another bowl, whisk eggs with vanilla. In a medium microwave-safe bowl, microwave mozzarella and cream cheese in 30-second bursts, stirring between each burst, until the cheese mixture is mostly melted. Whisk together until smooth. Add egg mixture and melted cheese mixture to dry mixture and knead well to combine.

Place the dough between two sheets of greaseproof paper and roll out to a 40 x 25cm rectangle. Brush dough with 2 tablespoons melted butter and sprinkle with brown sugar replacement and cinnamon. Starting from the long end, roll dough into a log. Chill for 10 minutes.

Slice the log into 12 equal pieces and arrange in the prepared baking dish. Brush tops of scrolls with remaining 1 tablespoon melted butter.

Bake for 30 minutes until scrolls are golden. Let cool slightly. Serve with cream cheese icing.

CHEESECAKE WITH BLACKBERRY JAM

700g cream cheese, room temperature
75g butter, softened
⅔ cup (140g) erythritol
3 large eggs, room temperature
¾ cup (185ml) sour cream
1 lemon, to make 1 tbsp lemon zest + 1 tbsp lemon juice
2 tsps vanilla essence
5 cups (700g) blackberries, fresh or frozen
Pinch of stevia powder

To make the cheesecake, preheat the oven to 150°C and grease and line a 22cm springform tin with baking paper.

Place the cream cheese and butter in a mixer and beat until smooth. Mix in the erythritol, then the eggs, one at a time. Mix through the sour cream, 1 teaspoon of the lemon zest and 1 teaspoon of the lemon juice and the vanilla essence.

Pour the mixture into the cake tin and smooth the top into an even layer. Bake for 90 minutes until pale yellow on top and a skewer inserted into the middle comes out clean. Let cool for at least 2 hours.

Meanwhile, to make the jam, place all the remaining ingredients into a saucepan and bring to a boil. Reduce to a low simmer and cook for at least 30 minutes, until thickened and reduced by nearly half. Stir frequently and break up the berries. Add more stevia to taste, if needed, and remove from the heat.

Let cool to room temperature and serve drizzled over the cake.

STRAWBERRY ICE CREAM

1¼ cups (250g) strawberries
⅓ cup (65g) xylitol
2 tbsps vodka (optional)
1 cup (250ml) sour cream
1 tsp vanilla extract
1 cup (250ml) thickened cream
⅓ cup (55g) powdered erythritol

Place strawberries, xylitol and vodka, if using, in a blender and blend until almost smooth, with some chunks remaining.

Transfer to a large bowl and add sour cream and vanilla extract, whisking to combine.

In another large bowl, whip the cream with the powdered erythritol until it holds stiff peaks. Gently fold the whipped cream into the strawberry mixture.

Transfer to an airtight container and freeze for at least 6 hours, until firm.

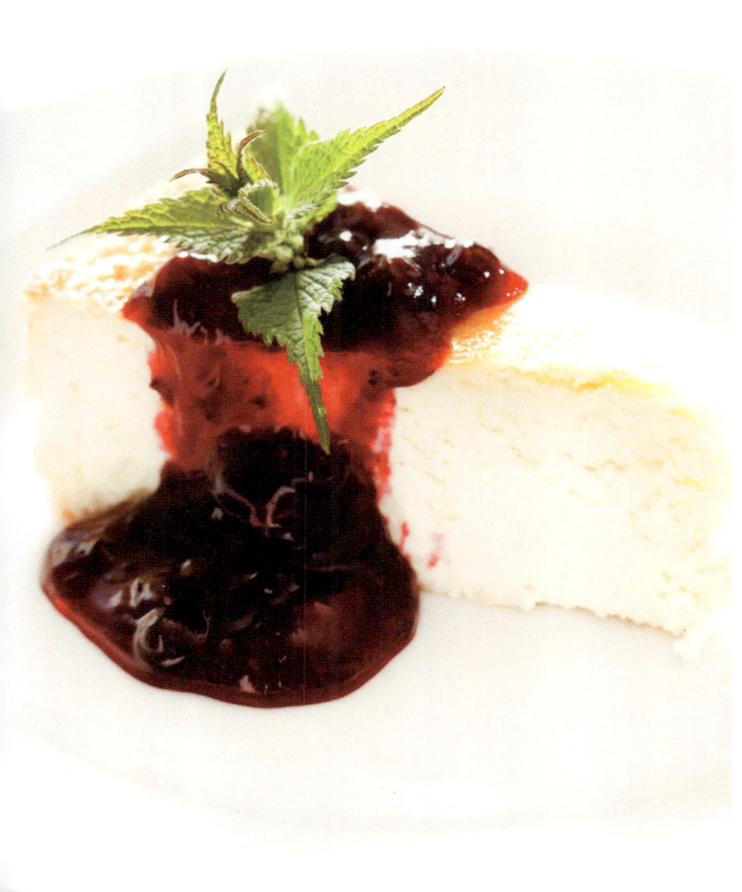

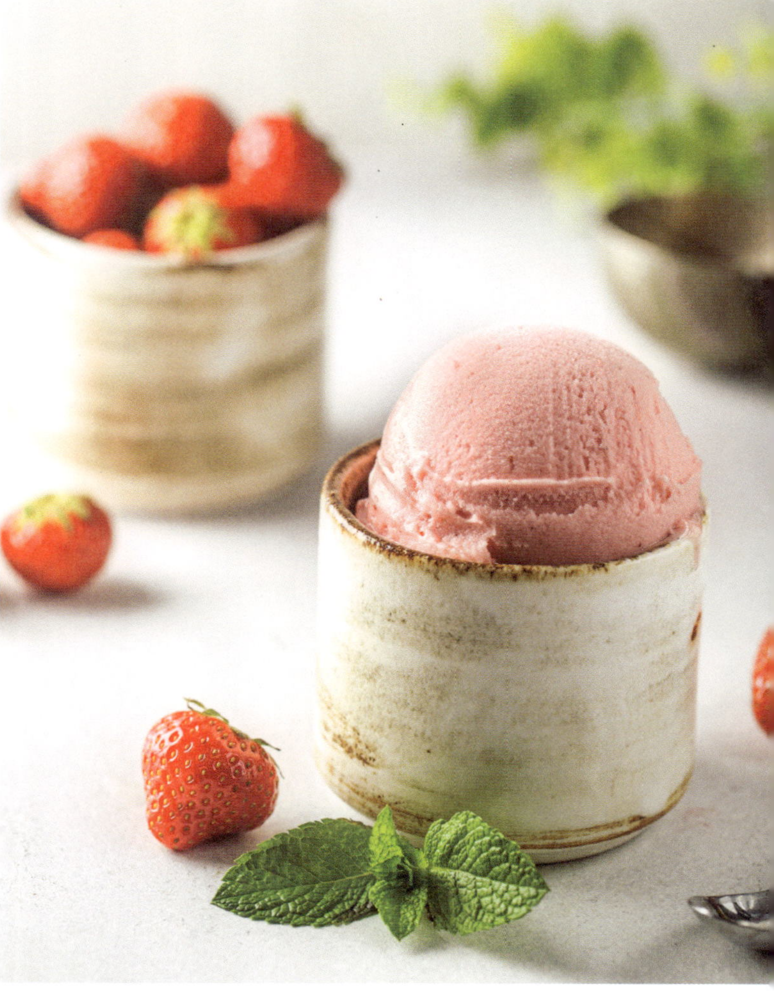

Cheesecake with Blackberry Jam

SERVES 10

PREP + COOK TIME: 1 HOUR 40 MINS + COOLING

VEG • GLUTEN FREE

Strawberry Ice Cream

SERVES 8

PREP + COOK TIME: 20 MINS + FREEZING

VEG • GLUTEN FREE

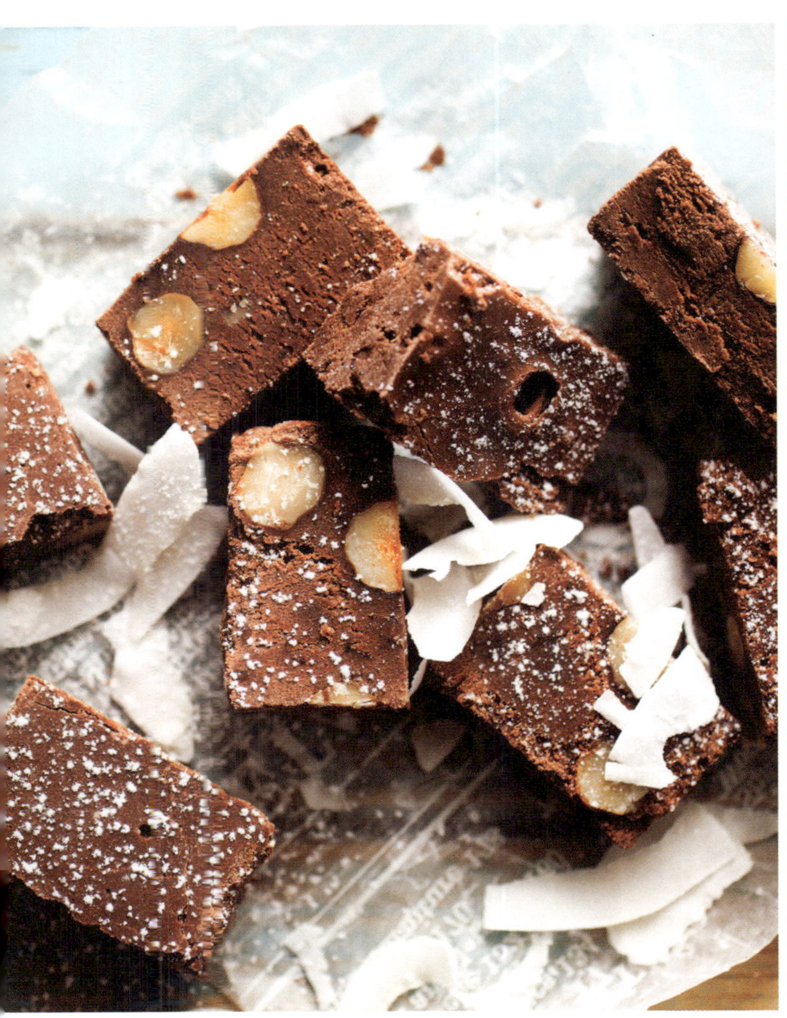

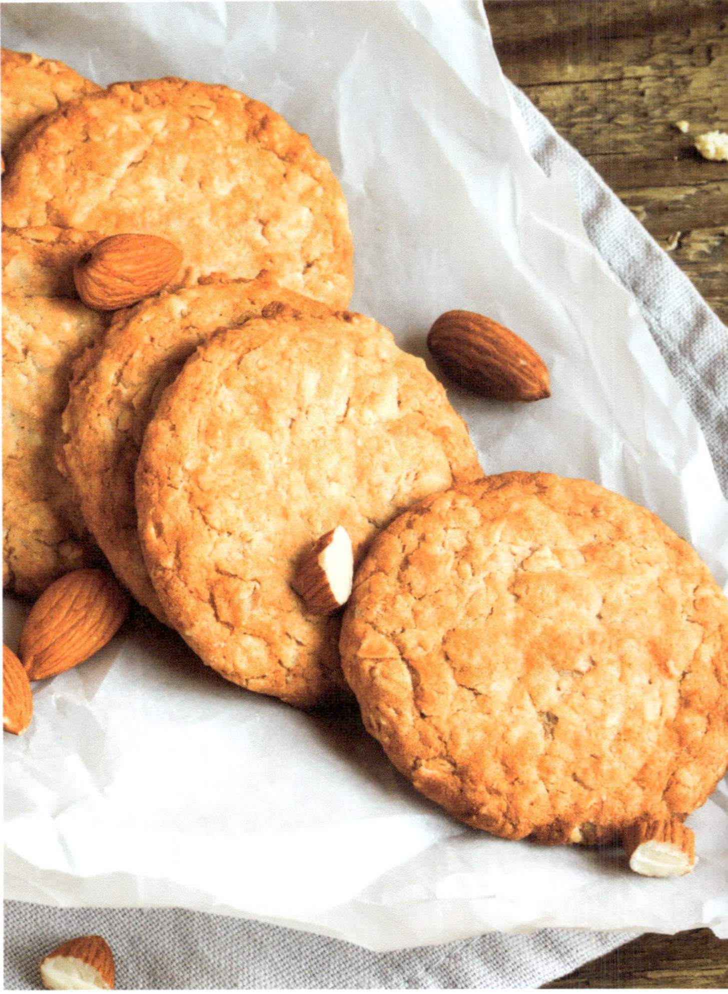

Chocolate Macadamia Fudge

MAKES 12 SQUARES

PREP + COOK TIME: 20 MINS + CHILLING

VEG • GLUTEN FREE

Almond Cookies

MAKES 18

PREP + COOK TIME: 45 MINS

VEG • GLUTEN FREE

CHOCOLATE MACADAMIA FUDGE

¼ cup (50g) cacao paste (or spread)
¼ cup (50g) raw cacao butter
⅓ cup (60g) powdered erythritol
30g butter
1½ tbsps coconut oil
½ tsp vanilla extract
½ tsp ground cinnamon
10 macadamia nuts, roughly chopped

Bring a medium saucepan of water to a boil over a high heat. Add the cacao paste and cacao butter to a large, heatproof bowl. Place the bowl over the boiling water, ensuring that the bottom of the bowl does not touch the water.

Reduce heat to medium-low. Stir continually until just melted, then add in the erythritol, butter, oil, vanilla and cinnamon. Taste and add more powdered sweetener if needed.

Remove from the heat. Add the macadamias and stir until just combined. Pour into a small heat-resistant tray.

Transfer to the fridge to chill for 2 hours (or longer) until set.

ALMOND COOKIES

1 cup (125g) almonds, finely chopped
2 tsps gelatin powder
120g butter, room temperature, roughly chopped
1 cup (100g) almond flour
1 tsp stevia or ⅔ cup (140g) erythritol
⅓ cup (30g) coconut flour
1 tsp vanilla essence

Preheat oven to 180°C. Lightly grease and line two large, flat baking trays.

Place all the ingredients in a stand mixer and mix together until well combined.

Remove from the mixing bowl and form into a log. Cut into 18 pieces and roll each into a flattened disc. Place these on the trays, leaving approximately 4cm of space between each.

Bake for 18 minutes until just golden on the edges.

Remove to a wire rack to cool.

Carrot & Nut Cookies

MAKES 40
PREP + COOK TIME: 30 MINS
VEG • GLUTEN FREE

1 cup (125g) almonds
½ cup (125g) almond butter
⅓ cup (60g) monkfruit sweetener
¼ cup (60ml) cream
2 tbsps butter
2 egg whites
1 tsp cinnamon
1 tsp baking powder
¾ cup (80g) shredded carrots
¼ cup (35g) chopped mixed nuts
½ cup (45g) coconut flakes

CREAM CHEESE ICING

125g cream cheese
½ cup (100g) monkfruit sweetener
2 tbsps butter
1 tsp cream
½ tsp vanilla

OPTIONAL TOPPINGS

Lemon zest, walnuts and pumpkin seeds

Preheat oven to 180°C. Line two baking trays with greaseproof paper.

Process the almonds in a food processor until they start to break down and clump. Add the almond butter, sweetener, cream, butter, egg whites, cinnamon and baking powder. Process until smooth. Stir in the carrots, chopped nuts and coconut flakes.

Scoop out heaped tablespoons of the mixture and place on the prepared trays, to make about 40 cookies.

Transfer to the oven and bake for 15 minutes or until firm to the touch and golden around the edges. Cool completely.

Meanwhile, cream together the icing ingredients with an electric hand mixer until smooth. Transfer to a piping bag or a ziplock bag with the corner cut off and pipe the icing over the cooled cookies.

Serve immediately or decorate with optional toppings, if desired.

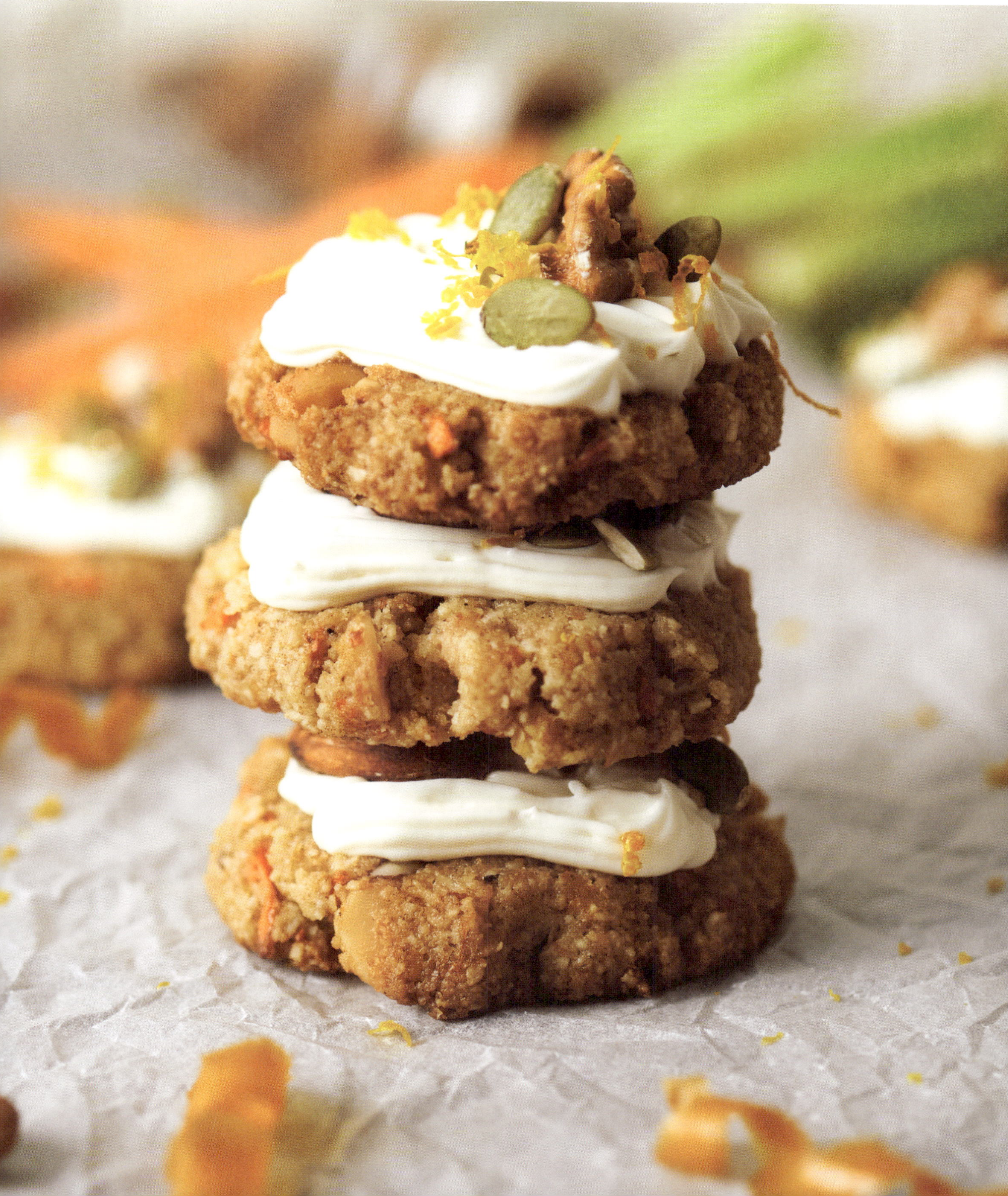

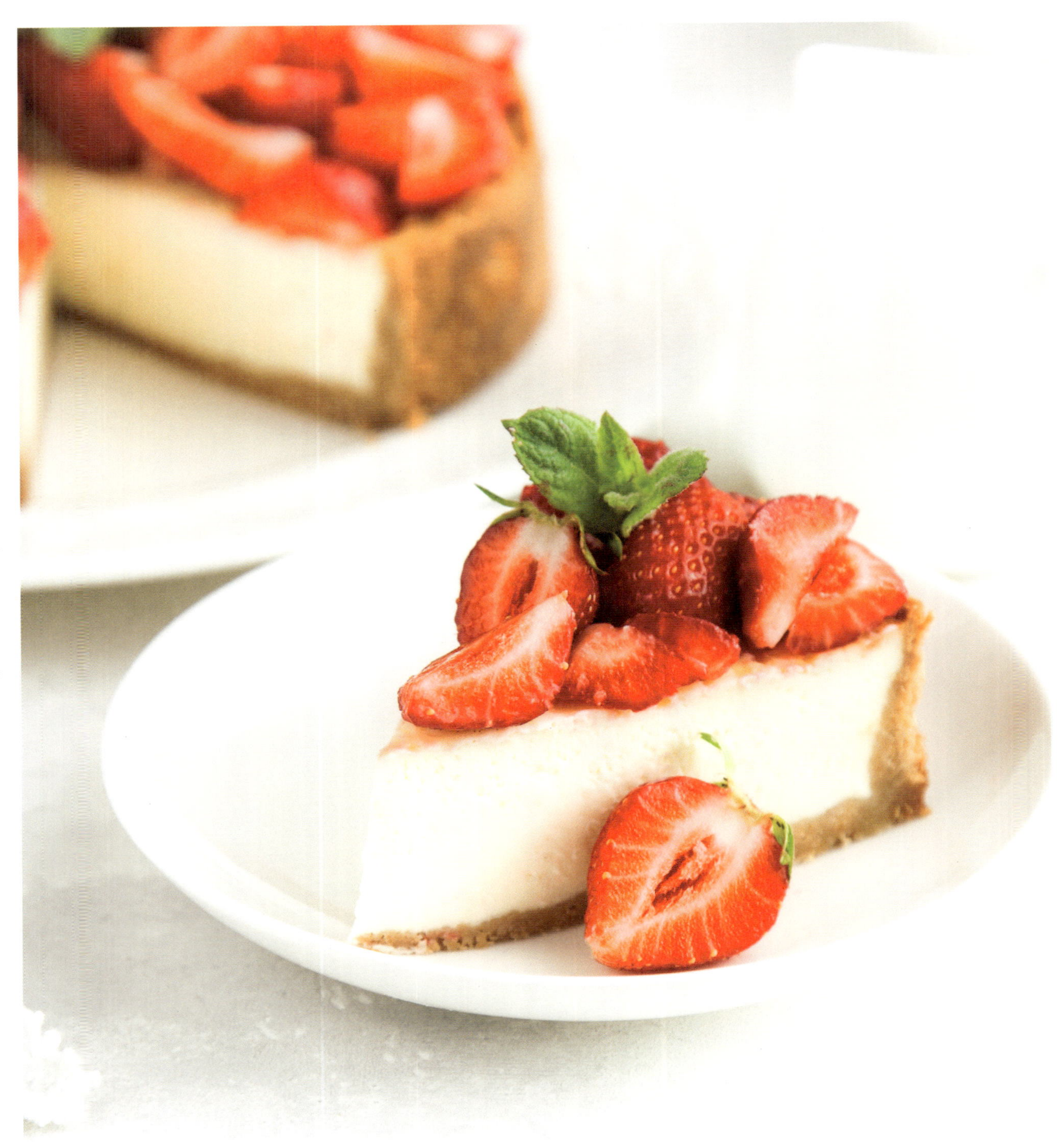

Strawberry Cheesecake

SERVES 12

PREP + COOK TIME: 30 MINS + FREEZING

VEG • GLUTEN FREE

STRAWBERRY CHEESECAKE

BASE

1½ cups (180g) almond meal

½ cup (60g) chopped cashews

85g unsalted butter, melted

3 tbsps monkfruit sweetener

1 tsp vanilla extract

Pinch of salt

CHEESECAKE

2½ cups (500g) fresh strawberries, hulled + more to decorate

⅔ cup (120g) powdered monkfruit sweetener or keto-friendly sweetener of choice

900g cream cheese

½ cup (125ml) sour cream

½ tbsp vanilla extract

1 tsp fresh lemon juice

½ cup (125ml) thickened cream, chilled

Grease and line a 22cm springform tin.

In a large bowl, mix together the almond meal, cashews, melted butter, monkfruit sweetener, vanilla and salt. Using your hands, press dough firmly into the springform tin. Transfer to the freezer while you prepare the filling.

Puree strawberries in a blender until smooth. Pass the mixture through a fine sieve and return to the blender. Add sweetener and cream cheese and blend until smooth. Add the sour cream, vanilla and lemon juice and continue to blend until no lumps remain.

In a separate bowl beat the cream until stiff peaks form. Fold the strawberry mixture into the cream bowl until combined.

Remove base from freezer and pour filling over the prepared base. Cover with plastic wrap and chill in the fridge for at least 5 hours or overnight (or freeze for 2-3 hours) before serving.

Run a sharp knife along the inside of the tin to release the cake before you remove the tin. Decorate with strawberries as desired.

Lemon Bars

MAKES 24

PREP + COOK TIME: 1 HOUR + CHILLING

VEG • GLUTEN FREE • DAIRY FREE

¼ cup (30g) almond meal
½ cup (125ml) coconut oil
Pinch of stevia powder
Pinch of salt
1 cup (100g) + 2½ tsps coconut flour
½ cup (125ml) lemon juice
½ cup (110g) erythritol
2 tsps lemon zest
4 large eggs, room temperature + 1 large egg yolk
1 tbsp arrowroot flour

Preheat oven to 180°C and grease and line a 15 x 20cm slice tin with baking paper.

To make the crust, mix together the almond meal, coconut oil, stevia powder and salt until well combined. Mix through the 1 cup of coconut flour until combined.

Press into the bottom of the slice tin and bake for 12 minutes until slightly browned on top. Remove from the oven and let cool while making the topping.

Place the lemon juice and erythritol in a saucepan and heat over low heat until the erythritol has dissolved. Remove from the heat and lightly whisk in the remaining coconut flour, then the lemon zest, eggs and egg yolk.

Pour the topping mix over the cooked base. Bake for 25 minutes at 160°C until the top is just set.

Remove from the oven and let cool for at least 1 hour. Then chill in the refrigerator for at least 4 hours, preferably overnight.

Before serving, dust the arrowroot flour over the top and cut into squares.

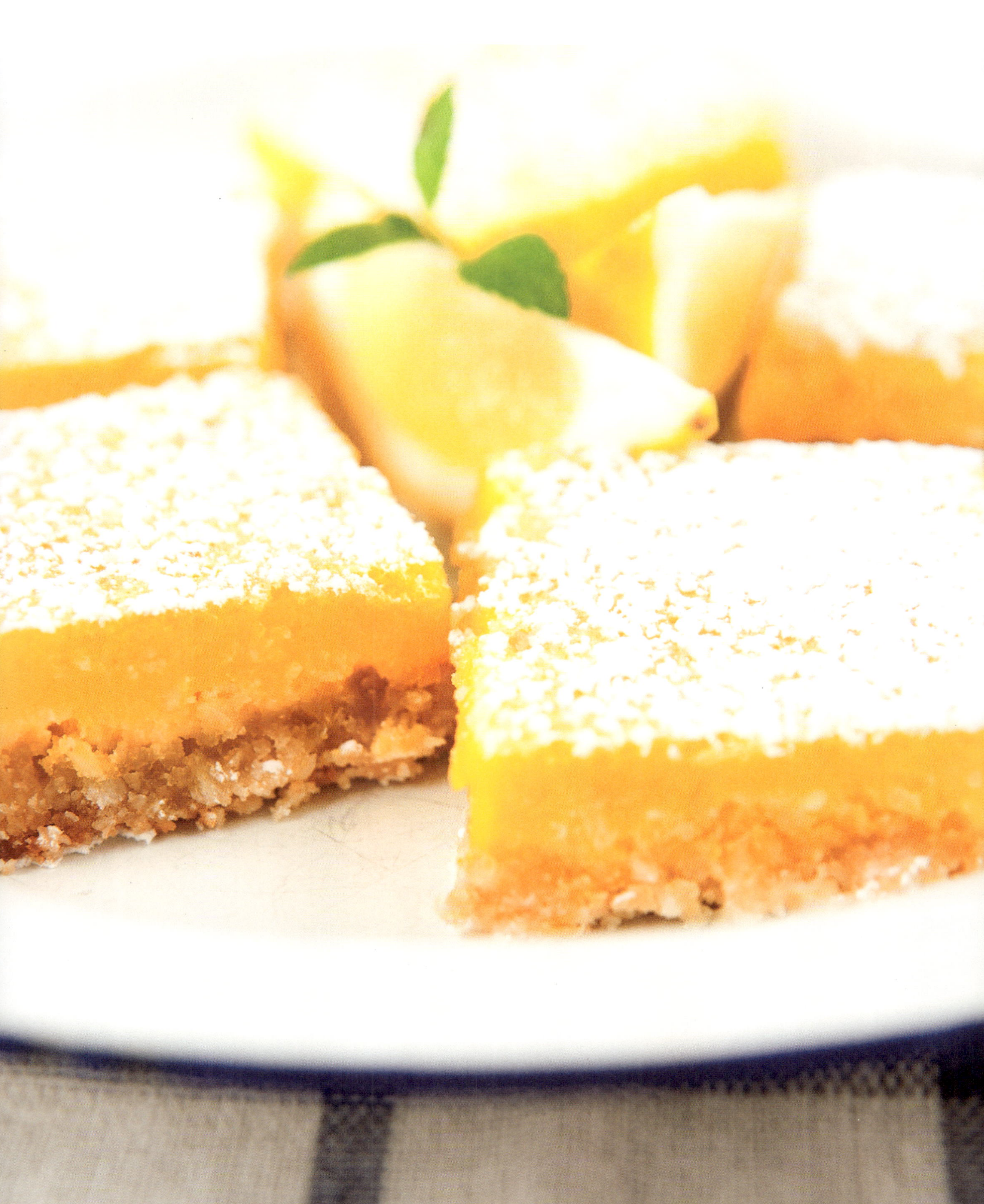

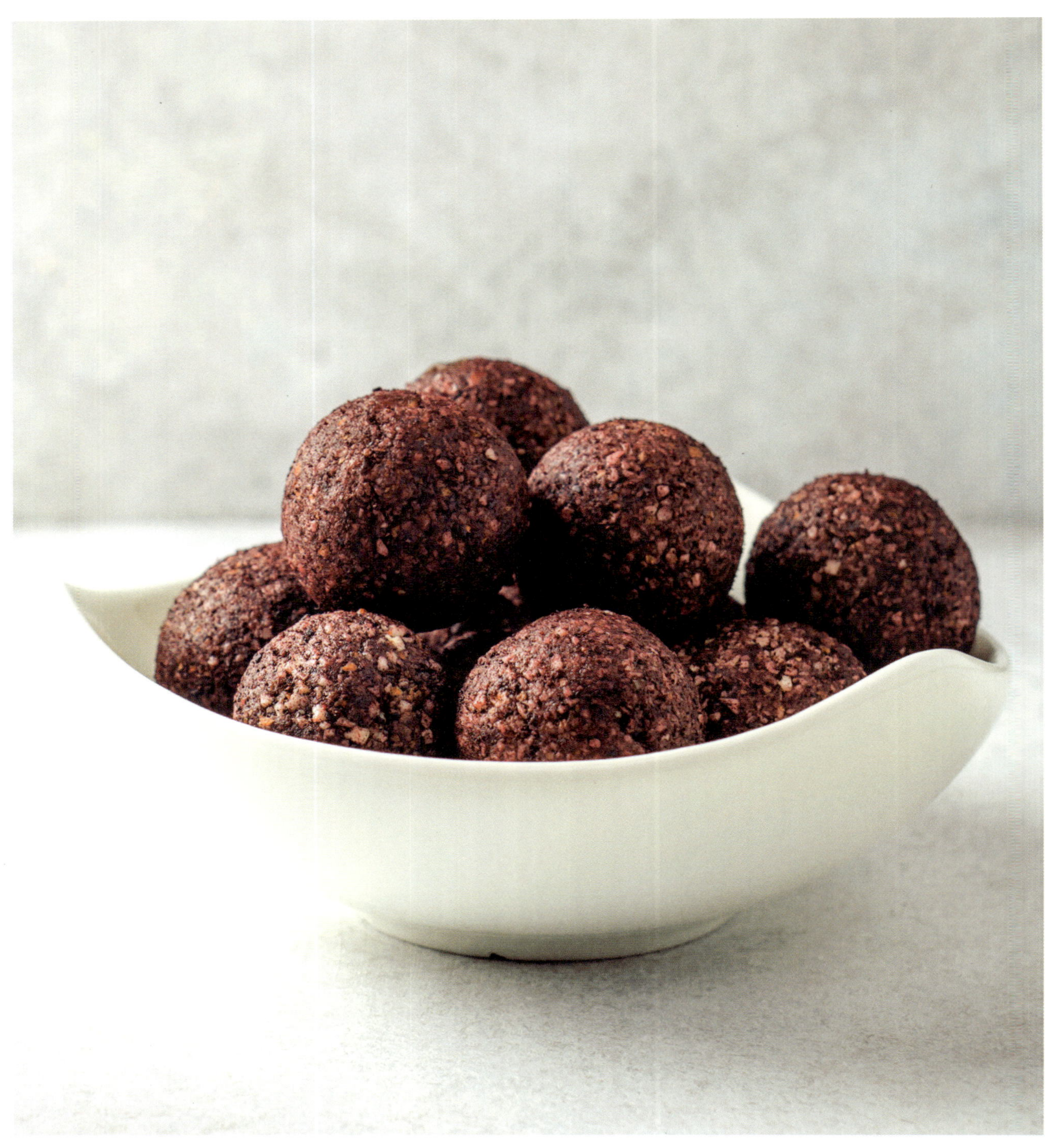

Acai Protein Balls

MAKES 10-12

PREP + COOK TIME: 15 MINS + CHILLING

VEG • GLUTEN FREE • DAIRY FREE

ACAI PROTEIN BALLS

8 tbsps vanilla collagen powder
8 tbsps acai berry powder
⅓ cup (40g) almond meal
4 tbsps MCT oil
2 tbsps almond butter
2 tsps cacao powder
1 tbsp monkfruit powder
1 tbsp water

Place all of the ingredients in a food processor or high-speed blender and pulse to combine.

Transfer to a large mixing bowl and knead for 3-4 minutes to bring the mixture together. Add a bit more water if needed.

Use your hands to roll into walnut-sized balls.

Place in the fridge for 30 minutes before eating.

Once refrigerated eat straight away or store in an airtight container in the freezer.

Lemon Cream Pie

SERVES 6 • PREP + COOK TIME: 45 MINS + CHILLING
VEG • GLUTEN FREE

CRUST

1½ cups (180g) almond meal
3 tbsps coconut flour
¼ cup (50g) erythritol
110g butter, chilled and diced
Pinch of salt
Zest of 1 lemon

LEMON CREAM

2 eggs
Juice of 2 lemons
¾ cup (200ml) thickened cream
½ cup (95g) powdered erythritol
Zest of 1 lemon
2 tbsps butter
250g mascarpone cheese
1 tbsp vanilla extract

TOPPING

¾ cup (200ml) thickened cream
1 tsp vanilla extract
Lemon zest and slices

Preheat the oven to 180°C. Grease a 25cm pie dish.

Place the almond meal, coconut flour and erythritol into a food processor. Add the diced butter and pulse until the mixture starts to form a dough.

Press the dough into the greased pie dish.

Transfer to the oven and bake for 15-20 minutes or until golden brown.

Leave to rest while you prepare the lemon cream.

In a large heavy saucepan over a medium-high heat whisk the eggs with lemon juice, cream and erythritol.

When the mixture starts to boil, reduce the heat to medium and continue whisking for 2-3 minutes until it just starts to thicken. Remove from the heat immediately. Add lemon zest and butter and whisk until butter is melted. Add mascarpone cheese and continue mixing until smooth and silky.

Pour the cream onto the crust and refrigerate for 8-12 hours to firm up.

For the topping, whisk the cream with vanilla until stiff. Smooth on top of the pie. Decorate with extra zest and lemon slices if desired and serve cold.

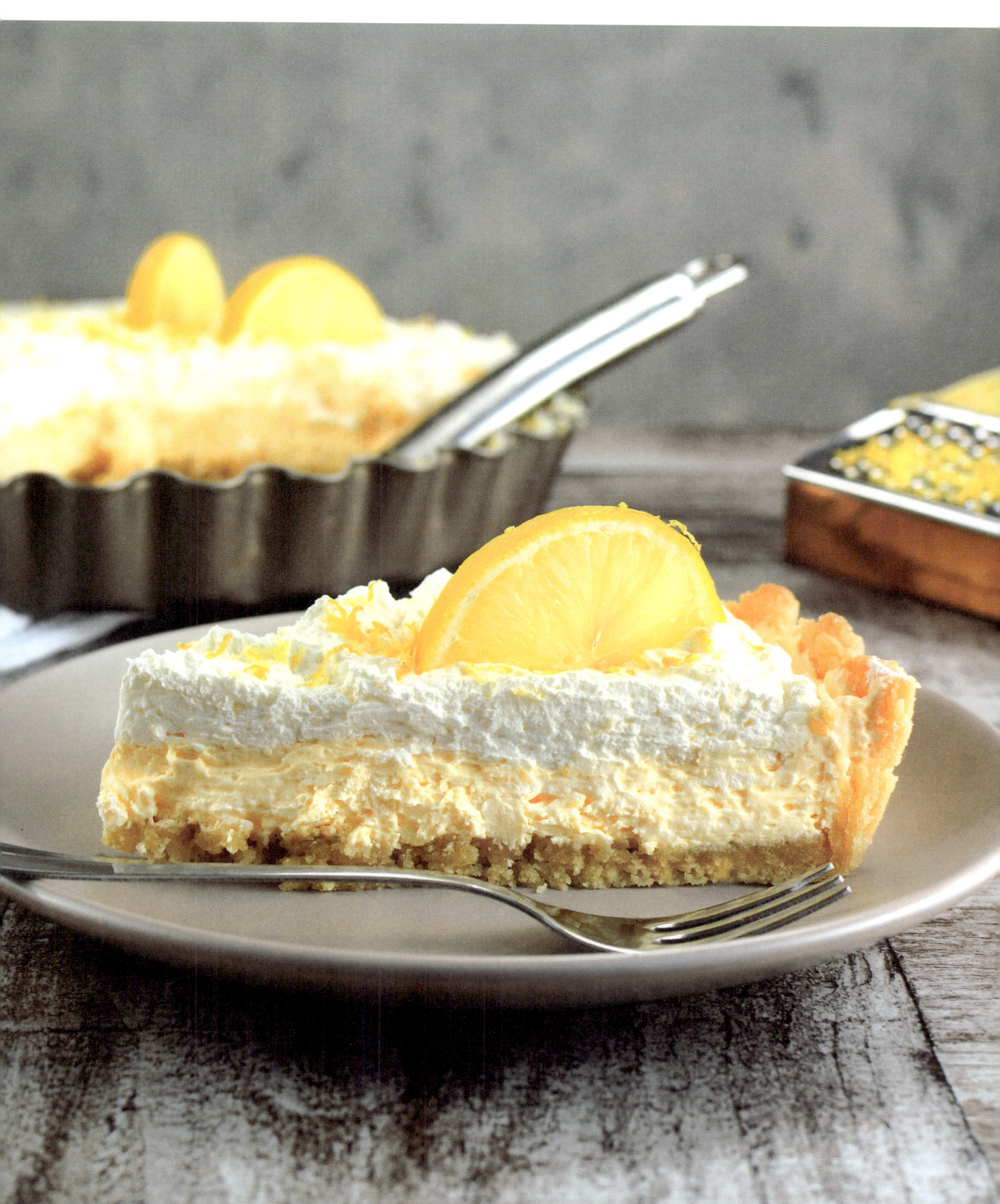

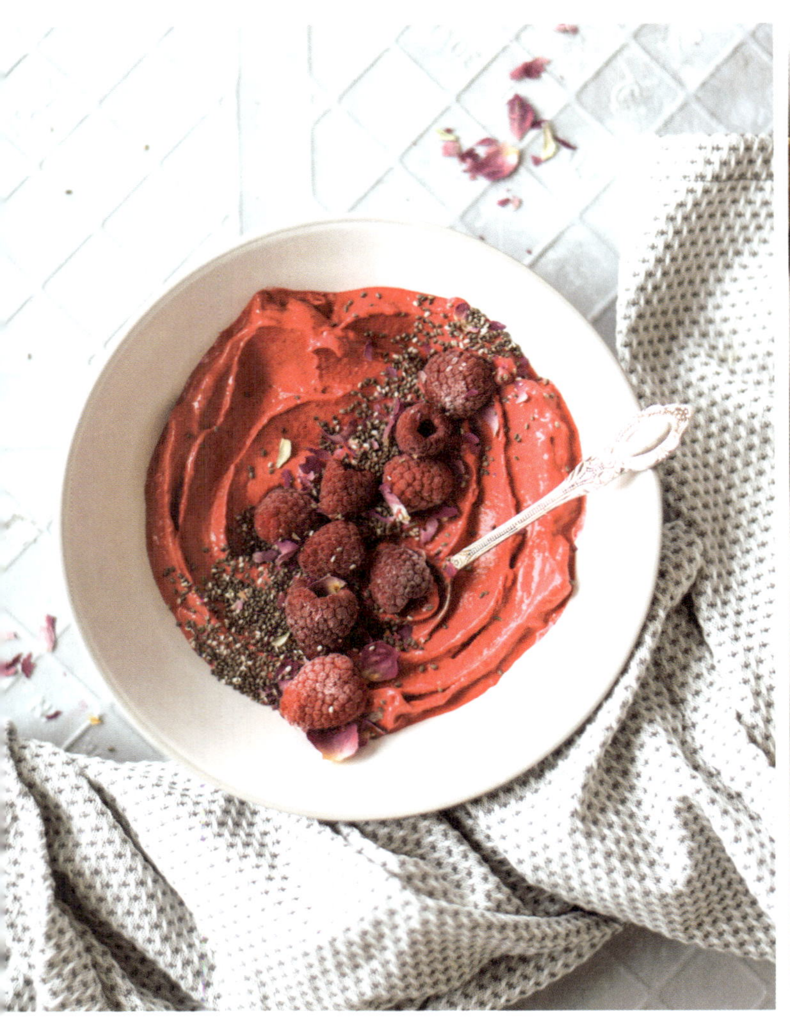

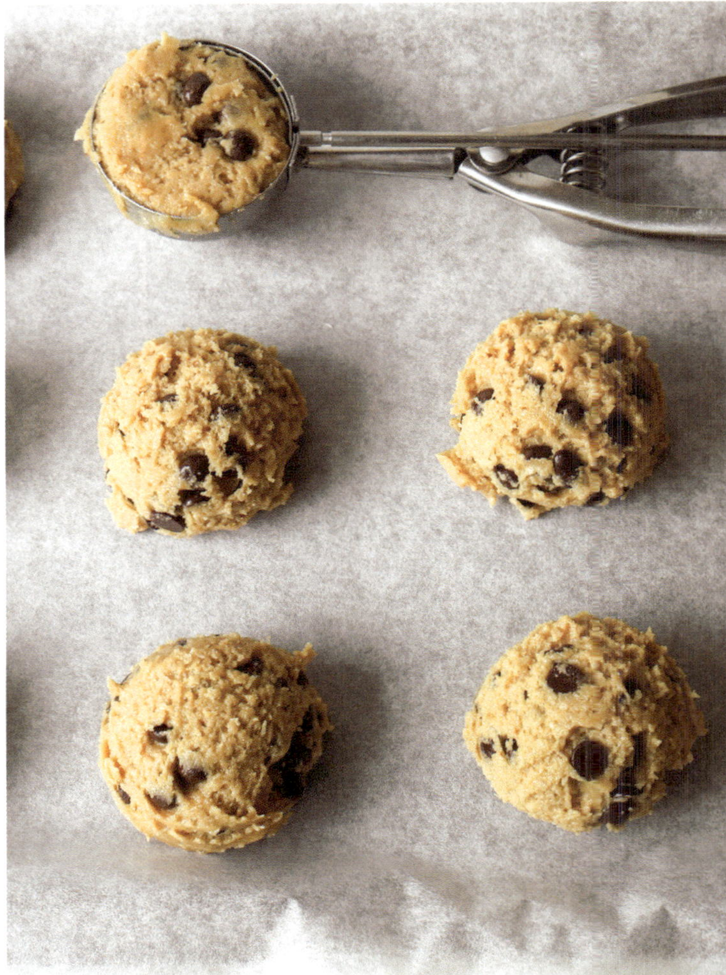

Raspberry Smoothie Bowl

SERVES 1

PREP + COOK TIME: 10 MINS

VEG • GLUTEN FREE • DAIRY FREE

Chocolate Chip Fat Bombs

MAKES 30

PREP + COOK TIME: 30 MINS

VEG • GLUTEN FREE

RASPBERRY SMOOTHIE BOWL

½ avocado, chopped
½ cup (125ml) almond milk
¾ cup (90g) frozen raspberries + more to serve
1 tbsp MCT oil or coconut oil
2 tbsps low-carb vanilla protein powder
1 tsp chia seeds, to serve

Place avocado, almond milk, raspberries, MCT or coconut oil and protein powder into a blender and process until smooth.

Serve in bowls topped with chia seeds and additional frozen raspberries.

CHOCOLATE CHIP FAT BOMBS

115g butter, softened
⅓ cup (55g) keto-friendly icing sugar replacement
½ tsp vanilla extract
½ tsp salt
2 cups (240g) finely ground almond meal
⅔ cup (100g) sugar-free dark chocolate chips

In a large bowl, beat butter with an electric hand mixer until light and fluffy.

Add sweetener, vanilla and salt and beat well to combine.

Slowly add in the almond meal, beating continuously until incorporated.

Fold in chocolate chips.

Cover and place in the fridge for 15-20 minutes to firm up.

Using a small cookie scoop, scoop dough into small balls.

Store in the fridge for up to a week, or in the freezer for up to 1 month.

Strawberry Tart

SERVES 10

PREP + COOK TIME: 40 MINS + COOLING

VEG • GLUTEN FREE

- 5 egg whites
- ⅓ cup (65g) xylitol
- 1½ cups (180g) finely ground almond meal
- Zest of 1 lemon
- 1 tsp vanilla extract
- 1 tsp baking powder
- 100g butter, melted and cooled
- 2 cups (400g) strawberries; 1¼ cups (250g) sliced + ¾ cup (150g) halved
- ½ cup (125ml) thickened cream
- 2 tbsps keto-friendly powdered sweetener

Preheat the oven to 190°C. Grease and line a rectangular tart tin.

In a large bowl whisk the egg whites until foamy. Add the xylitol and whisk until soft peaks begin to form. Add the almond meal, lemon zest, vanilla extract, baking powder and melted butter. Gently fold through to combine.

Transfer the mixture to the prepared tart tin, then scatter with sliced strawberries. Transfer to the oven and bake for 18-20 minutes until golden brown. Remove from the tin and set aside on a wire rack to cool completely.

When cool, whisk the cream until stiff peaks form. Transfer the cream to a piping bag with a star shaped nozzle. Pipe cream rosettes over the centre of the tart. Top the tart with halved strawberries, then dust with powdered sweetener.

Slice and serve immediately.

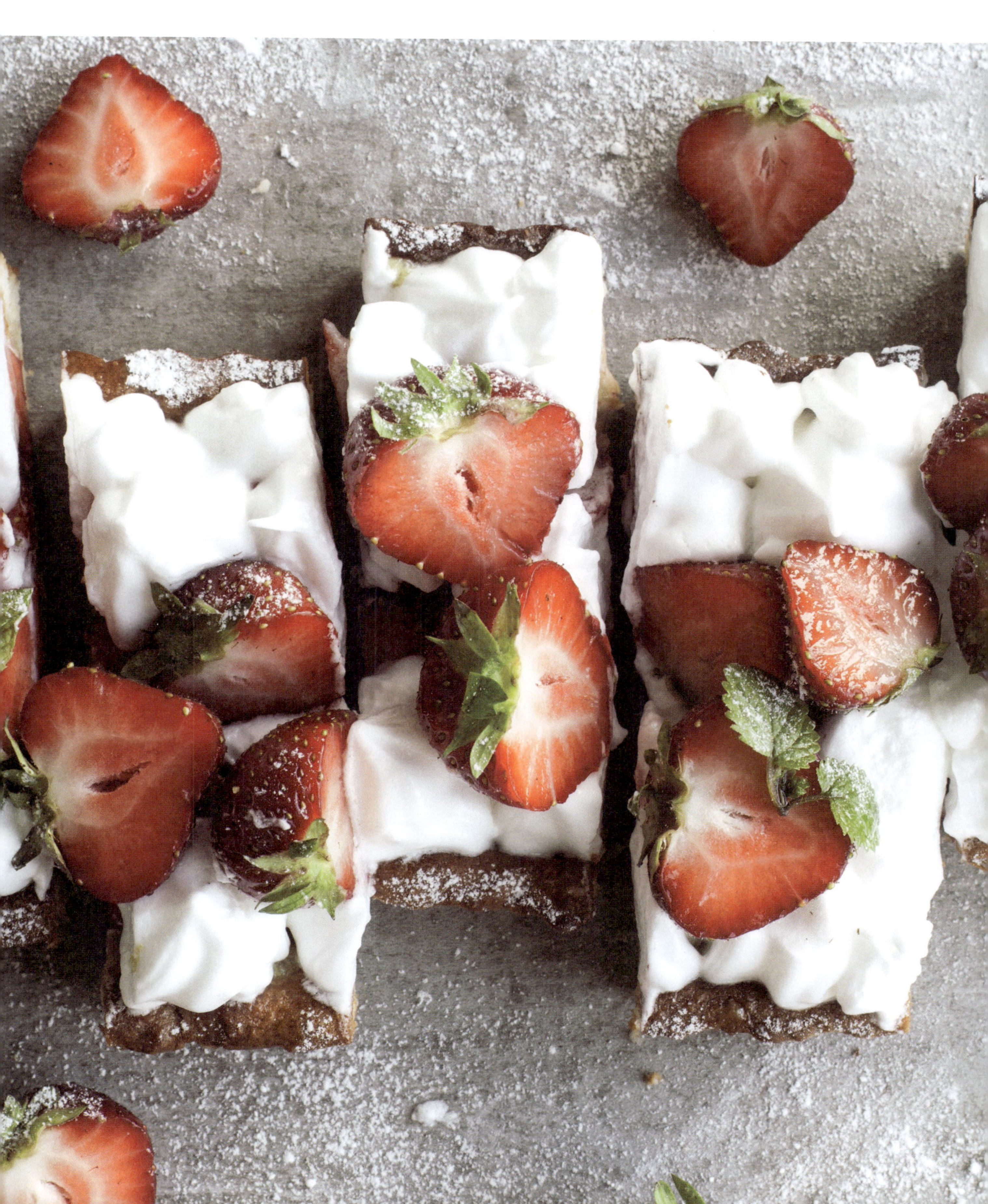

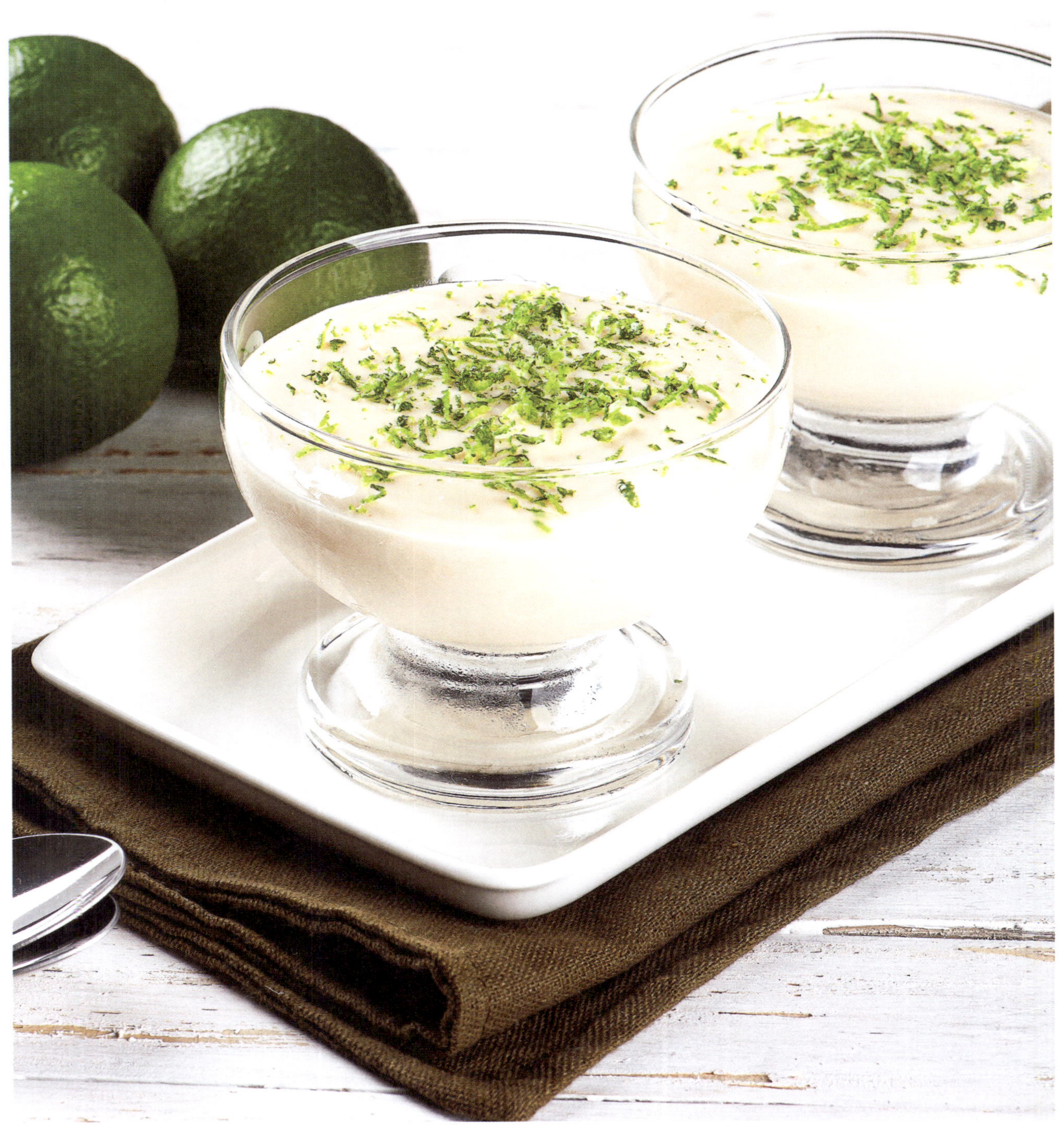

Lime Mousse

SERVES 8

PREP + COOK TIME: 15 MINS + CHILLING

GLUTEN FREE

LIME MOUSSE

2½ tsps gelatin powder
¼ cup (60ml) cold water
⅓ cup (80ml) boiling water
½ cup (100g) granulated erythritol
1 tbsp lime zest + more to serve
2 cups (500ml) cold thickened cream
⅔ cup (160ml) lime juice

Sprinkle gelatin over cold water in small bowl. Let stand for 2 minutes to soften. Add boiling water; stir until gelatin is completely dissolved and mixture is clear. Cool slightly.

Combine sweetener and lime zest in large bowl. Add thickened cream and beat with an electric mixer until stiff peaks form. Pour in gelatin mixture and lime juice. Beat again to combine.

Spoon into eight serving glasses then refrigerate for at least 2 hours or until set.

Scatter with lime zest to serve.

Tres Leches Cake

SERVES 12
PREP + COOK TIME: 1 HOUR + COOLING
VEG • GLUTEN FREE

CONDENSED CREAM

1 tbsp butter
2 tbsps erythritol or xylitol
1 tsp vanilla extract
1 cup (250ml) double cream

CAKE

¼ cup (60ml) double cream
2 eggs
100g butter, melted
1 tsp vanilla extract
¼ cup (50g) erythritol or xylitol
2 cups (200g) almond meal
1 tsp baking powder

TRES LECHES MIX

Condensed cream (see above)
¼ cup (60ml) cream
¼ cup (60ml) double cream

TOPPING

1 cup (250ml) thickened cream
1 tsp vanilla extract
4 tbsps erythritol or xylitol
Cocoa powder, for dusting

Preheat oven to 180°C. Grease and line a 22 x 30cm rectangular cake tin or casserole dish.

Melt butter and sweetener in a pan over medium heat. Add in vanilla and double cream. Bring the mixture to a boil and then turn down to low. Stir until the mixture is gently simmering.

Continue to simmer, stirring regularly, for 10-15 minutes until the mixture is reduced by half and is thick enough to cover the back of a spoon.

Set aside and allow to cool.

To make the cake whisk together all the cake ingredients in a large mixing bowl. Pour batter into prepared cake tin or casserole dish.

Transfer to the oven and bake for 20 minutes until an inserted skewer comes out clean.

While the cake is baking pour the prepared condensed cream into a large mixing bowl. Add the cream and double cream and whisk together to create the tres leches mix.

When the cake is ready remove from the oven and use a fork or skewer and poke several holes.

Pour the tres leches mixture onto the cake and use a spoon to spread it around gently so the cream fills the holes.

Set aside to cool for at least 3 hours.

Just before serving, whip together cream, vanilla and sweetener. Spread over the top of the cake and dust with cocoa powder.

Cut into squares to serve.

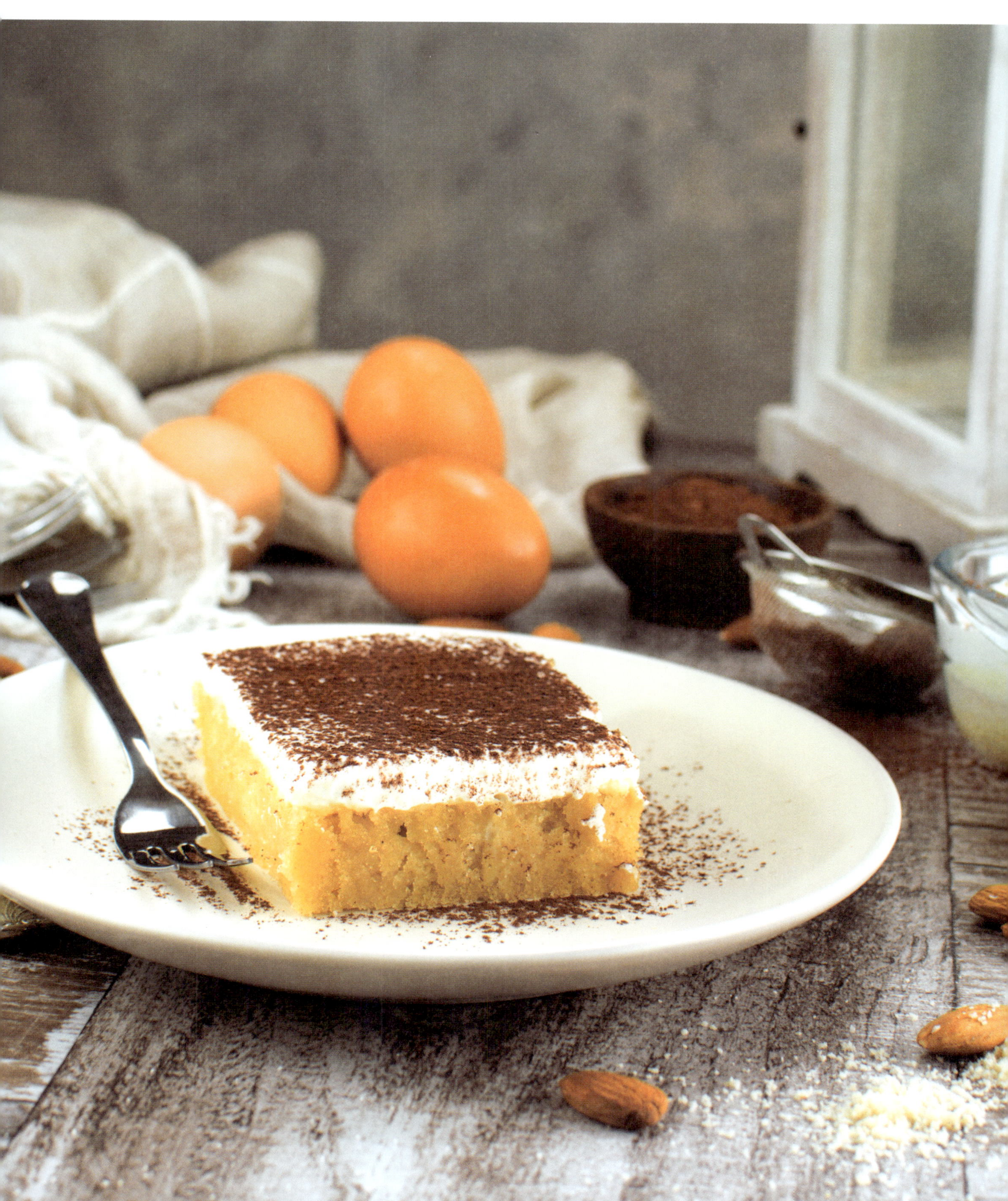

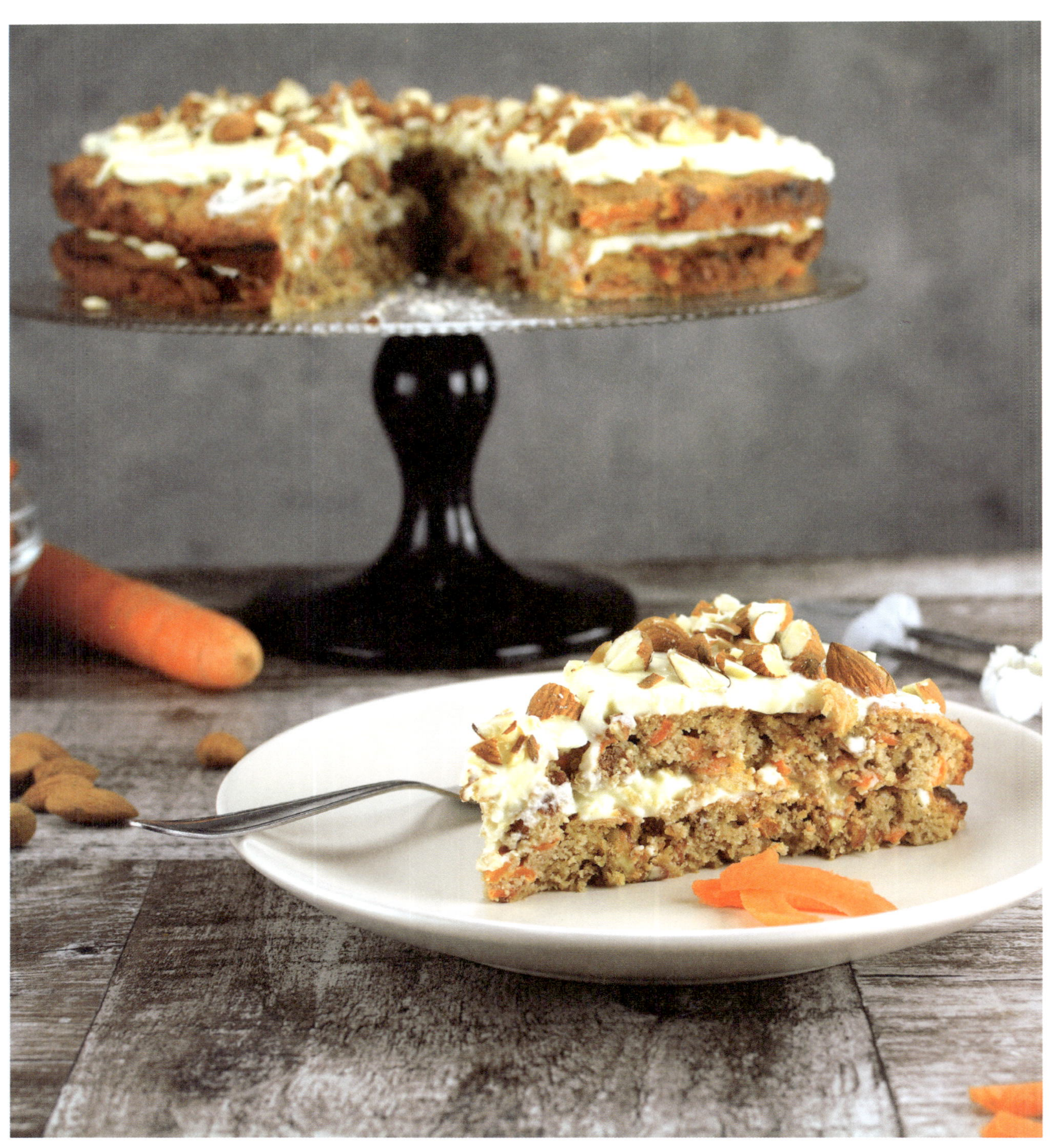

Carrot Cake

SERVES 8

PREP + COOK TIME: 1 HOUR + COOLING

VEG • GLUTEN FREE

CARROT CAKE

1½ cups (180g) almond meal

½ cup (100g) granulated erythritol or keto-friendly sweetener of choice

¼ cup (40g) keto-friendly brown sugar substitute

1½ tsps baking powder

¼ tsp bicarbonate of soda

½ tsp salt

1¼ tsps cinnamon

½ tsp nutmeg

⅛ tsp ground cloves

1 cup (110g) grated carrots

4 eggs

4 tbsps butter, melted

½ tsp vanilla extract

½ cup (60g) chopped almonds + ¼ cup (30g) roughly chopped, to serve

CREAM CHEESE ICING

250g cream cheese, softened

5 tbsps butter, softened

½ tsp vanilla extract

1 tbsp sour cream

½ cup (80g) powdered erythritol

Preheat the oven to 180°C. Grease and line two 20cm round cake tins with greaseproof paper.

In a large bowl whisk together the almond meal, granulated erythritol, brown sugar substitute, baking powder, bicarb, salt, cinnamon, nutmeg and cloves. Add the carrot, eggs, butter and vanilla and mix to combine. Stir in the chopped nuts. Pour into the prepared cake tins and transfer to the oven.

Bake for 22-25 minutes until set in the centre. Set aside on a wire rack to cool completely before icing.

Use an electric hand mixer to beat together the cream cheese, butter, vanilla and sour cream. Slowly add in the powdered erythritol and continue to whip for another 2-3 minutes or until fluffy.

Spread the icing on top of both cakes and sandwich the cakes together. Scatter with chopped almonds to serve.

Index

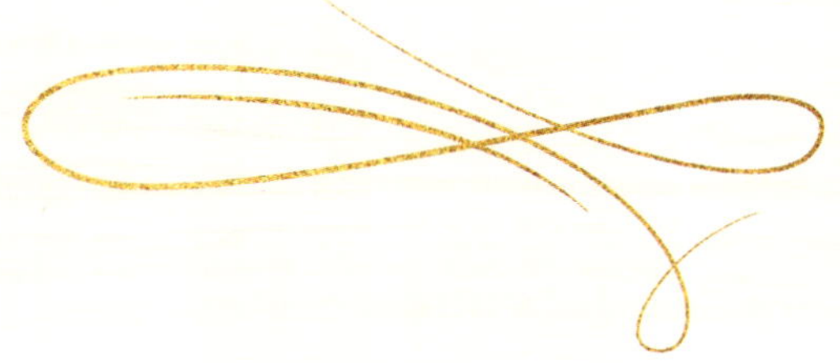

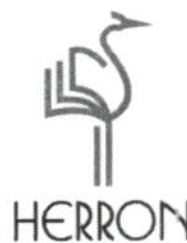

HERRON

First Published in 2023 by Herron Book Distributors Pty Ltd
14 Manton St
Morningside
QLD 4170
www.herronbooks.com

Captain Honey

Custom book production by Captain Honey Pty Ltd
12 Station St
Bangalow
NSW 2479
www.captainhoney.com.au

Recipes in this book were previously published in: *6 Ingredients: Keto* (2019), *Easy Keto* (2020), *10 Ways: The Keto Kitchen* (2022), *Best Ever: Keto Cookbook* (2022)

Cataloguing-in-Publication. A catalogue record for this book is available from the National Library of Australia

ISBN 978-1-922944-40-5

All images used under license from Shutterstock.com
Printed and bound in China

5 4 3 2 1 23 24 25 26 27

NOTES FOR THE READER

All reasonable efforts have been made to ensure the accuracy of the content in this book. Information in this book is not intended as a substitute for medical advice. The author and publisher cannot and do not accept any legal duty of care or responsibility in relation to the content in this book, and disclaim any liabilities relating to its use.

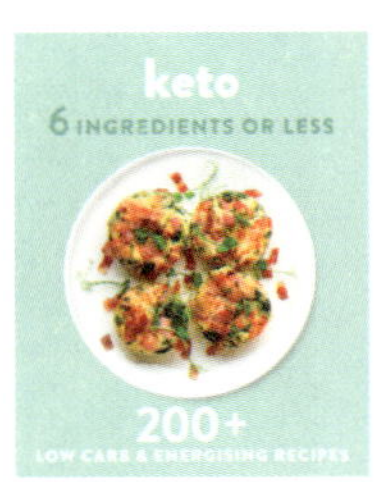

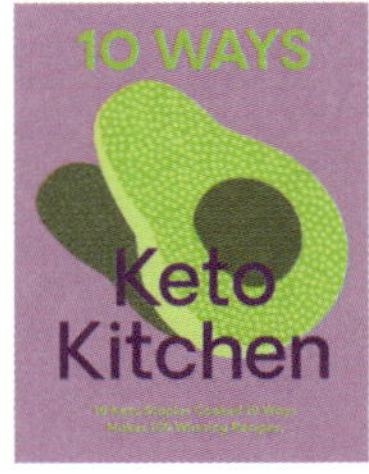

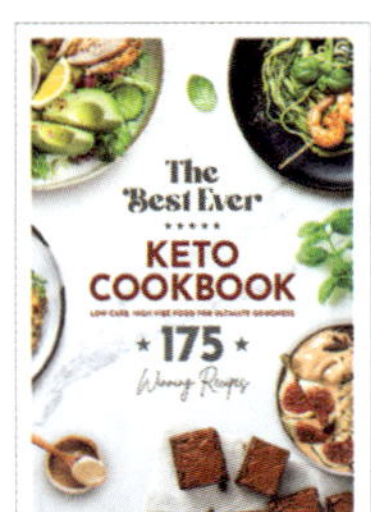

NOTE ABOUT REVIEWS

Thanks to the many customers who sent in complimentary comments about our keto cookbooks, or left great reviews on the websites of our key retailers like Kmart.

With thanks, we feature a few of these reviews on the back cover of this book. We appreciate your support and are excited that you loved the recipes.